WD

Genetic Disorders Sourcebook,
  1st Edition
Genetic Disorders Sourcebook,
  2nd Edition
Head Trauma Sourcebook
Headache Sourcebook
Health Insurance Sourcebook
Health Reference Series Cumulative
  Index 1999
Healthy Aging Sourcebook
Healthy Children Sourcebook
Healthy Heart Sourcebook for Women
Heart Diseases & Disorders
  Sourcebook, 2nd Edition
Household Safety Sourcebook
Immune System Disorders Sourcebook
Infant & Toddler Health Sourcebook
Injury & Trauma Sourcebook
Kidney & Urinary Tract Diseases &
  Disorders Sourcebook
Learning Disabilities Sourcebook,
  1st Edition
Learning Disabilities Sourcebook,
  2nd Edition
Liver Disorders Sourcebook
Leukemia Sourcebook
Lung Disorders Sourcebook
Medical Tests Sourcebook
Men's Health Concerns Sourcebook
Mental Health Disorders Sourcebook,
  1st Edition
Mental Health Disorders Sourcebook,
  2nd Edition
Mental Retardation Sourcebook
Movement Disorders Sourcebook
Obesity Sourcebook
Ophthalmic Disorders Sourcebook,
  1st Edition
Oral Health Sourcebook
Osteoporosis Sourcebook
Pain Sourcebook, 1st Edition
Pain Sourcebook, 2nd Edition
Pediatric Cancer Sourcebook
Physical & Mental Issues in Aging
  Sourcebook

Podiatry Sourcebook
Pregnancy & Birth Sourcebook
Prostate Cancer
Public Health Sourcebook
Reconstructive & Cosmetic Surgery
  Sourcebook
Rehabilitation Sourcebook
Respiratory Diseases & Disorders
  Sourcebook
Sexually Transmitted Diseases
  Sourcebook, 1st Edition
Sexually Transmitted Diseases
  Sourcebook, 2nd Edition
Skin Disorders Sourcebook
Sleep Disorders Sourcebook
Sports Injuries Sourcebook, 1st Edition
Sports Injuries Sourcebook, 2nd Edition
Stress-Related Disorders Sourcebook
Stroke Sourcebook
Substance Abuse Sourcebook
Surgery Sourcebook
Transplantation Sourcebook
Traveler's Health Sourcebook
Vegetarian Sourcebook
Women's Health Concerns Sourcebook
Workplace Health & Safety Sourcebook
Worldwide Health Sourcebook

Teen Health Series

Diet Information for Teens
Drug Information for Teens
Mental Health Information
  for Teens
Sexual Health Information
  for Teens
Skin Health Information
  for Teens
Sports Injuries Information
  for Teens

Environmental Health
SOURCEBOOK

Second Edition

Health Reference Series

Second Edition

Environmental Health
SOURCEBOOK

Basic Consumer Health Information about the Environment and Its Effect on Human Health, Including the Effects of Air Pollution, Water Pollution, Hazardous Chemicals, Food Hazards, Radiation Hazards, Biological Agents, Household Hazards, Such as Radon, Asbestos, Carbon Monoxide, and Mold, and Information about Associated Diseases and Disorders, Including Cancer, Allergies, Respiratory Problems, and Skin Disorders

Along with Information about Environmental Concerns for Specific Populations, a Glossary of Related Terms, and Resources for Further Help and Information

Edited by
Dawn D. Matthews

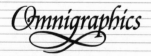

Omnigraphics

615 Griswold Street • Detroit, MI 48226

Bibliographic Note

Because this page cannot legibly accommodate all the copyright notices, the Bibliographic Note portion of the Preface constitutes an extension of the copyright notice.

Edited by Dawn D. Matthews

Health Reference Series

Karen Bellenir, *Managing Editor*
David A. Cooke, MD, *Medical Consultant*
Elizabeth Barbour, *Permissions Associate*
Dawn Matthews, *Verification Assistant*
Laura Pleva Nielsen, *Index Editor*
EdIndex, Services for Publishers, *Indexers*

* * *

Omnigraphics, Inc.

Matthew P. Barbour, *Senior Vice President*
Kay Gill, *Vice President—Directories*
Kevin Hayes, *Operations Manager*
Leif Gruenberg, *Development Manager*
David P. Bianco, *Marketing Consultant*

* * *

Peter E. Ruffner, *Publisher*

Frederick G. Ruffner, Jr., *Chairman*

Copyright © 2003 Omnigraphics, Inc.

ISBN

Library of Congress Cataloging-in-Publication Data

Environmental health sourcebook : basic consumer health information about the environment and its effect on human health, including the effects of air pollution, water pollution, hazardous chemicals, food hazards, radiation hazards, biological agents, household hazards ... / edited by Dawn D. Matthews.-- 2nd ed.
      p. cm. -- (Health reference series)
   Previous ed. published with title: Environmentally induced disorders sourcebook.
   Includes bibliographical references and index.
   ISBN 0-7808-0632-8 (lib. bdg. : alk. paper)
   1. Environmental health. 2. Environmentally induced diseases. 3. Environmental toxicology. I. Matthews, Dawn D. II. Environmentally induced disorders sourcebook. III. Health reference series (Unnumbered)

RA565.E484 2003
616.9'8--dc21
                                                            2003053601

∞

This book is printed on acid-free paper meeting the ANSI Z39.48 Standard. The infinity symbol that appears above indicates that the paper in this book meets that standard.

Printed in the United States

Table of Contents

Preface ix

Part I: Understanding the Health Effects of Environmental Hazards

Chapter 1—Environmental Hazards and Your Health 3

Chapter 2—Environmental Diseases from A to Z 17

Chapter 3—Asthma and Its Environmental Triggers 25

Chapter 4—Cancer Clusters 29

Chapter 5—Reducing Risk from Hazardous Waste 33

Chapter 6—A Family Guide to Environmental Health 59

Chapter 7—Environmental Genome Project 67

Chapter 8—Environmental Public Health Tracking
            Program 73

Chapter 9—The Emergency Planning and Community
            Right-to-Know Act (EPCRA) 77

Part II: Airborne Hazards

Chapter 10—An Introduction to Indoor Air Quality 89

Chapter 11—Asbestos: A Source of Indoor Air Pollution 95

Chapter 12—Carbon Monoxide 99

Chapter 13—Combustion Appliances and Indoor Air
        Pollution 103

Chapter 14—Formaldehyde in Indoor Air 115

Chapter 15—Mold, Moisture, and Indoor Air Quality 123

Chapter 16—Environmental Tobacco Smoke 131

Chapter 17—Air Ducts and Indoor Air Quality 133

Chapter 18—Outdoor Air Quality: The Six Common Air
        Pollutants 149

Chapter 19—Acid Rain 157

Chapter 20—Ozone 163

Chapter 21—Understanding the Air Quality Index 175

Part III: Waterborne Hazards

Chapter 22—Drinking Water and Your Health 191

Chapter 23—Drinking Water Standards 197

Chapter 24—Contaminants in Drinking Water 213

Chapter 25—Chlorination of Drinking Water: Its
        Benefits and Risks 219

Chapter 26—Lead in Drinking Water 223

Chapter 27—MTBE (Methyl-*Tert*-Butyl Ether) in
        Drinking Water 227

Chapter 28—Drinking Water: Microbial and Disinfection
        Byproducts 233

Chapter 29—Drinking Water from Household Wells 241

Chapter 30—Swimming Water Hazards 257

Part IV: Chemical Hazards

Chapter 31—Dioxins 263

Chapter 32—Lead and Your Health 267

Chapter 33—Health Hazards of Malathion 275

Chapter 34—Health Hazards of Mercury 279

Chapter 35—Pesticides 283

Chapter 36—Protecting People Who Work with
        Pesticides 295

Chapter 37—Pesticides and Mosquito Control 299

Chapter 38—DEET (N,N-Diethyl-Meta-Toluamide) 303

Chapter 39—Chemical Hazards in the Workplace 309

Chapter 40—Multiple Chemical Sensitivity Syndrome
(MCS) 327

Part V: Radiation and Electromagnetic Field Hazards

Chapter 41—Understanding the Health Effects of
Radiation Exposure 333

Chapter 42—Radon 341

Chapter 43—Managing Radioactive Materials and Waste 353

Chapter 44—Microwave Oven Radiation 357

Chapter 45—Smoke Detectors and Radiation 363

Chapter 46—Television Radiation 365

Chapter 47—Hazards of Electric and Magnetic Fields 369

Chapter 48—Cell Phones and Wireless Phones: Are They
Safe? 391

Part VI: Biological Hazards

Chapter 49—Anthrax 409

Chapter 50—Botulism 425

Chapter 51—Brucellosis 429

Chapter 52—Pneumonic Plague 433

Chapter 53—Smallpox 439

Chapter 54—Tularemia 445

Chapter 55—Viral Hemorrhagic Fevers 449

Part VII: Foodborne Hazards

Chapter 56—Preventing Foodborne Illness 457

Chapter 57—Parasites and Foodborne Illness 467

Chapter 58—*Escherichia Coli* 479

Chapter 59—Salmonellosis 483

Chapter 60—Shigellosis 489

Chapter 61—Shellfish-Associated Toxins 495

Chapter 62—Hepatitis A Virus 499

Chapter 63—Color Additives 503

Chapter 64—Are Bioengineered Foods Safe? 513

Part VIII: Environmental Hazards to Specific Populations

Chapter 65—Children's Environmental Health 523

Chapter 66—Ten Tips to Protect Children from
Pesticide and Lead Poisonings around the
Home 543

Chapter 67—Women's Health and the Environment 545

Chapter 68—Workers and Noise Hazards 551

Chapter 69—Prioritizing Environmental Health
Threats to Older Persons 555

Chapter 70—Environmental Health: Are Minority
Populations at Greater Risk? 557

Part IX: Additional Help and Information

Chapter 71—Glossary of Environmental Health Terms 585

Chapter 72—Environmental Agencies and Advocate
Groups 595

Chapter 73—Environmental Resources on the Internet 601

Chapter 74—Environmental Hotlines 605

Chapter 75—Environmental Protection Agency (EPA)
Compliance and Enforcement Information 619

Index 625

Preface

About This Book

The environment, which includes both natural and man-made components, is a critical component of human health. Exposure to hazardous substances in the air we breathe, the water we drink, the food we eat, and the soil where we live, work, and play is a major contributor to illness, disability, and death. In fact, the World Health Organization estimates that poor environmental quality is directly responsible for about 25 percent of all preventable ill health in the world.

This *Sourcebook* contains information about the heath effects of exposure to harmful substances in the environment. It includes facts about air pollution, water pollution, chemicals, foodborne hazards, radiation, biological hazards, and other contaminants that may be found inside homes, schools, and businesses. It explains the link between the environment and specific diseases, such as cancer, allergies, and skin disorders, and risks to specific populations, such as the very young and the elderly. A glossary of related terms and directories of resources provide additional help and information.

How to Use This Book

This book is divided into parts and chapters. Parts focus on broad areas of interest. Chapters are devoted to single topics within a part.

Part I: Understanding the Health Effects of Environmental Hazards explains the link between the environment and human health. It includes information about specific diseases with environmental triggers and offers tips for minimizing risks. Recent efforts to begin tracking environmental health hazards and to understand the genetic susceptibility to those hazards are also described.

Part II: Airborne Hazards contains information about indoor and outdoor air pollutants, including asbestos, carbon monoxide, formaldehyde, mold spores, environmental tobacco smoke, acid rain, and ozone. It also describes the Air Quality Index, a tool used to report on daily air quality.

Part III: Waterborne Hazards discusses drinking water purity, sources of water contamination, and the safety of water used for recreation. It includes facts about chemical and biological water pollutants, such as lead, methyl-*tert*-butyl ether (MTBE), bacteria, and parasites, and explains disinfection methods and the health effects of disinfection byproducts.

Part IV: Chemical Hazards describes the sources and health effects of chemicals such as dioxin, lead, malathion, mercury, pesticides, and repellants. Special problems associated with chemical exposures in the workplace and the concerns of people with multiple chemical sensitivity syndrome (MCS) are also discussed.

Part V: Radiation and Electromagnetic Field Hazards provides information about the health effects of radiation exposure and facts about some sources of environmental radiation, including radon, radioactive materials, and microwaves. It also explains the controversies surrounding low-level exposure to non-ionizing radiation.

Part VI: Biological Hazards contains information about the threat to human health from diseases that could result from the intentional release of biological agents into the environment. These include anthrax, botulism, pneumonic plague, smallpox, and others.

Part VII: Foodborne Hazards describes various types of bacterial, parasitic, viral, and chemical food contamination. It also discusses food additives and bioengineered foods.

Part VIII: Environmental Hazards to Specific Populations provides information about the special risks encountered by children, women, the elderly, and minority populations. Noise, often encountered by many workers in a variety of workplaces, is also addressed.

Part IX: Additional Help and Information includes a glossary of related terms, resource lists of environmental agencies and advocacy groups, and a chapter with information about the U.S. Environmental Protection Agency (EPA)'s compliance and enforcement program.

Bibliographic Note

This volume contains documents and excerpts from publications issued by the following U.S. government agencies: Agency for Toxic Substances and Disease Registry (ATSDR); Centers for Disease Control and Prevention (CDC); Consumer Product Safety Commission (CPSC); National Institute of Environmental Health Sciences (NIEHS); National Institutes of Health (NIH); South Carolina Department of Health and Environmental Control; U.S. Department of Agriculture; U.S. Department of Health and Human Services (DHHS); U.S. Department of Labor; U.S. Environmental Protection Agency (EPA); and the U.S. Food and Drug Administration (FDA).

In addition, this volume contains copyrighted documents from the following organizations and individuals: Alchemy Environmental Laboratories; California Occupational Health Branch; *Marin Independent Journal*; National Pesticide Information Center (NPIC); National Safety Council; New York State Department of Health; and UE United Electrical Radio and Machine Workers of America.

Acknowledgements

Special thanks go to the many organizations, agencies, and individuals who have contributed material for this *Sourcebook* and to the managing editor Karen Bellenir and permissions specialist Liz Barbour.

Note from the Editor

This book is part of Omnigraphics' *Health Reference Series*. The *Series* provides basic information about a broad range of medical concerns. It is not intended to serve as a tool for diagnosing illness, in prescribing treatments, or as a substitute for the physician/patient relationship. All persons concerned about medical symptoms or the possibility of disease are encouraged to seek professional care from an appropriate health care provider.

Our Advisory Board

The *Health Reference Series* is reviewed by an Advisory Board comprised of librarians from public, academic, and medical libraries. We would like to thank the following board members for providing guidance to the development of this series:

Medical Consultant

Medical consultation services are provided to the *Health Reference Series* editors by David A. Cooke, MD. Dr. Cooke is a graduate of Brandeis University, and he received his M.D. degree from the University of Michigan. He completed residency training at the University of Wisconsin Hospital and Clinics. He is board-certified in Internal Medicine. Dr. Cooke currently works as part of the University of Michigan Health System and practices in Brighton, MI. In his free time, he enjoys writing, science fiction, and spending time with his family.

Health Reference Series *Update Policy*

The inaugural book in the *Health Reference Series* was the first edition of *Cancer Sourcebook* published in 1989. Since then, the *Series* has been enthusiastically received by librarians and in the medical community. In order to maintain the standard of providing high-quality health information for the layperson the editorial staff at Omnigraphics felt it was necessary to implement a policy of updating volumes when warranted.

Medical researchers have been making tremendous strides, and it is the purpose of the *Health Reference Series* to stay current with the most recent advances. Each decision to update a volume will be made on an individual basis. Some of the considerations will include how much new information is available and the feedback we receive from people who use the books. If there is a topic you would like to see added to the update list, or an area of medical concern you feel has not been adequately addressed, please write to:

Editor
Health Reference Series
Omnigraphics, Inc.
615 Griswold Street
Detroit, MI 48226
E-mail: editorial@omnigraphics.com

Part One

Understanding the Health Effects of Environmental Hazards

Chapter 1

Environmental Hazards and Your Health

According to the World Health Organization, "In its broadest sense, environmental health comprises those aspects of human health, disease, and injury that are determined or influenced by factors in the environment. This includes the study of both the direct pathological effects of various chemical, physical, and biological agents, as well as the effects on health of the broad physical and social environment, which includes housing, urban development, land use and transportation, industry, and agriculture."[1] The term "environment" also may be used to refer to air, water, and soil. This more narrow definition ignores the manmade environment created by a society. Where and how a society chooses to grow and develop affects the quality of life by determining how long people spend traveling to work, shopping, or going to school. Where and how a society builds its houses, schools, parks, and roadways can also limit the ability of some people to move about and lead a normal life.

Because the impact of the environment on human health is so great, protecting the environment has long been a mainstay of public health practice. National, State, and local efforts to ensure clean air and safe supplies of food and water, to manage sewage and municipal wastes, and to control or eliminate vector-borne illnesses have contributed a great deal to improvements in public health in the

From "Chapter 8: Environmental Health," *Healthy People 2010: Volume 1, 2nd Edition*, U.S. Department of Health and Human Services (DHHS), Washington, DC: U.S. Government Printing Office, November 2000. Available online at http://www.health.gov/healthypeople/document/html/volume1/08environmental.htm.

3

United States. Unfortunately, in spite of the billions of dollars spent to manage and clean up hazardous waste sites in the Nation each year, little money has been spent evaluating the health risks associated with chronic, low-level exposures to hazardous substances. This imbalance results in an inadequate amount of useful information to evaluate and manage these sites effectively and to evaluate the health status of people who live near the sites.[2] In the past, research in environmental epidemiology and toxicology has often been based on limited information. New knowledge about the interactions between specific genetic variations among individuals and specific environmental factors provides enormous opportunity for further developing modifications in environmental exposures that contribute to disease. Further research is needed to address these and other problems and to improve the science and management of health effects on people exposed to environmental hazards.[3]

Issues

Environmental factors play a central role in human development, health, and disease. Broadly defined, the environment, including infectious agents, is one of three primary factors that affect human health. The other two are genetic factors and personal behavior.

Human exposures to hazardous agents in the air, water, soil, and food and to physical hazards in the environment are major contributors to illness, disability, and death worldwide. Furthermore, deterioration of environmental conditions in many parts of the world slows sustainable development. Poor environmental quality is estimated to be directly responsible for approximately 25 percent of all preventable ill health in the world, with diarrheal diseases and respiratory infections heading the list.[4] Ill health resulting from poor environmental quality varies considerably among countries. Poor environmental quality has its greatest impact on people whose health status already may be at risk.

Because the effect of the environment on human health is so great, protecting the environment has been a mainstay of public health practice since 1878.[5] National, Tribal, State, and local efforts to ensure clean air and safe supplies of food and water, to manage sewage and municipal wastes, and to control or eliminate vector-borne illnesses have contributed significantly to improvements in public health in the United States. However, the public's awareness of the environment's role in health is more recent. Publication of Rachel Carson's *Silent Spring* in the early 1960s, followed by the well-publicized poor health of residents of Love Canal in western New York, a significant toxic waste site, awakened public consciousness to environmental issues. The result of these and other similar events is the so-called environmental movement that has led to the introduction into everyday life of such terms as Superfund sites, water quality, clean air, ozone, urban sprawl, and agricultural runoff.

In 1993 alone, over $109 billion was spent on pollution abatement and control in the United States.[6] However, many hazardous sites still remain. Minimal research has been done to evaluate the health risks associated with chronic low-level exposures to hazardous substances, resulting in an inability to evaluate and manage such sites effectively and to evaluate the health status of residents living near such sites. Further environmental epidemiology and toxicology research is needed to address such problems and to improve the science and public health management of the health effects on people exposed to environmental hazards.

To address the broad range of human health issues affected by the environment, this chapter discusses six topics: outdoor air quality, water quality, toxics and waste, healthy homes and healthy communities, infrastructure and surveillance, and global environmental health issues.

Outdoor air quality. Air pollution continues to be a widespread public health and environmental problem in the United States, causing premature death, cancer, and long-term damage to respiratory and cardiovascular systems. Air pollution also reduces visibility, damages crops and buildings, and deposits pollutants on the soil and in bodies of water where they affect the chemistry of the water and the organisms living there. Approximately 113 million people live in U.S. areas designated as non-attainment areas by the U.S. Environmental Protection Agency (EPA) for one or more of the six commonly found air pollutants for which the Federal Government has established health-based standards.[7] The problem of air pollution is national— even international—in scope. Most of the U.S. population lives in expanding urban areas where air pollution crosses local and State lines and, in some cases, crosses U.S. borders with Canada and Mexico.[8,9]

Although some progress toward reducing unhealthy air emissions has been made, a substantial air pollution problem remains, with millions of tons of toxic air pollutants released into the air each year.[10] The presence of unacceptable levels of ground-level ozone is the largest problem, as determined by the number of people affected and the number of areas not meeting Federal standards.

Motor vehicles account for approximately one-fourth of emissions that produce ozone and one-third of nitrogen oxide emissions. Particulate and sulfur dioxide emissions from motor vehicles represent approximately 20 percent and 4 percent, respectively. Some 76.6 percent of carbon monoxide emissions are produced each year by transportation sources (for example, motor vehicles).[7]

Unhealthy air is expensive. The estimated annual health costs of human exposure to all outdoor air pollutants from all sources range from $40 billion to $50 billion, with an associated 50,000 premature deaths.[11]

Water quality. Providing drinking water free of disease-causing agents, whether biological or chemical, is the primary goal of all water supply systems. During the first half of the 20th century the causes for most waterborne disease outbreaks were bacteria; beginning in the 1970s protozoa and chemicals became the dominant causes.[12] Most outbreaks involve only a few individuals.[13,14,15] In 1993, however, more than 403,000 people became sick during a single episode of waterborne cryptosporidiosis.[15]

One problem in evaluating the relationship between drinking water and infectious diseases is the lack of adequate technology to detect parasitic contamination and to determine whether the organisms detected are alive and infectious. The development of new molecular technologies to detect and monitor water contamination will enhance water quality monitoring and surveillance.

Contamination of water can come from both point (for example, industrial sites) and nonpoint (for example, agricultural runoff) sources. Biological and chemical contamination significantly reduces the value of surface waters (streams, lakes, and estuaries) for fishing, swimming, and other recreational activities. For example, during the summer of 1997, blooms of *Pfiesteria piscicida* were implicated as the likely cause of fish kills in North Carolina and Maryland. The development of intensive animal feeding operations has worsened the discharge of improperly or inadequately treated wastes,[16] which presents an increased health threat in waters used either for recreation or for producing fish and shellfish.

Toxics and waste. Critical information on the levels of exposure to hazardous substances in the environment and their associated health effects often is lacking. As a result, efficient health-outcome measures of progress in eliminating health hazards in the environment are unavailable. The identification of toxic substances and waste, whether hazardous, industrial, or municipal, that pose an environmental health risk represents a significant achievement in itself. Public health strategies are aimed at tracking the Nation's success in eliminating these substances or minimizing their effects.

Toxic and hazardous substances, including low-level radioactive wastes, deposited on land often are carried far from their sources by air, groundwater, and surface water runoff into streams, lakes, and rivers where they can accumulate in the sediments beneath the waters. Ultimate decisions about the cleanup and management of these sites must be made keeping public health concerns in mind.

The introduction and widespread use of pesticides in the American landscape continues in agricultural, commercial, recreational, and home settings. As a result, these often very toxic substances pose a potential threat to people using them, especially if they are handled, mixed, or applied inappropriately or excessively. Furthermore, children are at increased risk for pesticide poisoning because of their smaller size and because pesticides may be stored improperly or applied to surfaces that are more readily accessible by children.

Healthy homes and communities. The public's health, particularly its environmental health, depends on the interaction of many factors. To provide a healthy environment within the Nation's communities, the places people spend the most time—their homes, schools, and offices—must be considered. Potential risks include indoor air pollution; inadequate heating, cooling, and sanitation; structural problems; electrical and fire hazards; and lead-based paint hazards. More than 6 million housing units across the country meet the Federal Government's definition of substandard housing.[17]

Many factors—including air quality; lead-based paint on walls, trim, floors, ceilings, etc.; and hazardous household substances such as cleaning products and pesticides—can affect health and safety. In 1996, the American Association of Poison Control Centers reported more than 2 million poison exposures from 67 participating poison control centers. The site of exposure was a residence in 91 percent of cases.[18]

Infrastructure and surveillance. Preventing health problems caused by environmental hazards requires: (1) having enough personnel and resources to investigate and respond to diseases and injuries potentially caused by environmental hazards; (2) monitoring the population and its environment to detect hazards, exposure of the public and individuals to hazards, and diseases potentially caused by these hazards; (3) monitoring the population and its environment to assess

7

the effectiveness of prevention programs; (4) educating the public and select populations on the relationship between health and the environment; (5) ensuring that laws, regulations, and practices protect the public and the environment from hazardous agents; (6) providing public access to understandable and useful information on hazards and their sources, distribution, and health effects; (7) coordinating the efforts of government agencies and nongovernmental groups responsible for environmental health; and (8) providing adequate resources to accomplish these tasks. Development of additional methods to measure environmental hazards in people will permit more careful assessments of exposures and health effects.

Global environmental health. Increased international travel and improvements in telecommunications and computer technology are making the world a smaller place. The term "global community" has real significance, as shared resources—air, water, and soil—draw people together. Actions in every country affect the environment and influence events around the world. Undoubtedly, the environment affects everyone's health. Sometimes benefits in one area inadvertently create worse conditions for people in different areas of the world. For example, in 1996, the United States exported more than $2.5 billion worth of pesticides.[19] Exported pesticides that are not registered, or pesticides that are restricted for use in the United States, are often used by developing countries. Their use not only endangers populations in those countries but also can contaminate food being exported from those countries to the United States. Sensitive populations, such as children and pregnant women, may be at risk from these environmental exposures. The United States can contribute to improving the health of people internationally, not only as part of a shared goal for humanity, but also because a healthy global population has positive social and economic benefits throughout the world.

Additionally, a number of countries have resources available to protect their populations from adverse health impacts, but because of inadequate information they are unable to do so. Lead abatement technology, for example, is one area where the United States can provide information to other countries. Likewise, consultation and assistance on numerous environmental health issues from lead poisoning to disaster preparedness will help reduce illness, disability, and death in countries with these problems, which can lead to a healthier global community.

The Nation should expand its efforts for improving environmental conditions to enhance the health of developing countries. It should also increase collaboration, coordination, and outreach efforts with the rest of the world to help close the gap between existing and attainable health status.

Trends

During the 1990s, progress in improving environmental health was mixed. The decline in childhood lead poisoning in the United States represents a public health success. In 1984, between 2 million and 3 million children aged 6 months to 5 years had blood lead levels (BLLs) greater than 15 mg/dL, and almost a quarter of a million had BLLs above 25 mg/dL,[20] a level that can affect vital organs and the brain. (Blood levels are measured in micrograms of lead found in a deciliter of blood.) By the early 1990s, fewer than 900,000 children had BLLs above 10mg/dL, the current standard for identifying children at risk.[21] This dramatic reduction is the result of research to identify persons at risk, professional and public education campaigns to spread the word, broad-based screening measures to find those at risk, and effective community efforts to clean up problem areas, namely, substandard housing units. However, despite the success achieved, more remains to be done before childhood lead poisoning becomes a disease of the past. Although childhood lead poisoning occurred in all population groups, the risk was higher for persons having low income, living in older housing, and belonging to certain racial and ethnic groups. For example, among non-Hispanic black children living in homes built before 1946, 22 percent had elevated BLLs. Because the risk for lead poisoning is not spread evenly throughout the population, efforts are continuing to identify children at risk and ensure that they receive preventive interventions.[22]

Unfortunately, not all trends for environmental health issues are as encouraging. Since the mid-1980s, asthma rates in the United States have risen to the level of an epidemic.[23] Asthma and other respiratory conditions often are triggered or worsened by substances found in the air, such as tobacco smoke, ozone, and other particles or chemicals. Based on existing data, an estimated 14.9 million people in the United States had asthma in 1995,[24] including more than 5 million children aged 17 years and under.[25] Between 1980 and 1993, the overall death rate for asthma increased 57 percent, from 12.8 to 20.1 deaths per million population;[23] for people aged 17 years and under, the death rate increased 67 percent, from 1.8 to 3.0 deaths per million population.[26] The direct economic and health care costs of asthma and other respiratory conditions can be large. In 1990, the estimated total cost of asthma was $6.2 billion; the total cost was projected to rise to $14.5 billion by the year 2000.[27] The indirect costs of asthma, measured in reduced quality of life and lost productivity, include the estimated 10 million school days each year that children miss. Lost productivity from missed work days of parents caring for children with asthma is estimated to be $1 billion—not including the cost of lost productivity from adults with asthma who miss work.[27]

Although successes in environmental public health are possible, they are difficult to achieve. Infectious and chemical agents still contaminate food and water. Animals continue to carry diseases to human populations, and outbreaks of once-common intestinal diseases (for example, typhoid fever), although less frequent, still occur. These outbreaks underscore the need to maintain and improve programs developed in the first half of the 20th century to ensure the safety of food and water. The challenge is to retain these basic capacities in the 21st century, with the added responsibilities for dealing with emerging hazards. The control of well-known hazards must coexist with ongoing research and the development of strategies and methods to understand and control new hazards. Another challenge is the need to help the public understand the link between human activity and the destruction of the environment.

Within the United States, significant strides toward a reduction in harmful air emissions can be achieved by individuals choosing not to drive their cars. People need to use public transit, walk, or bicycle more often. Laws can help improve street and highway design to facilitate pedestrians and bicyclists, and employers can embrace telecommuting, but the choice remains with the individual. Encouraging individuals to walk or bike also may play a role in reducing the problems of obesity and overweight individuals, which have risen to alarming levels in the U.S. population.

Urban sprawl has become an increasingly important concern in the United States for several reasons: increased outdoor air pollution in major urban areas, reduced quality of life due to the loss of free time and the stress of increased commuting time, and less green space in major metropolitan areas. Between 1983 and 1995, the average annual vehicle miles traveled increased 80 percent.[28]

These conditions lead to negative health conditions, such as asthma and injuries from road rage due to traffic-related stress.[29] In addition, sprawl diminishes the amount of land available for prime recreational and agricultural uses and can bring two land uses together that do not coexist well. For example, a residential development in an area that was previously agricultural may expose residents to environmental hazards, such as pesticides, which may pose a threat to their health.

On a global scale, the U.S.-Mexico border area illustrates how human activity can contribute to damaging the environment, affecting generations to come. Over the past 30 years, this region has experienced a dramatic surge in population and industrialization. The region has had great difficulty in supporting this growth and suffers from a lack of resources and expertise to manage solid waste properly, handle and store pesticides and other hazardous materials, supply sufficient drinking water, and support other sustainable development efforts.[8] Nations need to make choices about how to deal with such regions; offering technical assistance is an option to speed knowledge transfer and reduce environmental harm.

Disparities

Studies have linked race and socioeconomic status to increased exposure to environmental hazards, and information about gene-environment interactions improves the ability to determine who has increased risk of disease from these exposures. Table 1.1 and Table 1.2 summarize some inequities in the United States regarding exposure to selected potential environmental hazards.

Disparities exist in the environmental exposures certain populations face and in the health status of these populations. For example,

Table 1.1. Proportions of African American, Hispanic, and White Populations Living in Air-Quality Non-Attainment Areas, 1992.[30]

	Demographic Breakdowns		
Pollutant	African Americans	Hispanics	Whites
	Percent Living in Air-Quality Non-Attainment Areas		
Particulates	16.5	34.0	14.7
Carbon monoxide	46.0	57.1	33.6
Ozone	62.2	71.2	52.5
Sulfur dioxide	12.1	5.7	7.0
Lead	9.2	18.5	6.0

Table 1.2. Proportions of Certain Racial and Ethnic and Lower Socioeconomic Populations in Census Tracts Surrounding Waste Treatment, Storage, and Disposal Facilities (TSDF) Compared with the Proportions of These Groups in Other Census Tracts, 1994.[30]

	Demographic Breakdowns		
Location of TSDFs	African Americans	Hispanics	Persons Living Below the Poverty Line
	Percent		
Census tracts with either TSDFs or at least 50 percent of their area within 2.5miles of a tract with TSDF	24.7	10.7	19.0
Census tracts without TSDFs	13.6	7.3	13.1

in New York City, African American, Hispanic, and low-income populations have been found to have hospitalization and death rates from asthma three to five times higher than those for all New York City residents. African American children have been found to be three times more likely than white children to be hospitalized for asthma and asthma-related conditions and four to six times more likely to die from asthma.[30] With respect to BLL, children from certain racial and ethnic groups are disproportionately affected. While there are no studies to show rural and frontier dwellers are at increased risk to exposure to contaminated drinking water, the preponderance of this population depends on unregulated private wells for their drinking water. The U.S. Geological Survey (USGS) reports that 42.8 million persons in the United States (17 percent of the total population) were served by their own (self-supplied) water systems in 1990.[31]

Opportunities

An increase in public awareness of environmental health issues is key to achieving this chapter's goal and objectives. Education—at all levels—is a cornerstone of broad prevention efforts.

Improving the availability of environmental health data also will help meet the objectives. The Internet has increased dramatically access to environmental information. Databases such as TOXNET (at http://toxnet.nlm.nih.gov),[32] Internet Grateful Med (at http://igm.nlm.nih.gov),[33] and TRI (the Toxics Release Inventory www.epa.gov/ceisweb1/ceishome/ceisdata/xplor-tri/explorer.htm) may provide useful information about environmental hazards or other environmental problems in communities to health care providers, policymakers, and the public. Moreover, better dissemination of global environmental health information may reduce the occurrence of disease or exposure to harmful environmental agents for U.S. citizens traveling abroad.

To be successful, programs to improve environmental health must be based on scientific evidence. The complex relationship between human health and the acute and long-term effects of environmental exposures must be studied so prevention measures can be developed. Surveillance systems to track exposures to toxic substances such as commonly used pesticides and heavy metals must be developed and maintained. To the extent possible, these systems should use bio-monitoring data, which provide measurements of toxic substances in the human body. A mechanism is needed for tracking the export of pesticides restricted or not registered for use in the United States.

Environmental hazards are not limited by political boundaries. The scope of public and environmental health must be global if the Nation is to achieve good health for all persons in the United States. A global scope will help develop and achieve effective ways to prevent disease worldwide as well. The United States must work with other governments, nongovernmental organizations, and international organizations to help improve human health on a global scale.

Interim Progress Toward Year 2000 Objectives

Healthy People 2000 targets have been met for objectives dealing with outbreaks of waterborne diseases, with solid wastes, and with toxic substances released through industrial processes. Substantial progress has been made in objectives involving the proportion of people who live in counties that meet EPA air standards for air pollution, the number of States that require radon disclosures with real estate transactions, and the recycling of household hazardous waste. More moderate progress has taken place for the objectives involving radon and lead-based paint testing in homes, asthma hospitalizations, and States with laws to track environmental diseases. Mixed progress or movement away from the targets is being seen in objectives dealing with mental retardation and impaired surface waters (rivers, lakes, and estuaries). Data have been mixed or difficult to assess for

13

the cleanup of hazardous waste sites. The target for blood lead levels in children has not been met, though some progress has been made.

Note: Unless otherwise noted, data are from the Centers for Disease Control and Prevention, National Center for Health Statistics, *Healthy People 2000 Review*, 1998-99.

References

1. World Health Organization (WHO). Indicators for Policy and Decision Making in Environmental Health. (Draft). Geneva, Switzerland: WHO, 1997.

2. National Research Council. *Environmental Epidemiology: Public Health and Hazardous Wastes*. Vol. 1. Washington, DC: National Academy Press, 1991.

3. Agency for Toxic Substances and Disease Registry (ATSDR). Priority Health Conditions-An Integrated Strategy to Evaluate the Relationship Between Illness and Exposure to Hazardous Substances. Atlanta, GA: U.S. Department of Health and Human Services (HHS), 1993.

4. WHO. Fact Sheet 170. Geneva, Switzerland: WHO, 1997.

5. Commissioned Corps of the U.S. Public Health Service, HHS. http://www.os.dhhs.gov/phs/corps/direct1.html#history, June 14, 2000.

6. U.S. Bureau of Economic Analysis. Survey of Current Business. May 1995.

7. U.S. Environmental Protection Agency (EPA). National Air Quality and Trends Report. Washington, DC: EPA, Office of Air and Radiation, 1997.

8. EPA. U.S.-Mexico Border XXI Program: Framework Document. No. EPA 160. R-96-003. Washington, DC: EPA, 1996.

9. Thurston, G.D.; Gorczynski, J.E.; Currie, J.J.; et al. The nature and origins of acid summer haze air pollution in metropolitan Toronto, Ontario. *Environmental Research* 65(2):254-270, 1994.

10. EPA. 1997 National Toxics Inventory Report. Washington, DC: EPA, 1997.

11. American Lung Association. Health Costs of Air Pollution. 1990.

12. Craun, G.F. Statistics of waterbourne outbreaks in the U.S. (1920-1980). In: Craun, G.F., ed. *Waterborne Disease Outbreaks in the United States*. Boca Raton, FL: CRC Press, 1986.

13. Centers for Disease Control and Prevention (CDC). Surveillance for waterborne disease outbreaks—United States, 1991-1992. *Morbidity and Mortality Weekly Report* 42(SS-5):1-22, 1993. PubMed; PMID 8232179

14. CDC. Surveillance for waterborne disease outbreaks—United States, 1989-1990. *Morbidity and Mortality Weekly Report* 40(SS-3):1-21, 1991. PubMed; PMID 1770924

15. CDC. Surveillance for waterborne disease outbreaks—United States, 1993-1994. *Morbidity and Mortality Weekly Report* 45(SS-1):1-33, 1995.

16. Animal Waste Pollution in America: An Emerging Problem, Environmental Risks of Livestock and Poultry Production. Minority Staff Report for Senator Tom Harkin (D-IA), Ranking Member, U.S. Senate Committee on Agriculture, Nutrition, and Forestry. 1997.

17. U.S. Bureau of the Census. American Housing Survey for the United States in 1995. In: *Current Housing Reports*. H150/95RV. Washington, DC: U.S. Government Printing Office (GPO), 1997.

18. Litovitz, T.L.; Smilkstein, M.; Felberg, L.; et al. 1996 Annual Report of the American Association of Poison Control Centers: Toxic Exposure Surveillance System. *American Journal of Emergency Medicine* 15:447-500, 1997. PubMed; PMID 9270389

19. Chemical Economics Handbook. SRF International, September 1997. Retrieved April 10, 1998, from DIALOG database (#359).

20. ATSDR. The Nature and Extent of Childhood Lead Poisoning in Children in the United States: A Report to Congress. Washington, DC: HHS, 1988.

21. CDC. Screening Young Children for Lead Poisoning: Guidance for State and Local Public Health Officials. Atlanta, GA: CDC, 1997.

22. CDC. Update: Blood lead levels in the United States, 1991-1994. *Morbidity and Mortality Weekly Report* 46:143, 1997.

23. Mannino, D.M.; Homa, D.M.; Pertowski, C.A.; et al. Surveillance for asthma—United States, 1960-1995. In: CDC Surveillance Summaries, April 24, 1998. *Morbidity and Mortality Weekly Report* 47(SS-1):1-27, 1998. PubMed; PMID 9580746

24. National Heart, Lung, and Blood Institute. Data Fact Sheet. Asthma Statistics. Bethesda, MD: National Institutes of Health, Public Health Service, 1999.

25. President's Task Force on Environmental Health Risks and Safety Risks to Children. Asthma and the Environment: A Strategy to Protect Children. Washington, DC: the Task Force, 1998.

26. Redd, S. Chief, Air and Respiratory Branch, National Centers for Environmental Health, CDC. Personal communication.

27. Weiss, K.B.; Gergen, P.J.; and Hodgson, T.A. An economic evaluation of asthma in the United States. *New England Journal of Medicine* 326:862-866, 1992. PubMed; PMID 1542323

28. Hu, P.S. Summary of Travel Trends 1995 Nationwide Personal Transportation Survey. Washington, DC: U.S. Department of Transportation, 1999, 13.

29. Schmidt, C. Environmental Health Perspectives 106(6):1998.

30. Institute of Medicine. *Toward Environmental Justice—Research, Education, and Health Policy Needs*. Washington, DC: National Academy Press, 1999.

31. U.S. Geological Survey. U.S. Geological Survey: Estimated use of water in the United States in 1990. *USGS National Circular 1081*. Washington, DC: GPO, 1993.

32. Toxnet7, National Library of Medicine, Toxicology and Environmental Health Information Program, Bethesda, MD.

33. Internet Grateful Med, National Library of Medicine, Bethesda, MD.

Chapter 2

Environmental Diseases from A to Z

The air, the water, the sun, the dust, plants and animals, and the chemicals and metals of our world—they support life. They make it beautiful and fun. But, as wonderful as they are, they can also make some people sick. Following are some diseases that are related to your environment and some ideas for preventing or caring for them.

Allergies and Asthma

About 50 million people in the U.S.—one in five adults and kids—have allergies. They sneeze, their noses run and their eyes itch from pollen, dust and other substances. Some suffer sudden attacks that leave them breathless and gasping for air. This is allergic asthma. Asthma attacks often occur after periods of heavy exercise or during sudden changes in the weather. Some can be triggered by pollutants and other chemicals in the air and in the home. Doctors can test to find out which substances are causing reactions. They can also prescribe drugs to relieve the symptoms.

Birth Defects

Sometimes, when pregnant women are exposed to chemicals or drink a lot of alcohol, harmful substances reach the fetus. Some of

"Environmental Diseases from A to Z," a booklet produced by the National Institute of Environmental Health Sciences, 1996. Available online at http://www.niehs.nih.gov/external/a2z/prt-home.htm. Despite the older date of this document, it provides good descriptions of the types of diseases that can be caused by environmental sources.

these babies are born with an organ, tissue or body part that has not developed in a normal way. Aspirin and cigarette smoking can also cause birth problems. Each year, about 150,000 babies born in the United States have defects. Many of these could be prevented.

Cancer

Cancer occurs when a cell or group of cells begins to multiply more rapidly than normal. As the cancer cells spread, they affect nearby organs and tissues in the body. Eventually, the organs are not able to perform their normal functions. More than 8 million Americans have cancer. Some of these are caused by substances in the environment: cigarette smoke, asbestos, radiation, natural and man-made chemicals, alcohol, and sunlight. People can reduce their risk of getting cancer by limiting their exposure to these harmful agents.

Dermatitis

Dermatitis is a fancy name for inflamed, irritated skin. Many of us have experienced the oozing bumps and itching caused by poison ivy, oak and sumac. Some chemicals found in paints, dyes, cosmetics and detergents can also cause rashes and blisters. Too much wind and sun make the skin dry and chapped. Fabrics, foods, and certain medications can cause unusual reactions in some individuals. People can protect themselves from poison ivy by following a simple rule: "Leaves of three, leave them be." Smart folks know their poisons.

Emphysema

Air pollution and cigarette smoke can break down sensitive tissue in the lungs. Once this happens, the lungs cannot expand and contract properly. This condition is called emphysema. About 2 million Americans have this disease. For these people, each breath is hard work. Even moderate exercise is difficult. Some emphysema patients must breath from tanks of oxygen.

Fertility Problems

Fertility is the ability to produce children. However, one in eight couples has a problem. This can occur when a woman can't produce an egg, or when a man can't produce enough sperm. Infertility can be caused by infections that come from sexual diseases or from exposure to chemicals on the job or elsewhere in the environment. Researchers at the National Institute of Environmental Health Sciences (NIEHS) have shown that too much caffeine in the diet can temporarily reduce a woman's fertility. NIEHS scientists have also pinpointed the days when a woman is likely to be fertile.

Goiter

Sometimes people don't get enough iodine from the foods they eat. This can cause a small gland called the thyroid to grow larger. The thyroid can become so large that it looks like a baseball sticking out of the front of your neck. This is called goiter. Since the thyroid controls basic functions like growth and energy, goiter can produce a wide range of effects. Some goiter patients are unusually restless and nervous. Others tend to be sluggish and lethargic. Goiter became rare after public health officials decided that iodine should be added to salt.

Heart Disease

More than one in four Americans suffer from diseases of the heart and blood vessels. These diseases cause almost half of all deaths in the United States. While these may be due in part to poor eating habits and/or lack of exercise, environmental chemicals also play a role. While most chemicals that enter the body are broken down into harmless substances by the liver, some are converted into particles called free radicals that can react with proteins in the blood to form fatty deposits called plaques, which can clog blood vessels. A blockage can cut off the flow of blood to the heart, causing a heart attack.

Immune Deficiency Diseases

The immune system fights germs, viruses and poisons that attack the body. It is composed of white blood cells and other warrior cells. When a foreign particle enters the body, these cells surround and destroy this enemy. We have all heard of AIDS and the harm it does to the immune system. Some chemicals and drugs can also weaken the immune system by damaging its specialized cells. When this occurs, the body is more vulnerable to diseases and infections.

Job-Related Illnesses

Every job has certain hazards. Even a writer can get a paper cut. But did you know that about 137 workers die from job-related diseases

19

every day? This is more than eight times the number of people who die from job-related accidents. Many of these illnesses are caused by chemicals and other agents present in the workplace. Factories and scientific laboratories can contain poisonous chemicals, dyes and metals. Doctors and other health workers have to work with radiation. People who work in airports or play in rock concerts can suffer hearing loss from loud noise. Some jobs involve extreme heat or cold. Workers can protect themselves from hazards by wearing special suits and using goggles, gloves, ear plugs, and other equipment.

Kidney Diseases

About 3.5 million Americans have kidney diseases. These range from simple infections to total kidney failure. People with kidney failure cannot remove wastes and poisons from their blood. They depend on expensive kidney machines in order to stay alive. Some chemicals found in the environment can produce kidney damage. Some nonprescription drugs, when taken too often, can also cause kidney problems. Be sure to read the label and use drugs as directed.

Lead Poisoning

Sometimes, infants and children will pick up and eat paint chips and other objects that contain lead. Lead dust, fumes and lead-contaminated water can also introduce lead into the body. Lead can damage the brain, kidneys, liver, and other organs. Severe lead poisoning can produce headaches, cramps, convulsions, and even death. Even small amounts can cause learning problems and changes in behavior. Doctors can test for lead in the blood and recommend ways to reduce further exposure.

Mercury Poisoning

Mercury is a silvery metal that is extremely poisonous. Very small amounts can damage the kidneys, liver and brain. Years ago, workers in hat factories were poisoned by breathing the fumes from mercury used to shape the hats. Remember the "Mad Hatter" in Alice in Wonderland? Today, mercury exposure usually results from eating contaminated fish and other foods that contain small amounts of mercury compounds. Since the body cannot get rid of mercury, it gradually builds up inside the tissues. If it is not treated, mercury poisoning can eventually cause pain, numbness, weak muscles, loss of vision, paralysis and even death.

Nervous System Disorders

The nervous system, which includes the brain, spinal cord and nerves, commands and controls our thoughts, feelings, movements and behavior. The nervous system consists of billions of nerve cells. They carry messages and instructions from the brain and spinal cord to other parts of the body. When these cells are damaged by toxic chemicals, injury or disease, this information system breaks down. This can result in disorders ranging from mood changes and memory loss to blindness, paralysis and death. Proper use of safety devices such as seat belts, child restraints and bike helmets can prevent injuries and save lives.

Osteoporosis

When the body can't supply enough calcium, bones become thin and fragile. This is called osteoporosis. About 25 million Americans suffer from some kind of bone thinning. As people get older, back problems become more common, and bones in the spine, hips and wrists break more easily. Young people can lower their chances of getting osteoporosis in later years by exercising and eating calcium-rich foods like milk and yogurt.

Pneumoconiosis

Ordinary house and yard dusts do not pose a serious health hazard. But some airborne particles can be very dangerous. These include fibers from asbestos, cotton and hemp, and dusts from such compounds as silica, graphite, coal, iron and clay. These particles can damage sensitive areas of the lung, turning healthy tissue into scar tissue. This condition is called pneumoconiosis, or black lung. Chest pains and shortness of breath often progress to bronchitis, emphysema, and/or early death. Proper ventilation and the use of protective masks can greatly reduce the risk of lung disease.

Queensland Fever

People do not usually get diseases from farm animals. However, those who work with hides and animal products can get sick from breathing the infected dust around them. This illness is called Queensland fever because it was first discovered among cattle ranchers and dairy farmers in Queensland, Australia. It is caused by a tiny organism that infects livestock and then spreads to the milk and feces. Symptoms include fever, chills, and muscle aches and pains. Researchers have developed vaccines to protect livestock workers from this illness.

Reproductive Disorders

Beginning in the late 1940's, many women who were in danger of losing their unborn babies were prescribed a synthetic female hormone called DES (diethylstilbestrol). In 1971, scientists discovered that some of the daughters of these women were developing a very rare cancer of the reproductive organs. Since then, the use of DES and other synthetic hormones during pregnancy has been discontinued. NIEHS and other agencies are studying the possibility that some natural chemicals and man-made pesticides may cause similar problems. They are finding that some of these chemicals are so similar to female estrogen that they may actually mimic this important hormone. As a result, they may interfere with the development of male and female reproductive organs. This can lead to increased risk of early puberty, low sperm counts, ovarian cysts, and cancer of the breast or testicles.

Sunburn and Skin Cancer

Almost everyone has stayed in the sun too long and been burned. Too much sunlight can also produce the most common type of cancer—skin cancer. Some skin cancers are easy to treat because they do not spread beyond the surrounding tissue. Others, like melanoma, are much more dangerous because they spread to other parts of the body. Deaths due to melanoma are increasing by 4 percent each year. People can protect themselves from the sun's rays by applying sunscreen, wearing protective clothing, and, when possible, staying out of the sun between 10 a.m. and 2 p.m.

Tooth Decay

In the 1930's, health experts noticed that people who lived in areas where the water contained natural chemicals called fluorides had fewer cavities. Today, nearly half of all Americans drink water that is either naturally fluoridated or treated with fluorides. This has lowered the incidence of cavities as much as 65 percent. Dentists can also protect young teeth by applying special coatings called sealants.

Uranium Poisoning

Uranium is a dangerous element because it is radioactive. This means it gives off high-energy particles that can go through the body and damage living tissue. A single high dose of radiation can kill.

Small doses over a long period can also be harmful. For example, miners who are exposed to uranium dust are more likely to get lung cancer. Uranium poisoning can also damage the kidneys and interfere with the body's ability to fight infection. While most people will never come in contact with uranium, those who work with medical x-rays or radioactive compounds are also at risk. They should wear lead shields and follow recommended safety guidelines to protect themselves from unnecessary exposure.

Vision Problems

Our eyes are especially sensitive to the environment. Gases found in polluted air can irritate the eyes and produce a burning sensation. Tiny particles from smoke and soot can also cause redness and itching of the eyes. Airborne organisms like molds and fungus can cause infections of the eyes and eyelids. Too much exposure to the sun's rays can eventually produce a clouding of the lens called a cataract.

Waterborne Diseases

Even our clearest streams, rivers, and lakes can contain chemical pollutants. Heavy metals like lead and mercury can produce severe organ damage. Some chemicals can interfere with the development of organs and tissues, causing birth defects. Others can cause normal cells to become cancerous. Some of our waterways also contain human and animal wastes. The bacteria in the wastes can cause high fever, cramps, vomiting and diarrhea.

Xeroderma Pigmentosa

Xeroderma is a rare condition that people inherit from their parents. When these people are exposed to direct sunlight, their skin breaks out into tiny dark spots that look like freckles. If this condition is not treated, the spots can become cancerous. These areas must then be removed by a surgeon.

Yusho Poisoning

In 1968, more than one thousand people in western Japan became seriously ill. They suffered from fatigue, headache, cough, numbness in the arms and legs, and unusual skin sores. Pregnant women later delivered babies with birth defects. These people had eaten food that was cooked in contaminated rice oil. Toxic chemicals called PCB's (polychlorinated biphenyls) had accidentally leaked into the oil during the manufacturing process. Health experts now refer to this illness as Yusho, which means oil disease.

For years, PCB's were widely used in the manufacturing of paints, plastics and electrical equipment. When scientists discovered that low levels of PCB's could kill fish and other wildlife, their use was dramatically reduced. By this time, PCB's were already leaking into the environment from waste disposal sites and other sources. Today, small amounts of these compounds can still be found in our air, water, soil and some of the foods we eat.

Zinc Deficiency/Zinc Poisoning

Zinc is a mineral that the body needs to function properly. In rare cases, people can be poisoned if there is too much zinc in their food or water. However most people can take in large quantities without any harmful effects. In areas where nutrition is a problem, people may not get enough zinc from their diet. This can lead to retarded growth, skin sores, baldness, infertility and lower resistance to infections.

Chapter 3

Asthma and Its Environmental Triggers

What Is Asthma?

Asthma is a lung disease that can be life threatening.

Asthma is a chronic, or long-term disease, which can affect you for the rest of your life.

Asthma causes breathing problems. The airways in the lungs get blocked, causing the lungs to get less air than normal. Symptoms of an asthma attack can be difficulty with breathing, a tight feeling in the chest, coughing and wheezing. Asthma can develop quickly and it can range from being a mild discomfort to a life-threatening attack if breathing stops completely. Asthma problems are often separated by symptom-free periods.

What Happens in an Asthma Attack?

When asthma causes breathing problems, the breathing problems are called asthma attacks or episodes of asthma. During an asthma attack, three major changes that can take place in the lungs include:

1. Cells in the air tubes make more mucus than normal. This mucus is very thick and sticky, and tends to clog up the tubes.

"Asthma Facts," an undated fact sheet produced by the U.S. Environmental Protection Agency (EPA); available online at http://www.epa.gov/iaq/asthma/introduction.html. Cited February 2003.

2. Cells in the airways get inflamed, causing the air tubes to swell.

3. The muscles around the air tubes tighten.

These changes cause the air tubes to narrow which makes it hard to breathe.

Who Gets Asthma?

In the United States, about 15 million people of all age, race, and nationality have asthma. Asthma can occur at any age but is more common in children than adults.

Nearly 1 in 13 school-age children has asthma, and that rate is rising more rapidly in preschool-aged children than in any other group. Asthma is the leading cause of school absenteeism due to a chronic illness.

The impact of asthma falls disproportionately on African-American and certain Hispanic populations and appears to be particularly severe in urban inner cities. Many cases of asthma likely go undiagnosed.

How Are Children Affected by Asthma?

Asthma is the most common long-term childhood disease, affecting 4.8 million children. Nearly 1 in 13 school-aged children has asthma, and the percentage of children with asthma is rising more rapidly in preschool-aged children than in any other age group.

Asthma accounts for one-third of all pediatric emergency room visits and is the fourth most common cause for physician office visits. Asthma is one of the leading causes of school absenteeism, accounting for over 10 million missed school days per year. Asthma also accounts for many nights of interrupted sleep, limitation of activity, and disruptions of family and caregiver routines. Asthma symptoms that are not severe enough to require a visit to an emergency room or to a physician can still be severe enough to prevent a child with asthma from living a fully active life.

Children breathe more air, eat more food, and drink more liquid in proportion to their body weight than do adults. Their developing bodies may be more susceptible to environmental exposures than those of adults. In a typical day, children may be exposed to a wide array of environmental agents at home, in day care centers, schools and while playing outdoors.

What Triggers Asthma Attacks?

Asthma attacks can be caused by something that bothers the lungs. These are called asthma triggers. There are many kinds of asthma triggers. Two major categories of asthma triggers are allergens and irritants.

If you, or a loved one has asthma, it's important to learn which triggers are a problem. Ask your doctor to help. Your doctor may suggest keeping an asthma diary or recommend skin testing for allergies.

Once asthma triggers are known, actions can be taken to prevent asthma attacks. Cutting down exposure to your triggers may help in avoiding asthma attacks. When attacks occur, they will probably be less severe.

About Asthma Triggers

Allergens are substances that cause no problem for a majority of people but which trigger an allergic reaction in some people. During an allergy attack, the body releases chemicals called mediators. These mediators often trigger asthma episodes.

Irritants such as cold air, cigarette smoke, industrial chemicals, perfume, and paint and gasoline fumes can trigger asthma. These irritants probably trigger asthma symptoms by stimulating irritant receptors in the respiratory tract. These receptors, in turn, cause the muscles surrounding the airway to constrict, resulting in an asthma attack.

Viral infections are the leading cause of acute asthma attacks. Surprisingly, bacterial infections, with the exception of sinusitis, generally do not bring about asthma attacks. Since Americans spend up to 90% of their time indoors, exposure to indoor allergens and irritants may play a significant role in triggering asthma episodes.

The following is a list of some of the indoor environmental asthma triggers:

- Secondhand (cigarette) smoke
- Cockroaches
- Dust mites
- Molds
- Pets and other animals with fur or feathers
- House dust
- Ozone

- Combustion by-products
- Pollen (tree, grass and weed)

If I Have Asthma, What Can I Do?

If you have asthma, you probably want to know how to reduce your chances of having an asthma episode and what to do once you have an asthma episode. Your doctor will be able to assist you. Consult your physician to set up an asthma management plan. Your doctor can help you learn to monitor your asthma, take appropriate medication for your asthma, and identify and avoid your asthma triggers. Following your asthma management plan will help keep your asthma under control.

National Academy of Sciences Report— "Clearing the Air: Asthma and Indoor Air Exposures"

The Environmental Protection Agency (EPA) asked the National Academy of Sciences (NAS) to undertake an assessment of the role of indoor air quality in the growing asthma problem. EPA asked NAS to characterize the state of the science on health impacts and prevention strategies, and to provide recommendations on needed research. In response to this request, the National Academy of Sciences Institute of Medicine has issued a report, *Clearing the Air: Asthma and Indoor Air Exposures,* on the role of indoor environmental pollutants in the development and exacerbation of asthma. The report affirms the Administrator's asthma initiative to educate the public about the ways they can help control asthma by managing indoor air quality. The report concludes that exposure to indoor pollutants is an important contributor to the asthma problem in this nation. Asthma sufferers should consult with their doctor about reducing their exposure to secondhand smoke, dust mites, pet dander, molds, and cockroaches.

Chapter 4

Cancer Clusters

A cancer cluster is defined as a greater-than-expected number of cancer cases that occurs within a group of people in a geographic area over a period of time.

Challenges in Identifying

The complex nature of cancer makes it inherently challenging to identify, interpret, and address cancer clusters.

Cancer is a term representing many diseases with a variety of causes. The time between exposure to a cancer-causing agent, or the existence of other risk factors, and the development of cancer can be decades; therefore, causes are hard, and in some cases impossible, to identify.

Cancer in general is common. Since 1990, about 16 million new cancer cases have been diagnosed, according to the American Cancer Society (*Cancer Facts and Figures 2002*). About 1,284,900 new cancer cases were expected to be diagnosed in 2002.

Cancer rates vary by age, race, gender, risk-factors, and type. We know that risk for cancer increases with age and that cancer is caused by both external factors (e.g., tobacco, chemicals, radiation, and infectious organisms) and internal factors (e.g., inherited mutations, hormones, immune conditions). Nutrition, physical inactivity, obesity, and other lifestyle factors also play a role in cancer risk and outcomes.

"About Cancer Clusters," a fact sheet produced by the Centers for Disease Control and Prevention (CDC), reviewed 2002. Available online at http://www.cdc.gov/nceh/clusters/about%20clusters.htm.

These factors may act together or in sequence to initiate or promote cancer. Ten or more years often pass between exposures or mutations and detectable cancer.

Some racial and ethnic groups have a higher incidence of and deaths due to cancer. Such disparities may be due to multiple factors, such as late stage of disease at diagnosis, barriers to health care access, history of other diseases, biologic and genetic differences, health behaviors, differences in exposures to carcinogens in the environment and the workplace, and other risk factors.

Characteristics

What first appears to be a cancer cluster may not be one after all. A review of the situation may show that the number of new cancer cases is in the expected range for the population and therefore that the cases do not represent a cancer cluster. Cancer cases are more likely to represent a cancer cluster if they involve (1) one type of cancer, (2) a rare type of cancer, or (3) a type of cancer in a group not usually affected by that cancer, such as a cancer in children that is normally seen in adults. However, cases of common cancers are those most often perceived and reported by the public as being part of a cancer cluster.

Identification

The investigators develop a case definition, a time period of concern, and the population at risk. They then calculate the expected number of cases and compare them to the observed number. A cluster is confirmed when the observed/expected ratio is greater than 1.0, and the difference is statistically significant.

Usually, a local or state health department provides the first response to a suspected cancer cluster. The local or state health department gathers information about the suspected cancer cluster (e.g., types of cancer, number of cases, addresses and occupations of those people with cancer, possible causes), develops and applies the case definition, and determines whether there is a greater-than-expected number of cases.

Interpretation

Confirmation of a cancer cluster does not necessarily mean that there is any single, external cause or hazard that can be addressed. A confirmed cancer cluster could be the result of any of the following:

- chance

- miscalculation of the expected number of cancer cases (e.g., not considering a risk factor within the population at risk)

- differences in the case definition between observed cases and expected cases

- known causes of cancer (e.g., smoking)

- unknown cause(s) of cancer.

Follow-up investigations can be done, but can take years to complete and the results are generally inconclusive (e.g., usually, no cause is found).

Reporting

If you suspect a cancer cluster in your community or workplace, or if you'd like information such as cancer statistics or trends in your area, first contact your local or state health department or state cancer registry. For information about how to contact your state or local health department, go to http://www.cdc.gov/other.htm#states. For state cancer registry contact information, go to http://www.cdc.gov/cancer/npcr/statecon.htm#list.

Prevention and Early Detection

Concern about cancer and cancer clusters provides an opportunity for people to learn about how they can prevent cancer or identify it early. Sixty-five percent of public inquiries about cancer clusters involve cancers for which screening and preventive measures exist. The best steps that people can take regarding cancer are to (1) educate themselves about their personal risk and risk factors for cancer, (2) avoid these risks, and (3) take advantage of recommended cancer screenings.

The following organizations provide information on cancer in general, risk factors, and recommended screenings:

- American Cancer Society

- The Centers for Disease Control and Prevention (CDC)'s Cancer Prevention and Control Program

- The National Institutes of Health's National Cancer Institute (NCI)

Chapter 5

Reducing Risk from Hazardous Waste

As our society has changed over time, so have the amount and types of wastes we produce. Not only do households discard trash and garbage, but industrial and manufacturing processes create many different types of wastes as well. As technology has advanced, we have continually updated and improved our methods of waste treatment and management. Today, although many individuals, organizations, and businesses take steps to prevent or reduce the amount of waste they generate, it is inevitable that some materials still must be discarded. Environmental controls and sound management practices allow us to balance industrial growth with ecological and human health needs.

In 1965, to encourage environmentally sound methods for disposal of household, municipal, commercial, and industrial refuse, Congress passed the first federal law to require safeguards on these activities, the Solid Waste Disposal Act. Congress amended this law in 1976 by passing the Resource Conservation and Recovery Act (RCRA) (pronounced "Ric-ra"). The primary goals of RCRA are to:

- Protect human health and the environment from the potential hazards of waste disposal.

Excerpted from "RCRA: Reducing Risk from Waste," a booklet produced by the U.S. Environmental Protection Agency (EPA), EPA530-K-97-004, 1997. Despite the older date of this document it gives a good overview of the issues involved. Available online at http://www.epa.gov/epaoswer/general/risk/risk-1.pdf and http://www.epa.gov/epaoswer/general/risk/risk-2.pdf.

- Conserve energy and natural resources.
- Reduce the amount of waste generated.
- Ensure that wastes are managed in an environmentally sound manner.

As more information about the health and environmental impacts of waste disposal became available, Congress revised RCRA in 1980 and in 1984. The 1984 amendments are referred to as the Hazardous and Solid Waste Amendments.

RCRA is divided into sections called Subtitles. Subtitles C and D set forth a framework for the U.S. Environmental Protection Agency's (EPA's) comprehensive waste management program:

- EPA's Subtitle C program establishes a regulatory framework for managing hazardous waste from generation until ultimate disposal.

- EPA's Subtitle D program establishes a system for managing solid (primarily nonhazardous) waste, such as household waste.

RCRA also regulates underground storage tanks (USTs) that store petroleum or certain chemical products under Subtitle I. Requirements exist for the design and operation of these tanks and the development of systems to prevent accidental spills. Examples of facilities using these tanks include petroleum refineries, chemical plants, and commercial gas stations.

The Medical Waste Tracking Act of 1988 was a 2-year demonstration program that expired in June 1991. It created a Subtitle J program designed to track medical waste from generation to disposal. At present, no federal EPA tracking regulations are in effect for medical waste, but many states have adopted their own programs.

The Comprehensive Environmental Response, Compensation, and Liability Act (known as Superfund or CERCLA) is a related statute that deals with cleaning up inactive and abandoned hazardous waste sites. RCRA, on the other hand, deals with materials that are currently destined for disposal or recycling.

The term "RCRA" is often used interchangeably to refer to the law, regulations, and EPA policy and guidance. The law describes the waste management program mandated by Congress that gave EPA authority to develop the RCRA program.

EPA regulations carry out the Congressional intent by providing explicit, legally enforceable requirements for waste management.

These regulations can be found in Title 40 of the Code of Federal Regulations (CFR), Parts 238 through 282. EPA guidance documents and policy directives clarify issues related to the implementation of the regulations. These three elements are the primary parts of the RCRA program.

This chapter is intended to provide an overall perspective on how RCRA works, including the roles of EPA, states, tribes, the public, and the regulated community. It focuses primarily on Subtitle C and presents some information on Subtitle D as well. Additional information and publications can be obtained by calling the RCRA Hotline at 800-424-9346 or TDD (hearing impaired) 800-553-7672. From within the Washington, DC area, call 703-412-9810 or TDD 703-412-3323.

The Role of the States

In a given state, the hazardous waste regulatory program described in this document may be run by either EPA or a state hazardous waste agency. Both of these entities can be referred to as the "regulatory agency," depending on the state.

RCRA encourages states to assume primary responsibility for implementing the RCRA program, instead of EPA. States that want to adopt and implement the RCRA Subtitle C program must develop a program for the management of hazardous waste that is at least as stringent as the EPA program. State programs can be more stringent or broader in scope, however. This process ensures that minimum standards are met nationwide, while providing flexibility to states in implementing rules.

Subtitle C: What Is a Hazardous Waste?

Hazardous wastes come in many shapes and forms. They can be liquids, solids, contained gases, or sludges. They can be the byproducts of manufacturing processes or simply discarded commercial products, like cleaning fluids or pesticides. Whatever their form, proper management and disposal are essential to protect human health and the environment.

RCRA provides a general definition of the term "hazardous waste." EPA has defined by regulation which specific materials are considered hazardous waste under Subtitle C. Under this definition, the universe of potential hazardous wastes is extremely large and diverse. The regulatory definition evolves and changes as new information becomes available.

EPA works closely with industry and the public to determine which of these wastes should be subject to the RCRA hazardous waste regulations. The Agency developed four defining characteristics of hazardous waste and four lists of specific hazardous wastes.

According to EPA estimates, of the 13 billion tons of industrial, agricultural, commercial, and household wastes generated annually, more than 279 million tons (2 percent) are "hazardous," as defined by RCRA regulations.

Characteristic Wastes

A waste is hazardous if it exhibits one or more of the following characteristics:

- *Ignitability.* Ignitable wastes can create fires under certain conditions or are spontaneously combustible. Examples include waste oils and used solvents.

- *Corrosivity.* Corrosive wastes are acids or bases that are capable of corroding metal, such as storage tanks, containers, drums, and barrels. Battery acid is a good example.

- *Reactivity.* Reactive wastes are unstable under normal conditions. They can cause explosions, toxic fumes, gases, or vapors when mixed with water. Examples include lithium-sulfur batteries and explosives.

- *Toxicity.* Toxic wastes are harmful or fatal when ingested or absorbed. When toxic wastes are disposed of on land, contaminated liquid may drain (leach) from the waste and pollute ground water. Toxicity is defined through a laboratory procedure called the Toxicity Characteristic Leaching Procedure (TCLP). The TCLP helps identify wastes likely to leach concentrations of contaminants that may be harmful to human health or the environment. Certain chemical wastes and heavy metals are examples of potential toxic wastes.

Listed Wastes

By definition, EPA determined that some specific wastes are hazardous. These wastes are incorporated into lists published by the Agency. These lists are organized into three categories:

- *Source-specific wastes.* This list includes certain wastes from specific industries, such as petroleum refining or pesticide manufacturing. Certain sludges and wastewaters from treatment and production processes in these industries are examples of source-specific wastes.

- *Nonspecific source wastes.* This list identifies wastes from common manufacturing and industrial processes. These include solvents that have been used in cleaning or degreasing operations.

- *Commercial chemical products.* This list includes specific commercial chemical products in an unused form. Some pesticides and some pharmaceutical products become hazardous waste when discarded.

What Is a Hazardous Waste?

To be considered hazardous waste, materials must first meet the legal definition of solid waste. Solid waste is discarded material, including garbage, refuse, and sludge (solids, semisolids, liquids, or contained gaseous materials).

Solid wastes that meet any of the following criteria are considered hazardous and subject to EPA regulations. Hazardous wastes are those that:

- Possess one or more of the four characteristics of hazardous waste.

- Are included on an EPA list of hazardous waste.

- Are a mixture of nonhazardous and hazardous waste listed solely for a characteristic (e.g., dirty water mixed with spent solvents).

- Derive from the treatment, storage, or disposal of a hazardous waste (e.g., incineration ash or emission control dust).

- Are soil, ground water, or sediment (environmental media) contaminated with hazardous waste.

- Are either manufactured objects, plant or animal matter, or natural geological material (debris) containing hazardous waste that are intended for disposal (e.g., concrete, bricks, industrial equipment, rocks, and grass).

What Is Not a Regulated Hazardous Waste?

The following are some of the wastes that have been excluded from RCRA hazardous waste regulations:

- Domestic sewage.

- Irrigation waters or industrial discharges allowed under the Clean Water Act.

- Nuclear material regulated by the Atomic Energy Act.

- Household wastes, even when they include hazardous materials, such as paints and pesticides.

- Certain mining and mineral processing wastes.

Table 5.1. Typical Hazardous Wastes Generated by Selected Industries

Waste Generators	Waste Type
Chemical manufacturers	Strong acids and bases, Reactive wastes, Ignitable wastes, Discarded commercial chemical products
Vehicle maintenance shops	Paint wastes, Ignitable wastes, Spent solvents, Acids and bases
Printing industry	Photography waste with heavy metals, Heavy metal solutions, Waste inks, Spent solvents
Paper industry	Ignitable wastes, Corrosive wastes, Ink wastes, including solvents and metals
Construction industry	Ignitable wastes, Paint wastes, Spent solvents, Strong acids and bases
Cleaning agents and cosmetic manufacturing	Heavy metal dusts and sludges, Ignitable wastes, Solvents, Strong acids and bases
Furniture and wood manufacturing and refinishing	Ignitable wastes, Spent solvents, Paint wastes
Metal Manufacturing	Paint wastes containing heavy metals, Strong acids and bases, Cyanide wastes, Sludges containing heavy metals

All listed wastes are presumed to be hazardous regardless of the concentrations of their constituents. They must be handled according to EPA's Subtitle C hazardous waste regulations. If, however, a company can demonstrate that its specific waste is not hazardous, the waste may be delisted. Delisted wastes are no longer subject to Subtitle C regulations.

Expanding Definitions

RCRA regulations were written so that all characteristic and listed hazardous wastes are regulated under Subtitle C. As newer technologies have become available and new multimedia (land, air, and water) modeling tools have emerged, EPA has been able to better evaluate the risks posed by different hazardous constituent concentration levels. Consequently, RCRA regulations can be refined to more closely match the risk of a waste with the appropriate management approaches. The Agency is altering its current approach to managing hazardous wastes so that some wastes will not be subject to full regulation as hazardous wastes. Some may fall out of the realm of Subtitle C requirements and will be managed as nonhazardous solid waste instead.

Subtitle C: Controlling Hazardous Waste from Generation to Disposal

EPA designed the RCRA regulations to ensure proper management of hazardous waste from the moment the waste is generated until its ultimate disposal—cradle to grave. This step-by-step approach monitors and controls hazardous waste at every point in the waste cycle, thereby protecting human health and the environment from the dangers of mismanagement. This approach has two key elements:

- *Tracking.* A tracking system requires each facility handling waste to obtain an identification number. Generators must prepare a uniform manifest document to accompany any transported hazardous waste from the point of generation to the point of final disposal.

- *Permitting.* EPA or the states must issue a permit to facilities before they can treat, store, and dispose of hazardous waste. The permit prescribes enforceable management standards for the wastes.

The regulated community in this system includes those who generate, recycle, transport, treat, store, and dispose of hazardous wastes.

The Regulated Community

Generators: The hazardous waste management cycle begins with a generator—any person or business that produces hazardous waste or first causes hazardous waste to become subject to RCRA regulations. Examples of generators include owners and operators of large manufacturing facilities, small businesses, universities, and laboratories.

Under the RCRA regulations, generators are responsible for determining whether their waste is hazardous and accounting for the final disposal of their waste. Generators are regulated according to the amount of waste they produce and are categorized into three groups:

- *Large Quantity Generators (LQGs)* are those that generate the largest amount of hazardous waste—more than 2,200 pounds (1,000 kilograms) per calendar month, which is about five full 55-gallon drums. Since this category includes about 20,000 companies that produce the majority of the nation's waste, these generators are regulated more stringently than their counterparts who generate less waste. Examples of LQGs include pharmaceutical companies and chemical manufacturers.

- *Small Quantity Generators (SQGs)* are those that generate between 220 pounds (100 kilograms) and 2,200 pounds (1,000 kilograms) of hazardous waste per calendar month. Examples of SQGs include laboratories, printers, and dry cleaners.

- *Conditionally Exempt Small Quantity Generators (CESQGs)* are those that generate less than 220 pounds (100 kilograms) of hazardous waste per calendar month. Because these generators produce a small amount of hazardous waste and because full regulation would present an economic burden on businesses, CESQGs are subject to very minimal requirements. Examples of CESQGs include 1-hour photo labs and dental offices.

RCRA regulations apply to facilities that manage waste on site, as well as to those that ship waste off site. About 98 percent of the nation's hazardous waste is treated or disposed of by generators on site. These generators are typically large businesses that can afford treatment equipment and possess the necessary space for storage and disposal. Smaller firms, and those in crowded urban locations, are likely to transport their waste off site where it is managed by a commercial firm or a publicly owned and operated facility.

Generators that send their waste off site are required to package, mark, and label their waste properly for transportation. Proper packaging ensures that no hazardous waste will escape from containers during transport. Marking and labeling enables transporters and public officials, including those who respond to emergencies, to rapidly identify the waste and its hazards.

Transporters: Transporters pick up properly packaged and labeled hazardous waste from generators and transport it to designated facilities that recycle, treat, store, or dispose of the waste. They must put proper symbols on the transport vehicle to identify the type of waste being transported. The U.S. Department of Transportation (DOT) jointly regulates the transportation of hazardous waste. DOT specifies the markings, labels, and packaging required to ship hazardous waste. These symbols, like the labels on the hazardous waste containers, enable firefighters, police, and other officials to identify the potential hazards immediately in case of an emergency. Because an accident involving hazardous waste could create very serious problems, EPA regulations also require transporters to comply with procedures for hazardous waste spill cleanup.

Treatment, Storage, and Disposal Facilities: Treatment, storage, and disposal facilities (TSDFs) receive hazardous waste from generators or other TSDFs. Treatment facilities use various processes to alter the character or composition of a hazardous waste. Some treatment processes enable waste to be recovered and reused in manufacturing settings, while other treatment processes reduce the volume or hazard of waste to facilitate further storage or disposal. Storage facilities hold hazardous waste temporarily until it is treated or disposed of. Treatment and storage activities take place in various units such as tanks, containers, incinerators, surface impoundments, containment buildings, and waste piles. Disposal facilities usually place hazardous waste in landfills or surface impoundments after it has been treated properly.

One common method of treatment (and disposal) of hazardous waste is incineration, or combustion. In the United States, almost 300 facilities burn almost 4 million tons of hazardous waste in incinerators each year. Another 1 million is disposed of in other types of combustion facilities, known as boilers and industrial furnaces. These units offer an effective technology for managing much hazardous waste. The RCRA program specifically subjects these units to strict emissions controls and other requirements. In addition, all new units must receive a permit from the state or federal permitting agency to operate and must pass a test known as a trial burn, before operation begins to ensure that these units will not endanger human health or the environment. EPA continually evaluates the safety of hazardous waste combustion by examining and revising emissions standards.

Hazardous Waste Minimization

Proper hazardous waste management requires a waste minimization plan. To reduce the amount or toxicity of hazardous waste that must be managed (and therefore the amount of waste subject to regulation), many generators reduce, reuse, or recycle as part of their everyday practices. The most environmentally sound and economically efficient way of managing any waste is not to generate it in the first place (source reduction). Facilities can avoid creating hazardous wastes, or limit the amount created, by not mixing hazardous and nonhazardous wastes, by changing some materials or processes, and by safely storing hazardous products and containers to avoid spills and leaks.

If hazardous wastes are generated, they often can be recycled in an environmentally sound manner. In the context of hazardous waste management, there are certain practices or activities that are defined as recycling. A recycled material is one that is used, reused, or reclaimed. For example, cleaning solvents that become dirty through use can be filtered (reclaimed) and used again instead of being disposed of. The term "waste minimization" includes source reduction and environmentally sound recycling.

Wastes that cannot be recycled must be treated to reduce the toxicity of the hazardous constituents and the ability of the constituents to move throughout the environment. Treatment residues must be disposed of in an environmentally sound manner.

Approaches to Waste Minimization

- Substitution of raw materials might offer the greatest opportunity for waste minimization. By replacing a raw material that generates a large amount of hazardous waste during its processing with one that generates little or none, manufacturers can substantially reduce their waste volume.

- Manufacturing process changes consist of either eliminating a process that produces a hazardous waste or altering a process so that it no longer produces the waste.

- Substitution of products can also be effective. For example, citrus-based solvents often can be used instead of chlorinated solvents for cleaning or coating.

- Recycling (also referred to as recovery and reuse) is the process of removing reusable elements from a waste and returning them to productive use. Generators commonly recycle solvents, acids, and metals.

- Source separation (or segregation) keeps hazardous waste from contaminating nonhazardous waste through management practices that prevent the wastes from coming into contact with each other. This is the cheapest and easiest method of reducing the volume of hazardous waste to be disposed of and is widely used by industry. In addition to reducing disposal costs, source separation reduces handling and transportation costs.

Land Disposal Restrictions

About 23 million tons of hazardous waste are land disposed annually. This widespread disposal of hazardous waste in units located directly on the land has the potential to contaminate soil and ground water. To adequately protect public health and safety, hazardous wastes must be treated to minimize any risks before they can be disposed of in land disposal units.

RCRA's Land Disposal Restriction (LDR) program sets treatment standards and requires that hazardous wastes be treated before they are land disposed to destroy or immobilize hazardous constituents. All hazardous waste must be treated so that the concentration of hazardous constituents is below a certain level established for each waste. There are numerous treatment technologies available and new ones continually being developed.

Types of Land Disposal

- Landfills are disposal facilities where hazardous waste is placed in or on land. Properly designed and operated landfills are double-lined to prevent leakage. They also are equipped with systems that collect surface water runoff (like rain) that can come in contact with waste and become contaminated.

- Surface impoundments are double-lined natural or fabricated depressions or diked areas that can be used to treat, store, or dispose of hazardous waste. Surface impoundments may be any shape and any size (from a few hundred square feet to hundreds of acres in area). Surface impoundments are often referred to as pits, ponds, lagoons, and basins.

- Underground injection wells are steel and concrete-encased shafts into which hazardous wastes are deposited by force and under pressure. Liquid hazardous wastes are commonly disposed of in underground injection wells. Injecting wastes into encased wells deep in underground land formations protects ground-water aquifers from risk of contamination.

- Waste piles are noncontainerized, lined accumulations of solid, nonflowing hazardous waste. While some are used for final disposal, many waste piles are used for temporary storage until the waste is transferred to its final disposal site.

- Land treatment is a disposal process in which hazardous waste is applied onto or incorporated into the soil surface. Natural microbes in the soil break down or immobilize the hazardous constituents. Land treatment facilities are also called land application or land farming facilities.

Used Oil Management Standards

EPA has established a set of required practices, or management standards, for recycling used oil and burning it for energy recovery. These are commonsense, good-business practices designed to maximize recycling and minimize disposal of used oil, as well as to ensure its safe handling. Used oil comes from automotive crankcases, machine lubricants, and industrial processes. During normal use, impurities, such as dirt, metal scrapings, water, or chemicals, can get mixed in with the oil so that in time the oil no longer performs well. Eventually, this oil must be replaced with virgin or re-refined oil to do the job at hand. Then, used oil must be either disposed of, recycled, or burned for energy recovery.

Used oil can be treated to remove hazardous contaminants and reused as a new lubricating oil or as a fuel. An estimated 380 million gallons of used oil are recycled each year. It takes 42 gallons of crude oil, but only 1 gallon of used oil, to produce 2-1/2 quarts of new, high-quality lubricating oil.

The used oil management system is designed to minimize the potential risks associated with used oil. These standards impose requirements on used oil generators, collection centers, transporters, and processors. The used oil program also imposes standards on used oil burners and marketers to ensure that the burning of used oil for energy recovery is conducted in a manner that is protective of the environment. For example, used oil destined for burning must be tested for hazardous contaminants and burned in units that can control hazardous air emissions. Used oil generators also can burn used oil in space heaters used at their place of business.

The RCRA Structure

The Tracking System: To assist in tracking shipments of waste, EPA requires LQGs, SQGs, transporters, and TSDFs to obtain EPA identification numbers. LQGs and SQGs must also prepare Uniform Hazardous Waste Manifests for each shipment of hazardous waste. A

Table 5.2. Common Hazardous Waste Treatment Technologies

Several processes exist for making hazardous wastes less hazardous:

Biological treatment uses micro-organisms to break down hazardous organic compounds in a waste stream and make the waste less toxic.

Carbon adsorption is a chemical process that removes hazardous substances from the waste using specially treated carbon. This method is particularly effective in removing organic compounds from liquid waste.

Dechlorination removes chlorine from a substance to make it less toxic.

Glycolate dehalogenation uses chemical substances to react with hazardous contaminants to change their structure and toxicity.

Incineration (or combustion) destroys waste or makes it less hazardous through burning. Incineration is frequently used to destroy organic wastes.

Thermal treatment uses elevated temperatures as the primary means of changing the chemical, physical, or biological character of a waste. (Examples include wet air oxidation, molten salt pyrolysis, and calcination.)

Neutralization makes certain substances less acidic and other substances less alkaline.

Oxidation makes a waste less toxic by combining it with oxygen.

Precipitation removes solids from a liquid waste so that the hazardous solid portion can be disposed of safely.

Soil washing uses water or a washing solution in mechanical processes to scrub soils and remove hazardous contaminants.

Solidification and stabilization removes wastewater from a waste or changes it chemically, making it less likely to be transported by water.

Solvent extraction separates hazardous constituents from oily wastes, oils, sludges, and sediments to reduce the volume of waste that must be disposed of.

manifest is a form containing copies for all participants involved in the waste shipment. It identifies the type and quantity of waste and the generator, transporter, and facility to which the waste is being shipped. Generators must also certify on the manifest that they are minimizing the amount and toxicity of their waste and that the method of treatment, storage, or disposal they have chosen will minimize the risk to human health and the environment. When the waste reaches its final destination, the owner of that facility returns a copy of the manifest to the generator to confirm that the waste has arrived.

If the waste does not arrive as scheduled, generators must immediately notify EPA or the authorized state agency so that it can investigate and take appropriate action. Generators, transporters, and TSDFs must retain copies of the manifest for 3 years. Every other year, generators also must provide information on their activities to their authorized state agency or EPA.

The Permitting System: Owners or operators of TSDFs must obtain a permit in order to operate. A permit specifically allows a facility to treat, store, or dispose of hazardous waste and outlines the precautions that must be taken to manage the waste in a manner that adequately protects human health and the environment.

New TSDFs must receive a permit before they begin construction. Operating TSDFs with expiring permits must submit new permit applications 6 months before their existing permits run out. TSDFs operating under interim status must also apply for a permit. Congress granted interim status to facilities that already existed when RCRA was enacted or that were already operating when new wastes were listed. Interim status allows facilities to continue operating while their permit applications are being reviewed by the federal or state permitting agency. While both permitted and interim status TSDFs are subject to similar standards, the interim status standards are designed to be self-implementing. Generally, permitted and interim status TSDFs must:

- Analyze and identify wastes prior to treatment, storage, and disposal.

- Prevent the entry of unauthorized personnel into the facility by installing fences and surveillance systems, and by posting warning signs.

- Inspect the facility on a periodic basis to determine if there are any problems.

46

- Train employees in safe use of equipment and emergency response procedures.

- Prepare a contingency plan for emergencies and establish other emergency response procedures.

- Comply with the manifest system and with various reporting and record keeping requirements.

- Comply with facility-specific standards as dictated in the permit.

In addition to these general requirements, all TSDFs must comply with specific design and operating standards for their hazardous waste treatment, storage, and disposal units. These standards are especially important for disposal units, which must ensure that disposed waste will not leach or otherwise escape into soil or ground water. Disposal unit standards:

- Ban liquids from landfills.

- Ban underground injection of hazardous waste within 1/4-mile of a drinking water well.

- Require stringent structural and design conditions, such as double liners, leachate collection systems, and ground-water monitoring.

- Limit facility sitings in unstable hydrogeologic areas.

EPA also established regulations to address air emissions from hazardous waste disposal since some hazardous waste compounds can evaporate into the air. To prevent such escapes into the atmosphere, EPA requires certain equipment to be used for recycling, treatment, storage, and disposal of some hazardous wastes.

Closure and Financial Assurance

RCRA regulations and permits set forth certain procedures that are designed to protect the environment and surrounding communities when owners and operators of hazardous waste facilities close their sites. In addition, RCRA sets standards for ground-water monitoring, disposal unit maintenance, and security measures that some owners and operators of hazardous waste facilities will need to follow for up to 30 years after the facility closes (known as postclosure care).

Closure activities can be expensive, and some facilities might not be able to cover these costs at the time of closure. For example, if a company undergoes bankruptcy and has little money left at the time of the closure of its TSDF, it might not be able to provide the required closure and postclosure care. To address this situation, RCRA regulations require owners and operators to:

- Establish separate, secure financial assurance mechanisms (such as trust funds, surety bonds, and letters of credit) to pay for completion of all closure and postclosure operations.

- Be prepared to pay for 30 years of ground-water monitoring, disposal unit maintenance, and security measures after the facility closes.

- Demonstrate financial assurance for third-party liability to cover any accidents or mismanagement that results in the release of hazardous waste. Such funds can be used to compensate citizens or other third parties for any damage to neighboring property or injury to human health.

State Authorization

The hazardous waste regulatory program described in this chapter may be run by EPA or a state hazardous waste agency. Currently 47 states and two territories have been granted authority to run Subtitle C RCRA programs. As EPA continues to promulgate new or revised rules, states must become authorized to implement those rules. Thus, state authorization is an ongoing process.

EPA's regional offices implement and enforce RCRA in states and territories that do not have authorized programs. In states that are authorized, EPA can step in to assist states in enforcing the law, if needed. Otherwise, states that are authorized to operate RCRA programs oversee the hazardous waste tracking system in their state, operate the permitting system for hazardous waste facilities, ensure public participation requirements are met, act as the enforcement arm in cases where individuals or companies practice illegal hazardous waste management, and implement all other aspects of the RCRA program.

In terms of permitting hazardous waste facilities, authorized states are generally considered to be the permitting agency.

Citizen Action and Public Participation

The public plays an important role in the permitting process for both hazardous and municipal solid waste facilities. Facilities applying for a permit must involve the public in some aspects of the process. Businesses and the state or federal permitting agency also must make information available to the public. The public has opportunities to submit comments and request public hearings.

The following are some of the ways in which the public can stay involved:

- When a business submits a permit application, it must hold an informal meeting with the public and advertise the meeting with signs and/or advertisements in the paper or radio. The business must explain the plans for the facility, including information about the proposed processes it will use and wastes it will handle. Members of the public can sign up on the facility's mailing list.

- When the permitting agency receives a permit application from the business, it sends a notice to everyone on the mailing list. The application is then available for public review.

- The permitting agency may require the business to set up a library for the public with available relevant documents, such as the permit application and reports.

- The permitting agency announces its decision about granting or denying the permit by sending a letter to everyone on the mailing list and placing a notice in a newspaper or broadcasting over the radio. It also issues a fact sheet to explain the decision. Once the notice is issued, the public has 45 days to comment on the decision. Citizens may request a public hearing by contacting the permitting agency.

- The permitting agency must consider and respond to all public comments when making its decision.

- The public has the right to appeal the final permit decision.

- The permitting agency must notify the public prior to a trial burn at a combustion facility by sending a notice to everyone on the facility mailing list.

Cleaning up hazardous waste facilities, known as corrective action, is also of concern to citizens and local communities. Since spills from TSDFs can affect entire municipalities, RCRA guarantees that the public will have a role in the facility cleanup process. For example, the corrective action process gives the public access to facility inspection information, requires public notice of remediation proceedings, and allows the opportunity for public comment and participation in the remedy selection process.

Public participation initiatives are also used to remedy the disproportionate effects of environmental pollution on particular groups, such as minority and low-income populations. For example, through efforts to ensure environmental justice, EPA is analyzing how to incorporate public participation into decisions concerning the siting of hazardous waste facilities and the prioritization of corrective action cleanups.

More Ways to Participate

Many avenues exist for citizens to learn about and participate in what is happening around them, in addition to those offered under the RCRA program. A related law, known as the Emergency Planning and Community Right-to-Know Act, establishes a citizen's right to obtain information about toxic and hazardous chemicals handled at facilities in the community. One such avenue is the Toxics Release Inventory (TRI). Through this program, facilities across the country are required to report the quantities of 643 different toxic chemicals that are released into the environment each year. Facilities must report whether these toxic chemicals were released into the air or water or disposed of in underground injection wells or landfills. Facilities also have to indicate which releases were sent to a commercial Subtitle C landfill.

Ground Water What Is It?

Ground water is water that naturally flows through and is retained in soil and rock bodies beneath the land. It is a major source of drinking water and of water used for agriculture in the United States. Almost half of this country's population depends upon ground water for some or all of its drinking water.

Ground-water contamination can occur when liquids (usually rainwater) move through waste disposal sites, carrying pollutants with them, and into the ground water. The resulting mixture of liquid and pollutant is called leachate. Once contaminated, ground water is expensive and difficult to clean up. All new hazardous waste disposal sites are equipped with leachate collection systems.

RCRA regulations require ground-water monitoring, which detects early signs of contaminants leaching from hazardous waste disposal facilities. The most common monitoring device is a well from which samples of water are taken and analyzed for hazardous constituents.

RCRA regulations also require hazardous waste landfill and sur-face impoundment facilities to install double liners to protect against ground-water contamination. Liners are continuous layers of natu-ral or synthetic materials, such as clay or plastic, that are placed be-neath or on the sides of a landfill or surface impoundment and restrict the escape of hazardous waste into ground water.

Subtitle D: Municipal and Industrial Solid Waste

RCRA also covers municipal solid waste (MSW) and nonhazard-ous industrial waste. MSW is common garbage or trash generated by homes, industries, and commercial and institutional offices. Industrial nonhazardous wastes are wastes and wastewaters generated by manufacturing processes that are not considered to be hazardous.

Communities across the United States currently generate more than 200 million tons of MSW every year. This amount averages to about 4 pounds per person per day. EPA encourages individuals and businesses to reduce, reuse, and recycle to decrease the amount of waste generated. EPA promotes a hierarchy of waste management options for businesses and municipalities, as follows:

1. The best option is to not generate waste in the first place or to reuse what you already have. This is known as source reduc-tion or waste prevention. For example, individuals can prevent waste by leaving grass clippings on the lawn and by buying items with less packaging, such as bulk foods. Reusing items, such as bags and containers, instead of throwing them away reduces waste. Companies can buy reusable items, such as pallets, instead of disposable ones.

2. The second best option is recycling or composting. Many types of glass, paper, plastic, metal, and other assorted materials are recyclable. That means that it is technologically feasible for these materials to be broken down and remade into new products. To make this type of manufacturing economically feasible, people also need to buy products that are made from recycled materials. Many companies are recycling these types of materials, and common consumer goods are available with recycled content. Many municipalities and companies are also producing compost, a soil amendment, from yard trimmings from residents.

51

3. The final option for those materials that are not easily recyclable or compostable is disposal, either landfilling or combustion (preferably with energy recovery).

Approximately 60 percent of MSW is disposed of in landfills. Unlike their hazardous waste counterparts, federal MSW regulations do not require the treatment of waste before disposal. Although much of MSW consists of paper, aluminum cans, plastics, and other nontoxic items, some components, including batteries, and certain household products, such as cleaners, paints, stains, and pesticides, can present potential risks when improperly disposed of.

The Subtitle D program focuses on establishing standards, or criteria, for municipal solid waste landfills to ensure the safe management of MSW. The federal standards address the design, operation, and closure of MSW landfills. They impose restrictions on where such landfills may be located (e.g., not in a floodplain), and they require liners and ground-water monitoring. In addition, when these landfills become full, their closure is governed by specific procedures, as well as financial assurance requirements to pay for such operations.

These federal standards are designed to be self-implementing by the owner or operator of a facility. State and tribal regulatory agencies provide the primary oversight and issue permits. EPA works with states and tribes to ensure that landfills continually minimize risks from waste.

Another category of Subtitle D waste is called industrial solid waste or industrial nonhazardous waste. This waste is not considered MSW or hazardous waste under Subtitle C. Each year, approximately 12,000 manufacturing facilities generate and manage an estimated 7.6 billion tons of industrial solid waste (about 97 percent in the form of wastewater) on site in surface impoundments, landfills, land application units, and waste piles. Most nonhazardous industrial waste is managed in surface impoundments.

What Is in MSW?

Nationwide, MSW contains large percentages of paper and yard trimmings and a smaller percentage of metals, glass, plastics, food scraps, and other materials such as rubber, leather, textiles, and wood. Construction and demolition debris, automobile bodies, or municipal sewage are among the materials that are not considered MSW, according to the Agency's definition. Some states define the components somewhat differently.

Household Hazardous Waste (HHW)

Households often discard many common items that contain hazardous constituents, such as paints, stains, oven cleaner, motor oil, batteries, and pesticides. If these items were generated in large quantities by a business or manufacturing facility, they might be regulated as a hazardous waste. Individuals generating these types of waste from their homes are exempt, however, from the hazardous waste regulations. Certain other types of residences are exempt as well, such as motels, hotels, and campgrounds. The average household in the United States generates about 20 pounds of HHW per year.

To reduce the risks of disposing of these items in MSW landfills or incinerators, many communities have established HHW collection programs. These programs aggregate HHW and ensure its safe disposal in facilities designed to treat or dispose of hazardous waste. More than 3,000 collection programs have been documented in all 50 states.

Making RCRA Work

Three additional elements to the RCRA program provide strength and extra insurance to minimize risks from waste: monitoring, corrective action for environmental cleanups, and enforcement.

Monitoring

For EPA's Subtitle C program to be effective, all regulated groups must comply. To ensure compliance, state or federal officials inspect and monitor facilities regularly and take enforcement measures when necessary.

Inspection of a site is one of the RCRA program's most important monitoring tools. An inspection is required of all TSDFs at least once every 2 years and annually for state and federal facilities. During an inspection, regulatory personnel generally review the company's records, assess the facility's operating methods, and take waste samples, if needed. In particular, inspectors check for compliance with groundwater monitoring requirements, proper handling and labeling of wastes, and assurance of financial responsibility. If a facility is not complying with RCRA regulations, EPA or the state takes enforcement action.

Corrective Action

Despite RCRA's numerous precautions to prevent the release of hazardous waste into the environment, accidents still happen, and contamination persists from past mismanagement of these wastes. EPA estimates that between 50 and 70 percent of all TSDFs have some degree of environmental contamination requiring detailed investigation and perhaps cleanup. Under a program entitled Corrective Action, EPA has the statutory authority to require permitted and interim status TSDFs to clean up hazardous waste contamination. In addition, EPA also may use a catch-all statutory provision to require corrective action at any type of facility, such as generator sites, to ensure that all waste released into the environment is cleaned up in a timely manner.

To achieve necessary cleanups, facilities investigate environmental contamination and take remedial action to correct any problems associated with releases that may occur. Similarly, releases of materials from MSW landfills and USTs also occur. The RCRA regulations in these program areas also feature specific provisions and procedures to ensure necessary corrective action.

Enforcement

Enforcement may include civil and criminal penalties, orders to correct the violations, fines, and/or imprisonment. For minor violations, EPA or the state agency often notifies the facility through a letter or phone call that it is not in compliance and that legal actions will be taken if the owner or operator does not comply within a certain time period. For severe or recurrent violations, EPA or the state can levy a penalty on the owner or operator of up to $27,500 per day for each day the facility fails to comply past the specified deadline. EPA or the state can also suspend the facility's permit to operate and can bring a criminal suit against a facility's owner or operator. Examples of potential criminal violations of RCRA include falsifying information on a manifest, report, or permit; transporting waste either without a manifest or to a facility without a permit; and disposing of hazardous waste without a permit. Furthermore, if a facility deliberately violates RCRA, thus endangering human health and the environment, the violator could receive up to 15 years in prison and a maximum $250,000 fine.

On the other hand, to alleviate the use of time-consuming and expensive criminal and civil sanctions, EPA has established policies to allow more flexibility in the enforcement process, giving businesses the opportunity to mitigate penalties for noncompliance and offering incentives for self-policing and self-auditing. EPA's enforcement strategy gives states the flexibility to create their own enforcement policies up front. One of EPA's new initiatives encourages both large and small facilities to voluntarily audit themselves, to disclose instances of noncompliance, and to make good faith efforts to promptly correct the violations in return for a reduction of applicable penalties. Similarly, when EPA does take enforcement action against a business, the Agency may include in the settlement or enforcement action provisions allowing the facility to conduct supplemental and beneficial environmental projects in order to mitigate penalties for noncompliance.

Conclusion

RCRA is a response to a complex environmental management issue—one that is ultimately connected to the way our country operates, its heavy reliance on industrial production, and our technologically sophisticated lifestyles. As long as we demand the products that generate these wastes, we will need well-designed and well-operated facilities and sound alternatives for waste management. Technological change, population growth, and economic expansion present added environmental challenges. The cooperation of industry, government, and the public will ensure that these challenges are met.

The management of hazardous waste is a dynamic process that is continually being refined and updated based on new research, technology, and regulations. Since RCRA was enacted in 1976, substantial progress has been made in promoting a clean and safe environment while maintaining our nation's manufacturing and industrial strength. EPA continually works to protect the environment, while also achieving the following:

- Reduced administrative burdens on generators.

- Increased avenues for public participation.

- Increased flexibility to the regulated sectors for complying with RCRA requirements.

- Multimedia modeling, risk assessment technologies, and other state-of-the-art scientific practices.

We plan to continue pursuing partnerships with states, tribes, industry, and the public.

Regulated Environmental Laws

RCRA is one of a series of laws regulating potentially harmful substances in the environment. These laws were developed at different points in time and reflect concerns about particular issues such as ground-water protection, water quality, air quality, and worker safety. Some laws address the same hazardous substances at different points in their existence. For example, RCRA may regulate the disposal of a particular hazardous waste, while the Occupational Safety and Health Act (OSHA) protects workers who are exposed to that same substance in the workplace.

In another example, RCRA exempts certain wastewater treatment units from hazardous waste permit requirements, since these units are permitted under the Clean Water Act. Because the concerns addressed by these laws sometimes overlap, EPA works with the states and other federal agencies to help ensure that all aspects of environmental protection are well coordinated. EPA, in conjunction with other federal and state agencies, also attempts to identify and address areas not covered by existing laws.

Some of the environmental laws addressing hazardous substances include:

- Atomic Energy Act (EPA, U.S. Department of Energy, and U.S. Nuclear Regulatory Commission)—regulates nuclear energy production and nuclear waste disposal.

- Clean Air Act (EPA)—limits the emission of hazardous pollutants into the nation's air.

- Clean Water Act (EPA)—regulates the discharge of hazardous pollutants and sewage sludge into the nation's surface waters.

- Comprehensive Environmental Response, Compensation, and Liability Act (Superfund) (EPA)—provides for the cleanup of inactive and abandoned hazardous waste sites.

- Emergency Planning and Community Right-to-Know Act (EPA)—addresses the storage of chemicals in communities, planning for accidental releases, and the availability of information on releases of toxic wastes to the public.

- Federal Insecticide, Fungicide, and Rodenticide Act (EPA)— regulates the registration and use of pesticides.

- Hazardous Materials Transportation Act (DOT)—governs the transportation of hazardous waste and materials.

- Marine Protection, Research, and Sanctuaries Act (EPA)—addresses waste disposal at sea.

- Occupational Safety and Health Act (U.S. Occupational Safety and Health Administration)—regulates hazards in the workplace, including worker exposure to hazardous substances.

- Pollution Prevention Act (EPA)—focuses on reducing the amount of pollution at the source and promoting recycling.

- Safe Drinking Water Act (EPA)—limits contaminant levels in drinking water.

- Surface Mining Control and Reclamation Act (U.S. Department of the Interior)—regulates the environmental aspects of mining (particularly coal) and reclamation.

- Toxic Substance Control Act (EPA)—regulates the manufacture, use, and disposal of certain chemical substances.

Chapter 6

A Family Guide to Environmental Health

It's not too much of an exaggeration to say, your environment is your health. So to improve your health, see that your family's environment is a healthy one.

Of course, your environment isn't the only factor influencing your health. Genes play an important role, too, as your kids are sure to tell you. But, sorry, you can't choose your parents. You and your family can, on the other hand, do a lot about your personal environment—your surroundings, your exposures, your diet and your health habits—to extend your life and to improve your fitness and appearance.

For an example of how society has improved health by environmental action, you have to look no further than our protected reservoirs and water disinfection plants. The purification of city water supplies has been the most significant reason that the average life span has very nearly doubled over the past century or so. Millions and millions of us live longer and better because of clean water and because our country and industries have reduced our exposures to lead and other substances.

In addition to the environments we share, each of us has his or her own personal environment. Our personal environments can greatly

"A Family Guide: 20 Easy Steps to Personal Environmental Health Now," a health guide from the National Institute of Environmental Health Sciences (NIEHS), 1999. Available online at http://www.niehs.nih.gov/oc/factsheets/scene/adult/p-home.htm. Despite the older date of this document it will be helpful to reader seeking ways to ensure that their family's environment is a healthy one.

influence our lifespan and how healthy we feel and are. Following are simple some but important steps that you and your family can take—health-wise—about your environment:

Read the label on house and garden chemicals.

Before you point that spray can, get your spectacles out and see if the directions or warnings have changed. They do, frequently. In fact, before you even buy a household or garden chemical, you can compare labels to be sure you're buying the safest product for your intended use. (You also may decide a bug-less, weed-less lawn isn't all that important.) Note whether a product is for inside or outside use, and what protections—rubber gloves, respirators and such—are needed. What does the product do to birds, dogs and barefoot children?

Read the labels for dry-cleaning solutions and other household chemicals, too. If a label says, "Open windows and ventilate," there's a reason. Likewise, read drug labels for warnings, and food labels for ingredients that don't agree with you, as well as to avoid excess calories and fat. (A good rhyme to remember is: "Read the label, Mabel.") Labels have recently been added to some arts and craft supplies regarding ingredients posing a cancer risk. Charcoal has a new warning label.

Prescription and non-prescription drugs often get new warning labels when a new risk shows up during use.

Food labels were reformed in 1993 to be more informative about fats and calories. A reprint, "Food Label Close-Up," tells how to make best use of the new food label format. To have it sent to you, call your nearest Food and Drug Administration office listed in the U.S. section of your telephone book.

Turn down the volume.

While occasional loud noises may just reduce your hearing temporarily, continuous exposures or very loud noises can cause permanent damage. Musicians know about efficient ear plugs that extend the life of their ears and perhaps their professional lives as well. You can buy them for your teens and for yourself.

Your teens may relate to a story about a young rock musician's 40 percent hearing loss. "I was basically deaf for three years," says Kathy Peck of The Contractions. Her story is available at http://www.fda.gov/fdac/reprints/ots_ears.html.

In addition to loud music, firecrackers and small arms fire, if close enough, can damage hearing, immediately or over time. That is, hearing may decline and/or there may be ringing, buzzing or roaring in the ears or head. Additional information is available at the National Institute on Deafness and Other Communication Disorders Clearinghouse, 1-800-241-1044, or online at www.nidcd.nih.gov.

Put a carbon monoxide alarm in your home.

Carbon monoxide from cars in garages, space heaters and other home heating sources can be deadly. You need one or more smoke alarms, frequently checked of course, but they won't alert you to carbon monoxide. For that, you need at least one carbon monoxide alarm. A few dollars, a trip to the hardware and a few minutes' installation are all you need to forestall a possible tragedy.

Grow plants.

Plants, including house plants, are not only nice to look at, there's evidence they clean pollutants from the air.

Put drugs, drain openers, and vitamins out of kids' reach.

The iron-containing vitamins that many women take, as well as prescription and nonprescription drugs like aspirin or other pain relievers can kill kids who think they're candy. Lock them up or put them out of reach. Same with paint thinners, detergents, drain openers and other yard and home chemicals.

Look in your telephone book for your local Poison Control Center and ask for information and for "Mr. Yuk" telephone number stickers to place on your telephone for use in a poisoning emergency. Or you can get the location of your nearest center at http://www.poison.org/otherPC.

Getting this information now, before an emergency happens, can be a good family lesson in prevention by planning ahead.

Know the hazards of your job.

Wherever you and your family members work there are risks. They may be physical, like falling off a ladder or lifting heavy packages, or chemical risks from petroleum products and solvents. In other occupations, computer use and other repetitive tasks pose risks of carpal tunnel syndrome. Identify the risks of your work and take the necessary precautions—whether a particular respirator, gloves, goggles or a particular posture.

You say you work at home? Work is work. You can fall, spill corrosives on your skin or breathe toxic fumes, if you're not careful—and there may not be anyone around to help. When it comes to work accidents, you're not home free.

See if that cold might be an allergy.

You may think Johnny gets a lot of colds, but he may be allergic to dust mites, your cat, the pollen from trees, or cockroaches.

Plastic mattress and pillow covers, an exterminator and the elimination of dust-holders like curtains and rugs in your bedroom may help. Or, if it's trees and pollen that get to you, air conditioning and air filters may provide relief.

The allergy may affect only one person in the family. (Being allergic means reacting to substances that don't bother most other people.) The substance you react to can be natural substances such as molds or various manufactured chemicals.

Remember that lakes and streams aren't always pure.

A crystal clear stream or lake may be a nice place to wade or swim but may harbor bacteria that can turn your stomach inside out. When you and your family walk in the wild, take along your own drinking water or a disinfection kit.

To avoid waterborne diseases in less developed countries, you may need to avoid tap water (even ice cubes) and to stick to bottled water, to cooked foods or to fruit that you peel yourself, such as bananas or oranges.

Watch for lead, a continuing threat.

A lot has been done to reduce our contact with the mind and body-destroying lead in our environment. Lead-added paints and gasoline are a bad memory. (Lead content in paint was greatly reduced in the 1950s. Later, in 1978, the addition of lead was eliminated.) But there remain many deteriorating, pre-1950 buildings with flaking lead paint that contaminates the ground and ends up on children's hands and toys as dust. Your family may track in lead dust from a demolition site down the street.

If there's a chance a child in your family is being exposed to lead, a simple blood test can alert you before lead poisoning causes significant learning and behavior problems. More than one fifth of African-American children living in housing built before 1946 have elevated blood lead levels. For more information, talk to your doctor or call 1-800-LEAD-FYI. A short booklet called "Lead and Your Health" can be obtained by calling NIEHS at 919-541-3345 or by e-mailing your request to booklet@niehs.nih.gov.

Even low doses of lead can affect a child's development, causing problems with learning, remembering and concentrating. Keep the toddlers away from lead by cleaning up the flakes and dust regularly and either carefully removing the source or walling it in.

Good nutrition, including plenty of milk products and other sources of calcium, may offer some protection from lead.

Occasional high-level lead poisonings still occur from craft-style lead-glazed pottery cups and dishes. Questionable products are best used for display, rather than food or drink.

Test for radon.

Radon is a gas you can't smell in your home, but you can test for it. A naturally occurring gas that seeps out of rocks and soils, it comes from uranium buried in the earth and is itself radioactive. There is evidence of an elevated lung cancer risk among miners exposed to radon, especially miners who smoke. Radon also seeps into homes and collects in varying amounts. To assess the possible danger, the Institute of Medicine convened a panel of experts to review the data. These experts said the lung cancer risk from radon in homes is small compared to that from tobacco products. Of about 160,000 annual lung cancer deaths, radon-related deaths were estimated to probably total 15,400 to 21,800, mostly because of a synergism between smoking and radon. Fewer than 3,000 deaths were estimated as being radon-related among nonsmokers.

The Harvard Center for Risk Analysis argues that the weight of evidence is that radon in homes may pose a greater risk to more people, mostly smokers, than die of accidental falls, poisonings, home fires and burns, or accidental discharges of firearms. Though the risk can be debated, it is clear that a radon test is cheap, and that, when found, high radon levels can often be turned into low levels by simple ventilation.

Don't get badly overheated.

Exercise is a way to keep fit, but when you or a family member competes or runs the dog in hot weather, try to do it in the cooler hours and/or have water handy and drink plenty of it. Keep some available for Fido and the cats, too.

Heat is a serious threat: Nearly 1,700 people lost their lives from heat-related illnesses in a big heat wave in 1980, and the forecast is for global warming.

Know about ozone.

Ozone is a highly reactive form of oxygen—a linkage of three atoms of oxygen instead of the usual two—that occurs when there are a lot of vehicle exhaust and factory emissions. It accumulates when the air is stagnant.

Ozone can irritate and damage tissue in the lungs, nose and throat, and can make breathing hard, especially if you exercise outdoors during its peaks. Watch for ozone and other air quality alerts in your newspaper, TV and radio weathercasts. During alerts, jog in parks away from auto traffic, when possible. Especially if you have asthma, bronchitis or emphysema, limit the time you spend outdoors when ozone levels are high. Since evaporating gasoline adds to the ozone problem, when you service your car or mower, don't overfill the tank and spill the gasoline.

Wash your hands.

Whether you've been sneezing, handling chicken or other raw poultry or meat, have been to the toilet or changed a diaper, or are preparing to deliver a baby or perform brain surgery, washing your hands and environs (such as your cutting board in the kitchen) is a most important way to prevent the spread of germs and infection. In many of these situations, it is the most important preventive measure you can take. It's as simple as that.

You may not be doing surgery, but more than 6.5 million cases of stomach flu or worse occur each year, often because hands and food implements aren't washed often enough, especially after handling poultry. To start youngsters out with good hand-washing habits, your closest FDA office (listed in the U.S. government pages of the telephone book) can provide the "Food Safety Coloring Book" for your kids.

Watch pesticide drift.

If you spray your roses upwind of your tomatoes, you are likely to dose your family with unapproved pesticides. Some pesticides are for non-food use only and have not been proved safe for foods.

Eat a good diet.

Not just an apple but five or more servings of fruits and vegetables a day may help keep the doctor, and cancer and other disorders away.

Take a vitamin.

The federal government recommends all females of childbearing age take 400 micrograms (0.4 milligrams) of folic acid, one of the B vitamins, daily, to reduce the chances of having a child with a neural tube defect, a disorder in which the spine is open and easily damaged or even the child's brain is missing. The vitamin is needed regularly, before as well as during pregnancy, and it's hard to get the amount needed from an ordinary diet. But women and girls can get the additional folic acid they need by taking a multivitamin pill.

You can't avoid all accidents, but you can minimize the results.

Some good safety habits can save the lives and health of your family. Racecar drivers know that wearing seat and shoulder belts can reduce risk by 45-50 percent. Other injury-preventing habits that athletes and regular folks alike take: wearing bike helmets and other protective athletic gear, looking ahead of time for the fire exits in a theater or hotel, checking your smoke and CO detectors at home to make sure they beep, locking hunting rifles and other firearms away from kids and others who might misuse them, and avoiding unlit and dangerous areas (and lit and dangerous people.) Carry a first aid or snake bite kit when in the wild. Find a partner or two for climbing, swimming or other exploits—someone to get you out of a tight spot or to go for help.

Respect sex.

More than 13 million Americans—two thirds of them under age 25—have sexually transmitted diseases, including HIV infections. That's a pretty large monument to ignorance, as well as to youthful hormones and lack of restraint. For some young people, an infection may mean they'll never be able to have children. Other infections can lead to cervical cancer (cancer of the neck of the uterus, or womb) or, in the case of HIV infections, early death.

Young people can only be 100% safe if they avoid sex—waiting until they're prepared to have a lasting relationship with another uninfected individual. But sexually active teens and young adults can gain considerable protection by correctly and consistently using a latex condom. That's the advice of federal health agencies. You should discuss this with your kids before the fact—or at least see that they get responsible information. Some parents fear that they may promote sexual activity by discussing it. However, study after study shows that preparing children with good sex education does not promote earlier sex, and several studies suggest this preparation may delay the onset of sex.

Don't puff or chew.

Just when some adults are getting a second wind, others of the same age are dying of tobacco-related lung cancer, or are crippled by other heart and lung problems.

New smokers—young people—may worry more about the smell of their breath, about their teeth getting dark and about getting wrinkles than about dying. Yet, smoking cigarettes, cigars and pipe tobacco kills more people than AIDS, alcohol, drug abuse, car crashes, murders, suicides and fires combined. For many, there's also a feeling of helplessness, of an addiction they can't break, at least alone.

Watch out for the sun and the sunlamps.

It's not just the temporary pain of a sunburn you need to worry about. A youngster's burns may mean not only wrinkles but serious trouble, years later. Ordinary skin cancers can usually be surgically removed without difficulty, but melanomas (malignant moles) can kill, if not caught early.

Ultraviolet light from the sun or from sunlamps and sun beds are also linked to cataracts that dim vision. Hats and other covers and ultraviolet-blocking sunglasses all can help.

Chapter 7

Environmental Genome Project

The Environmental Genome Project (EGP) is a multicomponent project comprised of extramural and intramural research programs in four research areas:

- human DNA polymorphism discovery;
- functional analysis of human DNA polymorphism;
- population-based epidemiology studies of human DNA polymorphism;
- and technology development to support EGP related research.

The information gathered in these four research areas will help build understanding of the complex interrelationships between environmental exposure, genetic susceptibility, and human disease.

History

The EGP was announced as an NIEHS-sponsored initiative in September, 1997, when NIEHS made a public announcement inviting scientists to participate in planning the project. The EGP planning process and the concept of the EGP was first fully explored by the scientific community at a NIEHS-sponsored Symposium held at Masur Auditorium on the NIH campus on October 17-18, 1997. This

A fact sheet from the National Institute of Environmental Health Sciences (NIEHS), 2002. Available online at http://www.niehs.nih.gov/envgenom/egp.htm.

Symposium was co-chaired by Leland H. Hartwell (Fred Hutchinson Cancer Research Center), J. Carl Barrett (then Scientific Director of NIEHS) and Jack A. Taylor (NIEHS) and included discussions concerning gene-environment interactions, population sampling, DNA sequencing technology, functional analysis of polymorphism and the ethical legal and social issues raised by the EGP. In February 1998, Dr. Jose Velazquez (NIEHS) developed, presented, and got approval from the National Advisory Environmental Health Sciences Council of the concept document describing the EGP.

The concept of the EGP would not have been possible without The Human Genome Project (HGP) and its rapid progress in the early to mid-1990s. The HGP was conceived in the mid-1980s, when high-throughput DNA sequencing technology was rapidly being developed and optimized. In 1988, the NIH and the Department of Energy formalized a relationship to coordinate research and technical activities related to sequencing the human genome. In 1990, NIH-DOE published a joint 5-year research plan outlining the goals of the HGP. This and other efforts to sequence the human genome culminated with publication of the first complete drafts of the human genome sequence in 2001 [*Science 291, 1304* (2001); *Nature 409, 934* (2001)].

EGP-related research is dependent on the availability of human genome sequence information provided by the HGP and other human DNA sequencing projects. The EGP seeks to compare selected regions of the human genome sequence in different individuals to determine how much and where there is sequence variation, also called DNA polymorphism. Thus, the EGP is conceptually and historically linked to the HGP.

Overview

Experimental studies in molecular genetics, toxicology and other biomedical fields have shown that genetic differences between two individuals can determine the relative sensitivity of each individual to environmental chemicals or agents. Some human inherited disease susceptibilities are caused by a single inherited trait, and other disease susceptibilities may be determined by multiple genetic traits. For many diseases, the genetic blueprint of each individual does not in and of itself cause disease; instead, disease is the outcome of a complex interplay between multiple genetic and environmental factors.

The rationale of the EGP is that certain genes have a greater than average influence over human susceptibility to environmental agents. If we identify and characterize the polymorphism in those genes, we will increase our understanding of human disease susceptibility. This knowledge can be used to protect susceptible individuals from disease and to reduce adverse exposure and environmentally induced disease.

The EGP has identified a group of human genes that are likely to influence the outcome of environmental exposure. Polymorphic variants in these genes, called environmentally responsive genes, are being identified by systematic resequencing of a predefined diverse, randomly selected set of human DNA samples. The functional significance of specific gene variants is also being characterized to determine which gene variants are correlated with increased or decreased risk of disease. The EGP also carries out research on technologies that support its goals, epidemiology of genetic variation in human populations and the ethical, legal and social issues that are relevant to its studies.

Exposure-Disease Paradigm

All individuals are continually exposed to hazardous agents and chemicals in their environment. Thus, there is a defined probability that each individual will suffer an adverse effect, such as disease, as a result of such exposure. Effects of exposure can be observed within minutes or many years after exposure occurs, but it is well recognized that the outcome of exposure is determined by many variables. This process has been conceptualized by environmental health researchers and expressed as a paradigm that describes the continuum between exposure and disease.

Exposure can come from several external sources including the general physical environment (air, water, soil), the diet or from components specific to an individual's workplace/occupation. The route of exposure varies (air, water, food, soil) and the concentration of a hazardous compound in the environment varies continuously over time. Importantly, each individual receives a unique internal dose of the compound, which is determined by the individual's activities and movements while he/she is being exposed. Most biologically active agents have a much higher probability of causing an adverse effect in one or more target tissues in the human body (i.e., liver, skin, intestine, lung, blood, bone). Thus, the amount of a compound that actually reaches the target tissue is thought of as the biologically effective dose. A compound can reach this target tissue at a significant concentration and still have no biological consequences, if the compound is efficiently removed or destroyed by cellular defense systems before cellular damage occurs. However, if cellular damage occurs, the damage can have a biological effect that leads to sustained or permanent

69

changes in biological structures or functions. In many cases where no treatment or intervention is introduced, disease may develop and progress in these exposed individuals.

Genetic and Environmental Susceptibility

Every organism is exposed to hazardous agents in its environment on a continual basis. As a result organisms have evolved sophisticated pathways that can minimize the biological consequences of the exposures. These pathways constitute the environmental response machinery.

All genes are subject to genetic variability, which can be associated with the altered efficiency of a biological pathway. These genetic variations, or polymorphisms, can be associated with a person's risk for developing an illness as a result of environmental exposures. The biological components that influence the outcome of exposure include the following: cellular receptors for environmental compounds, enzymes that modify or activate chemical toxins, enzymes that repair DNA damage, factors that regulate cell cycle control, and factors that regulate cell division and cell death. Greater detail of this process is discussed later in this chapter. It is clear that variation in the genes that control these processes can influence the outcome of exposure, and this principle has guided development of the EGP research program.

Environmentally Responsive Genes

The outcome of environmental exposure is influenced by the function of many human genes. Not all of these genes or their functions are known at present. However, many genes have been identified that are likely to be important factors in genetic susceptibility to environmentally induced disease. These genes tend to fall into the following 8 categories: cell cycle, DNA repair, cell division, cell signaling, cell structure, gene expression, apoptosis and metabolism.

Cell cycle and cell division genes regulate the ability of a cell to proliferate, grow and differentiate. Changes in the progression of a cell through the cell cycle can increase the ability of a cell to survive stress; in most cases, a proliferating cell exposed to stress will enhance its survival by delaying the cell cycle so that cellular damage can be repaired prior to cell division. Cell signaling and gene expression pathways have profound effects on all cellular functions, including cell proliferation and differentiation. Some exogenous agents can activate these pathways in aberrant and deleterious ways (i.e., agents that mimic a biological component), and this can disrupt or alter normal cellular function.

Several genes that control metabolic pathways are crucial determinants of the outcome of exposure. In many cases, a compound enters a biological system in an inert innocuous form that is metabolically converted into a reactive species that causes cellular damage. The converse is also true: some metabolic pathways destroy toxic compounds by changing a compound's chemical structure (detoxification).

DNA repair genes influence the outcome of exposure to environmental agents that cause DNA damage. Individuals with higher or lower capacity for DNA repair have decreased or increased risk of certain types of environmentally induced disease, respectively. Heavily damaged cells often die by a process known as programmed cell death or apoptosis. This process protects the organism by removing aberrant cells and structures.

The EGP has generated a list of 554 environmentally responsive genes that are potential targets for resequencing in subgroups according to a phased timeline. This list was generated by the NIEHS scientific community. However, the list is not comprehensive and it is expected that more genes may be added over time. The first phase of resequencing extends from 1998 to 2001 and has been focused on polymorphic variants on a group of 123 genes. The second phase of resequencing, which will extend from 2001 to 2004, will focus on approximately 200 DNA repair and cell cycle control genes. Genes regulating metabolism, signal transduction, and apoptosis will also be targeted for resequencing.

Chapter 8

Environmental Public Health Tracking Program

The environment plays an important role in human development and health. Researchers have linked exposures to some environmental hazards with specific diseases. One example is the link between exposure to asbestos and lung cancer. Another example is the link between exposure to lead and decreased mental function in children. However, other links remain unproven, such as the suspected link between exposure to disinfectant byproducts (for example, chlorine from showerheads) and bladder cancer.

In 1988, in its report "The Future of Public Health," the Institute of Medicine noted that the removal of environmental health authority from public health agencies has led to fragmented responsibility, lack of coordination, and inadequate attention to the health dimensions of environmental problems.

In January 2001, the Pew Environmental Health Commission issued the report "America's Environmental Health Gap: Why the Country Needs a Nationwide Health Tracking Network." The report, which stated that the existing environmental health system is neither adequate nor well organized, recommended the creation of a "Nationwide Health Tracking Network" for disease and exposures.

Currently, no systems exist at the state or national level to track many of the exposures and health effects that may be related to environmental hazards. In addition, in most cases, existing environmental

A fact sheet from Centers for Disease Control and Prevention (CDC), National Center for Environmental Health (NCEH), 2002. Available online at http://www.cdc.gov/nceh/tracking/background.html.

hazard, exposure, and disease tracking systems are not linked together. Because existing systems are not linked, it is difficult to study and monitor relationships among hazards, exposures, and health effects.

CDC's Program

In fiscal year 2002, Congress provided the Centers for Disease Control and Prevention (CDC) with funding of $17.5 million to do the following:

- begin developing a nationwide environmental public health tracking network
- develop capacity in environmental health within state and local health departments

CDC's goal is to develop a tracking system that integrates data about environmental hazards and exposures with data about diseases that are possibly linked to the environment. This system will allow federal, state, and local agencies, and others to do the following:

- monitor and distribute information about environmental hazards and disease trends
- advance research on possible linkages between environmental hazards and disease
- develop, implement, and evaluate regulatory and public health actions to prevent or control environment-related diseases.

Planning for an environmental public health tracking network is an important priority for CDC because of the opportunity it provides to address some of the most challenging problems facing local, state, and national public health leaders. From the outset, this activity has involved substantial collaboration between CDC and its public health and environmental partners.

CDC assembled four workgroups to develop recommendations for the environmental public health tracking program. The workgroups included representatives from 30 organizations, including the following:

- Federal agencies
- State and local public health and environment agencies
- Non-governmental organizations

- Academic institutions.

The workgroups addressed the following topics:

- Organization and management
- Data technology and tracking methodology
- Tracking system inventory and needs assessment
- Translation, policy, and public health action.

Current Activities

CDC recently awarded grants to 20 state and local health departments and three Schools of Public Health to begin developing a national environmental health tracking network and to develop capacity in environmental health at the state and local levels.

The state and local health departments are being funded to:

- Build environmental public health capacity
- Increase collaboration between environmental and health agencies
- Identify and evaluate existing data systems
- Build partnerships with non-governmental organizations and communities
- Develop model systems that link data and can be applied to other states or localities.

The Schools of Public Health will support the efforts of state and local health departments and will investigate possible links between health effects and the environment.

Chapter 9

The Emergency Planning and Community Right-to-Know Act (EPCRA)

The Emergency Planning and Community Right-to-Know Act of 1986 (EPCRA) establishes requirements for Federal, State and local governments, Indian Tribes, and industry regarding emergency planning and Community Right-to-Know reporting on hazardous and toxic chemicals.

The Community Right-to-Know provisions help increase the public's knowledge and access to information on chemicals at individual facilities, their uses, and releases into the environment. States and communities, working with facilities, can use the information to improve chemical safety and protect public health and the environment.

What Does EPCRA Cover?

EPCRA has four major provisions:

- Emergency planning (Section 301-303),

- Emergency release notification (Section 304),

- Hazardous chemical storage reporting requirements (Sections 311-312), and

- Toxic chemical release inventory (Section 313).

"The Emergency Planning and Community Right-to-Know Act," a fact sheet produced by the Office of Solid Waste, U.S. Environmental Protection Agency (EPA), EPA550-F-00-004, 2000.

Information gleaned from these four requirements will help States and communities develop a broad perspective of chemical hazards for the entire community as well as for individual facilities.

Regulations implementing EPCRA are codified in Title 40 of the Code of Federal Regulations, parts 350 to 372. The chemicals covered by each of the sections are different, as are the quantities that trigger reporting. Table 9.1 on summarizes the chemicals and thresholds.

What Are Emergency Response Plans (Sections 301-303)?

Emergency response plans contain information that community officials can use at the time of a chemical accident. Community emergency response plans for chemical accidents were developed under section 303. The plans must:

- Identify facilities and transportation routes of extremely hazardous substances;

- Describe emergency response procedures, on and off site;

- Designate a community coordinator and facility coordinator(s) to implement the plan;

- Outline emergency notification procedures;

- Describe how to determine the probable affected area and population by releases;

- Describe local emergency equipment and facilities and the persons responsible for them;

- Outline evacuation plans;

- Provide a training program for emergency responders (including schedules); and,

- Provide methods and schedules for exercising emergency response plans.

Planning activities of Local Emergency Planning Committees (LEPCs) and facilities initially focused on, but were not limited to, the 356 extremely hazardous substances listed by EPA. The list includes the threshold planning quantities (minimum limits) for each substance. Any facility that has any of the listed chemicals at or above its threshold planning quantity must notify the State Emergency Response Commission (SERC) and LEPC within 60 days after they first receive a shipment or produce the substance on site.

What Are the Emergency Notification Requirements (Section 304)?

Facilities must immediately notify the LEPC and the SERC if there is a release into the environment of a hazardous substance that is equal to or exceeds the minimum reportable quantity set in the regulations. This requirement covers the 356 extremely hazardous substances as well as the more than 700 hazardous substances subject to the emergency notification requirements under CERCLA Section 103(a)(40 CFR 302.4). Some chemicals are common to both lists. Initial notification can be made by telephone, radio, or in person. Emergency notification requirements involving transportation incidents can be met by dialing 911, or in the absence of a 911 emergency number, calling the operator. This emergency notification needs to include:

- The chemical name;

- An indication of whether the substance is extremely hazardous;

- An estimate of the quantity released into the environment;

- The time and duration of the release;

- Whether the release occurred into air, water, and/or land;

- Any known or anticipated acute or chronic health risks associated with the emergency, and where necessary, advice regarding medical attention for exposed individuals;

- Proper precautions, such as evacuation or sheltering in place; and,

- Name and telephone number of contact person.

A written follow-up notice must be submitted to the SERC and LEPC as soon as practicable after the release. The follow-up notice must update information included in the initial notice and provide information on actual response actions taken and advice regarding medical attention necessary for citizens exposed.

What Are SERCs and LEPCs?

The Governor of each state designated a State Emergency Response Commission (SERC). The SERCs, in turn, designated about 3,500 local emergency planning districts and appointed Local Emergency Planning Committees (LEPCs) for each district. The SERC supervises and coordinates the activities of the LEPC, establishes procedures for receiving and processing public requests for information collected under EPCRA, and reviews local emergency response plans.

The LEPC membership must include, at a minimum, local officials including police, fire, civil defense, public health, transportation, and environmental professionals, as well as representatives of facilities subject to the emergency planning requirements, community groups, and the media. The LEPCs must develop an emergency response plan, review it at least annually, and provide information about chemicals in the community to citizens.

What Are the Community Right-to-Know Requirements (Sections 311/312)?

Under Occupational Safety and Health Administration (OSHA) regulations, employers must maintain a material safety data sheet

Table 9.1. EPCRA Chemicals and Reporting Thresholds

	Section 302	Section 304	Sections 311/312	Section 313
Chemicals Covered	356 extremely hazardous substances	>1,000 substances	500,000 products	650 toxic chemicals and categories
Thresholds	Threshold Planning Quantity, 1-10,000 pounds on site at any one time	Reportable quantity, 1-5,000 pounds, released in a 24-hour period	TPQ or 500 pounds for Section 302 chemicals; 10,000 pounds on site at any one time for other chemicals	25,000 pounds per year manufactured or processed; 10,000 pounds a year used; certain persistent bioaccumulative toxics have lower thresholds

(MSDS) for any hazardous chemicals stored or used in the work place. Approximately 500,000 products have MSDSs.

Section 311 requires facilities that have MSDSs for chemicals held above certain quantities to submit either copies of their MSDSs or a list of MSDS chemicals to the SERC, LEPC, and local fire department. If the facility owner or operator chooses to submit a list of MSDS chemicals, the list must include the chemical or common name of each substance and must identify the applicable hazard categories. These hazard categories are:

- Immediate (acute) health hazard;

- Delayed (chronic) health hazard;

- Fire hazard;

- Sudden release of pressure hazard; and

- Reactive hazard.

If a list is submitted, the facility must submit a copy of the MSDSs for any chemical on the list upon the request of the LEPC or SERC.

Facilities that start using a chemical or increase the quantity to exceed the thresholds must submit MSDSs or a list of MSDSs chemicals within three months after they become covered. Facilities must provide a revised MSDS to update the original MSDS if significant new information is discovered about the hazardous chemical.

Facilities covered by section 311 must, under section 312, submit annually an emergency and hazardous chemical inventory form to the LEPC, the SERC, and the local fire department. Facilities provide either a Tier I or Tier II form. Tier I forms include the following aggregate information for each applicable hazard category:

- An estimate (in ranges) of the maximum amount of chemicals for each category present at the facility at any time during the preceding calendar year;

- An estimate (in ranges) of the average daily amount of chemicals in each category; and,

- The general location of hazardous chemicals in each category.

The Tier II report contains basically the same information as the Tier I, but it must name the specific chemicals. Many states require Tier II information under state law. Tier II forms provide the following information for each substance:

- The chemical name or the common name as indicated on the MSDS;

- An estimate (in ranges) of the maximum amount of the chemical present at any time during the preceding calendar year and the average daily amount;

- A brief description of the manner of storage of the chemical;

- The location of the chemical at the facility; and

- An indication of whether the owner elects to withhold location information from disclosure to the public.

Because many SERCs have added requirements or incorporated the Federal contents in their own forms, Tier I/II forms should be obtained from the SERC. Section 312 information must be submitted on or before March 1 each year. The information submitted under sections 311 and 312 is available to the public from LEPCs and SERCs.

In 1999, EPA excluded gasoline held at most retail gas stations from EPCRA 311/312 reporting. EPA estimates that about 550,000 facilities are now covered by EPCRA 311/312 requirements.

What Is the Toxics Release Inventory (Section 313)?

EPCRA section 313 (commonly referred to as the Toxics Release Inventory or TRI) requires certain facilities to complete a Toxic Chemical Release Inventory Form annually for specified chemicals. The form must be submitted to EPA and the State on July 1 and cover releases

Table 9.2. Reporting Schedules

Section

302	One time notification to SERC
304	Each time a release above a reportable quantity occurs; to LEPC and SERC
311	One time submission; update only for new chemicals or information; to SERC, LEPC, fire department
312	Annually, by March 1 to SERC, LEPC, fire department
313	Annually, by July 1, to EPA and State Chemical Emergency Preparedness and Prevention Office

and other waste management of toxic chemicals that occurred during the preceding calendar year. One purpose of this reporting requirement is to inform the public and government officials about releases and other waste management of toxic chemicals. The following information is required on the form:

- The name, location and type of business;
- Whether the chemical is manufactured (including importation), processed, or otherwise used and the general categories of use of the chemical;
- An estimate (in ranges) of the maximum amounts of the toxic chemical present at the facility at any time during the preceding year;
- Quantity of the chemical entering the air, land, and water annually;
- Off-site locations to which the facility transfers toxic chemicals in waste for recycling, energy recovery, treatment or disposal; and
- Waste treatment/disposal methods and efficiency of methods for each waste stream;

In addition, the Pollution Prevention Act of 1990 requires collection of information on source reduction, recycling, and treatment. EPA maintains a national TRI database, available on the Internet.

What Else Does EPCRA Require?

Trade Secrets. EPCRA section 322 addresses trade secrets as they apply EPCRA sections 303, 311, 312, and 313 reporting; a facility cannot claim trade secrets under section 304 of the statute. Only chemical identity may be claimed as a trade secret, though a generic class for the chemical must be provided. The criteria a facility must meet to claim a chemical identity as a trade secret are in 40 CFR part 350. In practice, less than one percent of facilities have filed such claims.

Even if chemical identity information can be legally withheld from the public, EPCRA section 323 allows the information to be disclosed to health professionals who need the information for diagnostic and treatment purposes or local health officials who need the information for prevention and treatment activities. In non-emergency cases, the health professional must sign a confidentiality agreement with the facility and provide a written statement of need. In medical emergencies, the health professional, if requested by the facility, provides these documents as soon as circumstances permit.

Any person may challenge trade secret claims by petitioning EPA. The Agency must then review the claim and rule on its validity.

EPCRA Penalties. EPCRA Section 325 allows civil and administrative penalties ranging up to $10,000-$75,000 per violation or per day per violation when facilities fail to comply with the reporting requirements. Criminal penalties up to $50,000 or five years in prison apply to any person who knowingly and willfully fails to provide emergency release notification. Penalties of not more than $20,000 and/or up to one year in prison apply to any person who knowingly and willfully discloses any information entitled to protection as a trade secret.

Citizens Suits. EPCRA section 326 allows citizens to initiate civil actions against EPA, SERCs, and the owner or operator of a facility for failure to meet the EPCRA requirements. A SERC, LEPC, and State or local government may institute actions against facility owner/operators for failure to comply with EPCRA requirements. In addition, States may sue EPA for failure to provide trade secret information.

Who's Covered by TRI?

The TRI reporting requirement applies to facilities that have 10 or more full-time employees, that manufacture (including importing), process, or otherwise use a listed toxic chemical above threshold quantities, and that are in one of the following sectors:

- Manufacturing (Standard Industrial Classification (SIC) codes 20 through 39)
- Metal mining (SIC code 10, except for SIC codes 1011,1081, and 1094)
- Coal mining (SIC code 12, except for 1241 and extraction activities)
- Electrical utilities that combust coal and/or oil (SIC codes 4911, 4931, and 4939)
- Resource Conservation and Recovery Act (RCRA) Subtitle C hazardous waste treatment and disposal facilities (SIC code 4953)

- Chemicals and allied products wholesale distributors (SIC code 5169)

- Petroleum bulk plants and terminals (SIC code 5171)

- Solvent recovery services (SIC code 7389)

Where Can You Find EPCRA Information?

MSDSs, hazardous chemical inventory forms, follow-up emergency notices, and the emergency response plan are available from the SERC and LEPC.

MSDSs on hazardous chemicals are maintained by a number of universities and can be accessed through http://www.hazard.com.

EPA also provides fact sheets and other information on chemical properties through its website http://www.epa.gov. EPA has compiled a list of all chemicals covered by name under these regulations into a single list and published them as The Title III List of Lists available at www.epa.gov/ceppo/pubs/title3.pdf.

Profiles of extremely hazardous substances are available at http://www.epa.gov/swercepp/ehs/ehslist.html.

Each year, EPA publishes a report summarizing the TRI information that was submitted to EPA and States during the previous year. In addition, TRI data are available through EPA's Envirofacts database at http://www.epa.gov/enviro. TRI data are also available at http://www.epa.gov/tri, http://www.rtk.net, and http://www.scorecard.org.

All of these sites can be searched by facility, city, county, and state and provide access to basic TRI emissions data. The RTK-Net site, maintained by the public advocacy group OMB Watch, provides copies of the full TRI form for each facility. The Scorecard site, maintained by the Environmental Defense public advocacy group, ranks facilities, States, and counties on a number of parameters (e.g., total quantities of carcinogens released) as well as maps that show the locations of facilities in a county or city.

Are There Other Laws That Provide Similar Information?

The Oil Pollution Act (OPA) of 1990 includes national planning and preparedness provisions for oil spills that are similar to EPCRA provisions for extremely hazardous substances. Plans are developed at the local, State and Federal levels. The OPA plans offer an opportunity for LEPCs to coordinate their plans with area and facility oil spill plans covering the same geographical area.

The 1990 Clean Air Act Amendments require the EPA and OSHA to issue regulations for chemical accident prevention. Facilities that have certain chemical above specified threshold quantities are required to develop a risk management program to identify and evaluate hazards and manage those hazards safely. Facilities subject to EPA's risk management program rules must submit a risk management plan (RMP) summarizing its program. RMP information can be accessed through http://yosemite.epa.gov/oswer/ceppoweb.nsf/content/RMPS.htm.

Part Two

Airborne Hazards

Chapter 10

An Introduction to Indoor Air Quality

Indoor Air Quality

Good news and bad news about indoor air affects everyone. The bad news is that indoor air often contains higher concentrations of hazardous pollutants than outdoor air. However, the good news is that everyone can reduce indoor air pollution.

How can the air inside our homes be so bad for us?

Over the years, buildings have been made more airtight to conserve energy. A variety of methods have been employed to keep the hot or cool air from escaping from our homes: installing storm windows and insulation; applying caulk and weather stripping to seal cracks and other openings; and heating our homes with kerosene, wood, coal, and natural gas. Unfortunately, when we trap in hot or cool air, we also trap in pollutants and sometimes generate more.

This material is reprinted from "Indoor Air Quality," a fact sheet produced by the National Safety Council. © 2000. Permission to reprint granted by the National Safety Council (NSC), a membership organization dedicated to protecting life and promoting health. For more information, visit the website of the National Safety Council at www.nsc.org; And under the heading "Indoor Air: Frequent Questions," from "Frequent Questions: Indoor Air," an undated fact sheet produced by the U.S. Environmental Protection Agency (EPA), available online at http://www.epa.gov/iaq/ia_faqs.html. Cited February 2003.

Why is this an issue?

On average, people spend about 90 percent of their time indoors. Sixty-five percent of that is spent at home. To make matters worse, those who are most susceptible to indoor air pollution are the ones who are home the most: children, pregnant women, the elderly, and those with chronic illnesses. Children breathe in 50 percent more air per pound of body weight than adults do. U.S. Environmental Protection Agency (EPA) studies have found that pollutant levels inside can be two to five times higher than outdoors. After some activities, indoor air pollution levels can be 100 times higher than outdoors.

What are the sources of pollutants?

There are many sources of pollutants in the home. Obvious ones are chemicals, cleaning products, and pesticides. Less obvious are pollutants caused by such simple tasks as cooking, bathing, or heating the home. Fortunately, there are easy steps that everyone can take to reduce the potential for indoor air pollution and to improve the quality of the air they breathe.

How do you know if the air inside your home is dangerous to your health?

Often, it is difficult to determine which pollutant or pollutants are the sources of a person's ill health, or even if indoor air pollution is the problem. Many indoor air pollutants cannot be detected by our senses (e.g., smell) and the symptoms they produce can be vague and sometimes similar, making it hard to attribute them to a specific cause. Some symptoms may not show up until years later, making it even harder to discover the cause. Common symptoms of exposure to indoor air pollutants include: headaches, tiredness, dizziness, nausea, itchy nose, and scratchy throat. More serious effects are asthma and other breathing disorders and cancer.

How does this affect children?

Children may be more susceptible to environmental exposures than adults and, because of their developing systems, particularly vulnerable to their effects. Asthma is a case in point. About 4.2 million children in the United States, and more than 12.4 million people total, are affected by asthma each year. A recent study, published in the

American Journal of Respiratory and Critical Care Medicine concluded that 65 percent of asthma cases among elementary school-age children could be prevented by controlling exposure to indoor allergens and environmental tobacco smoke (ETS). By controlling biological contaminants (e.g., dust mites and cat allergens), asthma cases could be reduced by 55 to 60 percent.

Indoor Air: Frequent Questions

What causes indoor air problems?

Indoor pollution sources that release gases or particles into the air are the primary cause of indoor air quality problems in homes. Inadequate ventilation can increase indoor pollutant levels by not bringing in enough outdoor air to dilute emissions from indoor sources and by not carrying indoor air pollutants out of the home. High temperature and humidity levels can also increase concentrations of some pollutants.

Pollutant Sources

There are many sources of indoor air pollution in any home. These include combustion sources such as oil, gas, kerosene, coal, wood, and tobacco products; building materials and furnishings as diverse as deteriorated, asbestos-containing insulation, wet or damp carpet, and cabinetry or furniture made of certain pressed wood products; products for household cleaning and maintenance, personal care, or hobbies; central heating and cooling systems and humidification devices; and outdoor sources such as radon, pesticides, and outdoor air pollution.

The relative importance of any single source depends on how much of a given pollutant it emits and how hazardous those emissions are. In some cases, factors such as how old the source is and whether it is properly maintained are significant. For example, an improperly adjusted gas stove can emit significantly more carbon monoxide than one that is properly adjusted.

Some sources, such as building materials, furnishings, and household products like air fresheners, release pollutants more or less continuously. Other sources, related to activities carried out in the home, release pollutants intermittently. These include smoking, the use of unvented or malfunctioning stoves, furnaces, or space heaters, the use of solvents in cleaning and hobby activities, the use of paint strippers in redecorating activities, and the use of cleaning products and pesticides in housekeeping. High pollutant concentrations can remain in the air for long periods after some of these activities.

Amount of Ventilation

If too little outdoor air enters a home, pollutants can accumulate to levels that can pose health and comfort problems. Unless they are built with special mechanical means of ventilation, homes that are designed and constructed to minimize the amount of outdoor air that can leak into and out of the home may have higher pollutant levels than other homes. However, because some weather conditions can drastically reduce the amount of outdoor air that enters a home, pollutants can build up even in homes that are normally considered leaky.

How does outdoor air enter a house?

Outdoor air enters and leaves a house by: infiltration, natural ventilation, and mechanical ventilation. In a process known as infiltration, outdoor air flows into the house through openings, joints, and cracks in walls, floors, and ceilings, and around windows and doors. In natural ventilation, air moves through opened windows and doors. Air movement associated with infiltration and natural ventilation is caused by air temperature differences between indoors and outdoors and by wind. Finally, there are a number of mechanical ventilation devices, from outdoor-vented fans that intermittently remove air from a single room, such as bathrooms and kitchen, to air handling systems that use fans and duct work to continuously remove indoor air and distribute filtered and conditioned outdoor air to strategic points throughout the house. The rate at which outdoor air replaces indoor air is described as the air exchange rate. When there is little infiltration, natural ventilation, or mechanical ventilation, the air exchange rate is low and pollutant levels can increase.

What if you live in an apartment?

Apartments can have the same indoor air problems as single-family homes because many of the pollution sources, such as the interior building materials, furnishings, and household products, are similar. Indoor air problems similar to those in offices are caused by such sources as contaminated ventilation systems, improperly placed outdoor air intakes, or maintenance activities.

Solutions to air quality problems in apartments, as in homes and offices, involve such actions as: eliminating or controlling the sources of pollution, increasing ventilation, and installing air cleaning devices. Often a resident can take the appropriate action to improve the indoor air quality by removing a source, altering an activity, unblocking an air supply vent, or opening a window to temporarily increase the ventilation; in other cases, however, only the building owner or manager is in a position to remedy the problem. You can encourage building management to follow guidance in EPA and National Institute for Occupational Safety and Health (NIOSH)'s "Building Air Quality: A Guide for Building Owners and Facility Managers" (http://www.epa.gov/iaq/largebldgs/index.html).

Chapter 11

Asbestos: A Source of Indoor Air Pollution

This chapter answers the most frequently asked health questions about asbestos. For more information, you may call the ATSDR Information Center at 1-888-422-8737. This information is important because this substance may harm you. The effects of exposure to any hazardous substance depend on the dose, the duration, how you are exposed, individual susceptibility and personal habits, and whether other chemicals are present.

Exposure to asbestos usually occurs by breathing contaminated air in workplaces that make or use asbestos. Asbestos is also found in the air of buildings containing asbestos that are being torn down or renovated. Asbestos exposure can cause serious lung problems and cancer. This substance has been found in at least 83 of the 1,585 National Priorities List sites identified by the Environmental Protection Agency (EPA).

What is asbestos?

Asbestos is the name given to a group of six different fibrous minerals (amosite, chrysotile, crocidolite, and the fibrous varieties of tremolite, actinolite, and anthophyllite) that occur naturally in the environment. Asbestos minerals have separable long fibers that are strong and flexible enough to be spun and woven and are heat resistant.

"ToxFAQs for Asbestos," Agency for Toxic Substances and Disease Registry (ATSDR), CAS# 1332-21-4, 2001. Available online at http://www.atsdr.cdc.gov/ tfacts61.html.

Because of these characteristics, asbestos has been used for a wide range of manufactured goods, mostly in building materials (roofing shingles, ceiling and floor tiles, paper products, and asbestos cement products), friction products (automobile clutch, brake, and transmission parts), heat-resistant fabrics, packaging, gaskets, and coatings. Some vermiculite or talc products may contain asbestos.

What happens to asbestos when it enters the environment?

Asbestos fibers can enter the air or water from the breakdown of natural deposits and manufactured asbestos products. Asbestos fibers do not evaporate into air or dissolve in water. Small diameter fibers and particles may remain suspended in the air for a long time and be carried long distances by wind or water before settling down. Larger diameter fibers and particles tend to settle more quickly.

Asbestos fibers are not able to move through soil. Asbestos fibers are generally not broken down to other compounds and will remain virtually unchanged over long periods.

How might I be exposed to asbestos?

We are all exposed to low levels of asbestos in the air we breathe. These levels range from 0.00001 to 0.0001 fibers per milliliter of air and generally are highest in cities and industrial areas.

People working in industries that make or use asbestos products or who are involved in asbestos mining may be exposed to high levels of asbestos. People living near these industries may also be exposed to high levels of asbestos in air.

Asbestos fibers may be released into the air by the disturbance of asbestos-containing material during product use, demolition work, building or home maintenance, repair, and remodeling. In general, exposure may occur only when the asbestos-containing material is disturbed in some way to release particles and fibers into the air.

Drinking water may contain asbestos from natural sources or from asbestos-containing cement pipes.

How can asbestos affect my health?

Asbestos mainly affects the lungs and the membrane that surrounds the lungs. Breathing high levels of asbestos fibers for a long time may result in scar-like tissue in the lungs and in the pleural membrane (lining) that surrounds the lung. This disease is called asbestosis and is usually found in workers exposed to asbestos, but not in the general public. People with asbestosis have difficulty breathing, often a cough, and in severe cases heart enlargement. Asbestosis is a serious disease and can eventually lead to disability and death.

Breathing lower levels of asbestos may result in changes called plaques in the pleural membranes. Pleural plaques can occur in workers and sometimes in people living in areas with high environmental levels of asbestos. Effects on breathing from pleural plaques alone are not usually serious, but higher exposure can lead to a thickening of the pleural membrane that may restrict breathing.

How likely is asbestos to cause cancer?

The Department of Health and Human Services (DHHS), the World Health Organization (WHO), and the EPA have determined that asbestos is a human carcinogen.

It is known that breathing asbestos can increase the risk of cancer in people. There are two types of cancer caused by exposure to asbestos: lung cancer and mesothelioma. Mesothelioma is a cancer of the thin lining surrounding the lung (pleural membrane) or abdominal cavity (the peritoneum). Cancer from asbestos does not develop immediately, but shows up after a number of years. Studies of workers also suggest that breathing asbestos can increase chances of getting cancer in other parts of the body (stomach, intestines, esophagus, pancreas, and kidneys), but this is less certain. Early identification and treatment of any cancer can increase an individual's quality of life and survival.

Cigarette smoke and asbestos together significantly increase your chances of getting lung cancer. Therefore, if you have been exposed to asbestos you should stop smoking. This may be the most important action that you can take to improve your health and decrease your risk of cancer.

How can asbestos affect children?

We do not know if exposure to asbestos will result in birth defects or other developmental effects in people. Birth defects have not been observed in animals exposed to asbestos.

It is likely that health effects seen in children exposed to high levels of asbestos will be similar to the effects seen in adults.

How can families reduce the risk of exposure to asbestos?

Materials containing asbestos that are not disturbed or deteriorated do not, in general, pose a health risk and can be left alone. If you suspect that you may be exposed to asbestos in your home, contact your state or local health department or the regional offices of EPA to find out how to test your home and how to locate a company that is trained to remove or contain the fibers.

Is there a medical test to show whether I've been exposed to asbestos?

Low levels of asbestos fibers can be measured in urine, feces, mucus, or lung washings of the general public. Higher than average levels of asbestos fibers in tissue can confirm exposure but not determine whether you will experience any health effects.

A thorough history, physical exam, and diagnostic tests are needed to evaluate asbestos-related disease. Chest x-rays are the best screening tool to identify lung changes resulting from asbestos exposure. Lung function tests and CAT scans also assist in the diagnosis of asbestos-related disease.

Has the federal government made recommendations to protect human health?

In 1989, EPA banned all new uses of asbestos; uses established before this date are still allowed. EPA established regulations that require school systems to inspect for damaged asbestos and to eliminate or reduce the exposure by removing the asbestos or by covering it up. EPA regulates the release of asbestos from factories and during building demolition or renovation to prevent asbestos from getting into the environment.

EPA has proposed a concentration limit of 7 million fibers per liter of drinking water for long fibers.

The Occupational Safety and Health Administration has set limits of 100,000 fibers with lengths greater than or equal to 5 μm per cubic meter of workplace air for 8-hour shifts and 40-hour work weeks.

References

Agency for Toxic Substances and Disease Registry (ATSDR). 2001. Toxicological profile for asbestos. Update. Atlanta, GA: U.S. Department of Health and Human Services, Public Health Service.

Chapter 12

Carbon Monoxide

Carbon monoxide (CO) is an odorless, colorless gas that interferes with the delivery of oxygen in the blood to the rest of the body. It is produced by the incomplete combustion of fuels.

What are the major sources of CO?

Carbon monoxide is produced as a result of incomplete burning of carbon-containing fuels including coal, wood, charcoal, natural gas, and fuel oil. It can be emitted by combustion sources such as unvented kerosene and gas space heaters, furnaces, woodstoves, gas stoves, fireplaces and water heaters, automobile exhaust from attached garages, and tobacco smoke. Problems can arise as a result of improper installation, maintenance, or inadequate ventilation.

What are the health effects?

Carbon monoxide interferes with the distribution of oxygen in the blood to the rest of the body. Depending on the amount inhaled, this gas can impede coordination, worsen cardiovascular conditions, and produce fatigue, headache, weakness, confusion, disorientation, nausea, and dizziness. Very high levels can cause death.

This material is reprinted from "Carbon Monoxide," a fact sheet produced by the National Safety Council. © 2002. Permission to reprint granted by the National Safety Council (NSC), a membership organization dedicated to protecting life and promoting health. For more information, visit the website of the National Safety Council at www.nsc.org.

The symptoms are sometimes confused with the flu or food poisoning. Fetuses, infants, elderly, and people with heart and respiratory illnesses are particularly at high risk for the adverse health effects of carbon monoxide.

An estimated 1,000 people die each year as a result of carbon monoxide poisoning and thousands of others end up in hospital emergency rooms.

What can be done to prevent CO poisoning?

- Ensure that appliances are properly adjusted and working to manufacturers' instructions and local building codes.

- Obtain annual inspections for heating system, chimneys, and flues and have them cleaned by a qualified technician.

- Open flues when fireplaces are in use.

- Use proper fuel in kerosene space heaters.

- Do not use ovens and gas ranges to heat your home.

- Do not burn charcoal inside a home, cabin, recreational vehicle, or camper.

- Make sure stoves and heaters are vented to the outside and that exhaust systems do not leak.

- Do not use unvented gas or kerosene space heaters in enclosed spaces.

- Never leave a car or lawn mower engine running in a shed or garage, or in any enclosed space.

- Make sure your furnace has adequate intake of outside air.

What if I have carbon monoxide poisoning?

Don't ignore symptoms, especially if more than one person is feeling them. If you think you are suffering from carbon monoxide (CO) poisoning, you should:

- Get fresh air immediately. Open doors and windows. Turn off combustion appliances and leave the house.

- Go to an emergency room. Be sure to tell the physician that you suspect CO poisoning.

- Be prepared to answer the following questions: Is anyone else in your household complaining of similar symptoms? Did everyone's symptoms appear about the same time? Are you using any fuel-burning appliances in the home? Has anyone inspected your appliances lately? Are you certain they are working properly?

What about carbon monoxide detectors?

Carbon monoxide (CO) detectors can be used as a backup but not as a replacement for proper use and maintenance of your fuel-burning appliances. CO detector technology is still being developed and the detectors are not generally considered to be as reliable as the smoke detectors found in homes today. You should not choose a CO detector solely on the basis of cost; do some research on the different features available.

Carbon monoxide detectors should meet Underwriters Laboratories Inc. standards, have a long-term warranty, and be easily self-tested and reset to ensure proper functioning. For maximum effectiveness during sleeping hours, carbon monoxide detectors should be placed close to sleeping areas.

If your CO detector goes off, you should:

- Make sure it is the CO detector and not the smoke alarm.

- Check to see if any member of your household is experiencing symptoms.

- If they are, get them out of the house immediately and seek medical attention.

- If no one is feeling symptoms, ventilate the home with fresh air and turn off all potential sources of CO.

- Have a qualified technician inspect your fuel-burning appliances and chimneys to make sure they are operating correctly.

Chapter 13

Combustion Appliances and Indoor Air Pollution

Hazards may be associated with almost all types of appliances. The purpose of this chapter is to answer some common questions you may have about the potential for one specific type of hazard—indoor air pollution—associated with combustion appliances.

Combustion appliances are those which burn fuels for warmth, cooking, or decorative purposes. Typical fuels are gas, both natural and liquefied petroleum (LP); kerosene; oil; coal; and wood. Examples of the appliances are space heaters, ranges, ovens, stoves, furnaces, fireplaces, water heaters, and clothes dryers. These appliances are usually safe. However, under certain conditions, these appliances can produce combustion pollutants that can damage your health, or even kill you.

Possible health effects range from headaches, dizziness, sleepiness, and watery eyes to breathing difficulties or even death. Similar effects may also occur because of common medical problems or other indoor air pollutants.

The information in this chapter will:

1. encourage the proper use, maintenance, and installation of combustion appliances;

"What You Should Know about Combustion Appliances and Indoor Air Pollution," a booklet produced by the U.S. Consumer Product Safety Commission (CPSC), reviewed 1998. CPSC Document #452. Deemed current by the CPSC as of February 2003. Available online at http://www.cpsc.gov/cpscpub/pubs/452.html.

2. discuss the pollutants produced by these appliances;

3. describe how these pollutants can affect your health; and,

4. tell you how you can reduce your exposure to them.

What You Should Know about Indoor Air Pollution

Should I be concerned about indoor air pollution?

Yes. Studies have shown that the air in our homes can be even more polluted than the outdoor air in big cities. Because people spend a lot of time indoors, the quality of the air indoors can affect their health. Infants, young children and the elderly are a group shown to be more susceptible to pollutants. People with chronic respiratory or cardio-vascular illness or immune system diseases are also more susceptible than others to pollutants.

Many factors determine whether pollutants in your home will affect your health. They include the presence, use, and condition of pollutant sources, the level of pollutants both indoors and out, the amount of ventilation in your home, and your overall health.

Most homes have more than one source of indoor air pollution. For example, pollutants come from tobacco smoke, building materials, decorating products, home furnishings, and activities such as cooking, heating, cooling, and cleaning. Living in areas with high outdoor levels of pollutants usually results in high indoor levels. Combustion pollutants are one category of indoor air pollutants.

What are combustion pollutants?

Combustion pollutants are gases or particles that come from burning materials. The combustion pollutants discussed in this chapter come from burning fuels in appliances. The common fuels burned in these appliances are natural or LP gas, fuel oil, kerosene, wood, or coal. The types and amounts of pollutants produced depend upon the type of appliance, how well the appliance is installed, maintained, and vented, and the kind of fuel it uses. Some of the common pollutants produced from burning these fuels are carbon monoxide, nitrogen dioxide, particles, and sulfur dioxide. Particles can have hazardous chemicals attached to them. Other pollutants that can be produced by some appliances are unburned hydrocarbons and aldehydes.

Combustion always produces water vapor. Water vapor is not usually considered a pollutant, but it can act as one. It can result in high humidity and wet surfaces. These conditions encourage the growth of biological pollutants such as house dust mites, molds, and bacteria.

Where do combustion pollutants come from?

Combustion pollutants found indoors include: outdoor air, tobacco smoke, exhaust from car and lawn mower internal combustion engines, and some hobby activities such as welding, woodburning, and soldering. Combustion pollutants can also come from vented or unvented combustion appliances. These appliances include space heaters, gas ranges and ovens, furnaces, gas water heaters, gas clothes dryers, wood or coal-burning stoves, and fireplaces. As a group these are called combustion appliances.

What is a vented appliance? What is an unvented appliance?

Vented appliances are appliances designed to be used with a duct, chimney, pipe, or other device that carry the combustion pollutants outside the home. These appliances can release large amounts of pollutants directly into your home, if a vent is not properly installed, or is blocked or leaking.

Unvented appliances do not vent to the outside, so they release combustion pollutants directly into the home.

Table 13.1 gives typical appliance problems that cause the release of pollutants in your home. Many of these problems are hard for a homeowner to identify. A professional is needed.

Can I use charcoal grills or charcoal hibachis indoors?

No. Never use these appliances inside homes, trailers, truck-caps, or tents. Carbon monoxide from burning and smoldering charcoal can kill you if you use it indoors for cooking or heating. There are about 25 deaths each year from the use of charcoal grills and hibachis indoors.

NEVER burn charcoal inside homes, trailers, tents, or other enclosures. The carbon monoxide can kill you.

What are the health effects of combustion pollutants?

The health effects of combustion pollutants range from headaches and breathing difficulties to death. The health effects may show up immediately after exposure or occur after being exposed to the pollutants for a long time. The effects depend upon the type and amount of pollutants and the length of time of exposure to them. They also depend upon several factors related to the exposed person. These include the age and any existing health problems. There are still some questions about the level of pollutants or the period of exposure needed to produce specific health effects. Further studies to better define the release of pollutants from combustion appliances and their health effects are needed.

Table 13.1. Combustion Appliances and Potential Problems

Appliances	Fuel	Typical Potential Problems
Central Furnaces, Room Heaters, Fireplaces	Natural or Liquefied Petroleum Gas	Cracked heat exchanger; Not enough air to burn fuel properly; Defective/blocked flue; Maladjusted burner
Central Furnaces	Oil	Cracked heat exchanger; Not enough air to burn fuel properly; Defective/blocked flue; Maladjusted burner
Central Heaters, Room Heaters	Wood	Cracked heat exchanger; Not enough air to burn fuel properly; Defective/blocked flue; Green or treated wood
Central Furnaces, Stoves	Coal	Cracked heat exchanger; Not enough air to burn fuel properly; Defective grate
Room Heaters, Central Heaters	Kerosene	Improper adjustment; Wrong fuel (not-K-1); Wrong wick or wick height; Not enough air to burn fuel properly
Water Heaters	Natural or Liquefied Petroleum Gas	Not enough air to burn fuel properly; Defective/blocked flue; Maladjusted burner
Ranges, Ovens	Natural or Liquefied Petroleum Gas	Not enough air to burn fuel properly; Maladjusted burner; Misuse as a room heater
Stoves, Fireplaces	Wood, Coal	Not enough air to burn fuel properly; Defective/blocked flue; Green or treated wood; Cracked heat exchanger or firebox

The following sections discuss health problems associated with some common combustion pollutants. These pollutants include carbon monoxide, nitrogen dioxide, particles, and sulfur dioxide. Even if you are healthy, high levels of carbon monoxide can kill you within a short time. The health effects of the other pollutants are generally more subtle and are more likely to affect susceptible people. It is always a good idea to reduce exposure to combustion pollutants by using and maintaining combustion appliances properly.

Carbon Monoxide

Each year, according to CPSC, there are more than 200 carbon monoxide deaths related to the use of all types of combustion appliances in the home. Exposure to carbon monoxide reduces the blood's ability to carry oxygen. Often a person or an entire family may not recognize that carbon monoxide is poisoning them. The chemical is odorless and some of the symptoms are similar to common illnesses. This is particularly dangerous because carbon monoxide's deadly effects will not be recognized until it is too late to take action against them.

Carbon monoxide exposures especially affect unborn babies, infants, and people with anemia or a history of heart disease. Breathing low levels of the chemical can cause fatigue and increase chest pain in people with chronic heart disease. Breathing higher levels of carbon monoxide causes symptoms such as headaches, dizziness, and weakness in healthy people. Carbon monoxide also causes sleepiness, nausea, vomiting, confusion, and disorientation. At very high levels it causes loss of consciousness and death.

Nitrogen Dioxide

Breathing high levels of nitrogen dioxide causes irritation of the respiratory tract and causes shortness of breath. Compared to healthy people, children, and individuals with respiratory illnesses such as asthma, may be more susceptible to the effects of nitrogen dioxide.

Some studies have shown that children may have more colds and flu when exposed to low levels of nitrogen dioxide. When people with asthma inhale low levels of nitrogen dioxide while exercising, their lung airways can narrow and react more to inhaled materials.

Particles

Particles suspended in the air can cause eye, nose, throat, and lung irritation. They can increase respiratory symptoms, especially in people with chronic lung disease or heart problems. Certain chemicals attached to particles may cause lung cancer, if they are inhaled. The risk of lung cancer increases with the amount and length of exposure. The health effects from inhaling particles depend upon many factors, including the size of the particle and its chemical make-up.

Sulfur Dioxide

Sulfur dioxide at low levels of exposure can cause eye, nose, and respiratory tract irritation. At high exposure levels, it causes the lung airways to narrow. This causes wheezing, chest tightness, or breathing problems. People with asthma are particularly susceptible to the effects of sulfur dioxide. They may have symptoms at levels that are much lower than the rest of the population.

Other Pollutants

Combustion may release other pollutants. They include unburned hydrocarbons and aldehydes. Little is known about the levels of these pollutants in indoor air and the resulting health effects.

What do I do if I suspect that combustion pollutants are affecting my health?

If you suspect you are being subjected to carbon monoxide poisoning get fresh air immediately. Open windows and doors for more ventilation, turn off any combustion appliances, and leave the house. You could lose consciousness and die from carbon monoxide poisoning if you do nothing. It is also important to contact a doctor IMMEDIATELY for a proper diagnosis. Remember to tell your doctor that you suspect carbon monoxide poisoning is causing your problems. Prompt medical attention is important.

Remember that some symptoms from combustion pollutants—headaches, dizziness, sleepiness, coughing, and watery eyes—may also occur because of common medical problems. These medical problems include colds, the flu, or allergies. Similar symptoms may also occur because of other indoor air pollutants. Contact your doctor for a proper diagnosis.

To help your doctor make the correct diagnosis, try to have answers to the following questions:

- Do your symptoms occur only in the home? Do they disappear or decrease when you leave home, and reappear when you return?

- Is anyone else in your household complaining of similar symptoms, such as headaches, dizziness, or sleepiness? Are they complaining of nausea, watery eyes, coughing, or nose and throat irritation?

- Do you always have symptoms?

- Are your symptoms getting worse?

- Do you often catch colds or get the flu?

- Are you using any combustion appliances in your home?

- Has anyone inspected your appliances lately? Are you certain they are working properly?

Your doctor may take a blood sample to measure the level of carbon monoxide in your blood if he or she suspects carbon monoxide poisoning. This sample will help determine whether carbon monoxide is affecting your health.

Contact qualified appliance service people to have your appliances inspected and adjusted if needed. You should be able to find a qualified person by asking your appliance distributor or your fuel supplier. In some areas, the local fuel company may be able to inspect and adjust the appliance.

How can I reduce my exposure to combustion pollutants?

Proper selection, installation, inspection and maintenance of your appliances are extremely important in reducing your exposure to these pollutants. Providing good ventilation in your home and correctly using your appliance can also reduce your exposure to these pollutants.

Additionally, there are several different residential carbon monoxide detectors for sale. The CPSC is encouraging the development of detectors that will provide maximum protection. These detectors would warn consumers of harmful carbon monoxide levels in the home. They may soon be widely available to reduce deaths from carbon monoxide poisoning.

Appliance Selection

- Choose vented appliances whenever possible.

- Only buy combustion appliances that have been tested and certified to meet current safety standards. Examples of certifying organizations are Underwriters Laboratories (UL) and the

American Gas Association (AGA) Laboratories. Look for a label that clearly shows the certification.

- All currently manufactured vented gas heaters are required by industry safety standards to have a safety shut-off device. This device helps protect you from carbon monoxide poisoning by shutting off an improperly vented heater.

- Check your local and state building codes and fire ordinances to see if you can use an unvented space heater, if you consider purchasing one. They are not allowed to be used in some communities, dwellings, or certain rooms in the house.

- If you must replace an unvented gas space heater with another, make it a new one. Heaters made after 1982 have a pilot light safety system called an oxygen depletion sensor (ODS). This system shuts off the heater when there is not enough fresh air, before the heater begins producing large amounts of carbon monoxide. Look for the label that tells you that the appliance has this safety system. Older heaters will not have this protection system.

- Consider buying gas appliances that have electronic ignitions rather than pilot lights. These appliances are usually more energy efficient and eliminate the continuous low-level pollutants from pilot lights.

- Buy appliances that are the correct size for the area you want to heat. Using the wrong size heater may produce more pollutants in your home and is not an efficient use of energy.

- Talk to your dealer to determine the type and size of appliance you will need. You may wish to write to the appliance manufacturer or association for more information on the appliance.

- All new woodstoves are EPA-certified to limit the amounts of pollutants released into the outdoor air. For more information on selecting, installing, operating, and maintaining woodburning stoves, write to the EPA Wood Heater Program. Before buying a woodstove check your local laws about the installation and use of woodstoves.

Proper Installation

You should have your appliances professionally installed. Professionals should follow the installation directions and applicable building codes. Improperly installed appliances can release dangerous pollutants in your home and may create a fire hazard. Be sure that the installer checks for backdrafting on all vented appliances. A qualified installer knows how to do this.

Ventilation

To reduce indoor air pollution, a good supply of fresh outdoor air is needed. The movement of air into and out of your home is very important. Normally, air comes through cracks around doors and windows. This air helps reduce the level of pollutants indoors. This supply of fresh air is also important to help carry pollutants up the chimney, stovepipe, or flue to the outside.

Keep doors open to the rest of the house from the room where you are using an unvented gas space heater or kerosene heater, and crack open a window. This allows enough air for proper combustion and reduces the level of pollutants, especially carbon monoxide.

Use a hood fan, if you are using a range. They reduce the level of pollutants you breath, if they exhaust to the outside. Make sure that enough air is coming into the house when you use an exhaust fan. If needed, slightly open a door or window, especially if other appliances are in use. For proper operation of most combustion appliances and their venting system, the air pressure in the house should be greater than that outside. If not, the vented appliances could release combustion pollutants into the house rather than outdoors. If you suspect that you have this problem you may need the help of a qualified person to solve it.

Make sure that your vented appliance has the vent connected and that nothing is blocking it. Make sure there are no holes or cracks in the vent. Do not vent gas clothes dryers or water heaters into the house for heating. This is unsafe.

Open the stove's damper when adding wood. This allows more air into the stove. More air helps the wood burn properly and prevents pollutants from being drawn back into the house instead of going up the chimney. Visible smoke or a constant smoky odor inside the home when using a woodburning stove is a sign that the stove is not working properly. Soot on furniture in the rooms where you are using the stove also tells this. Smoke and soot are signs that the stove is releasing pollutants into the indoor air.

Correct Use

Read and follow the instructions for all appliances so you understand how they work. Keep the owner's manual in a convenient place to refer to when needed. Also, read and follow the warning labels because they tell you important safety information that you need to know. Reading and following the instructions and warning labels could save your life.

Always use the correct fuel for the appliance.

Only use water-clear ASTM 1-K kerosene for kerosene heaters. The use of kerosene other than 1-K could lead to a release of more pollutants in your home. Never use gasoline in a kerosene heater because it can cause a fire or an explosion. Using even small amounts of gasoline could cause a fire.

Use seasoned hardwoods (elm, maple, oak) instead of softwoods (cedar, fir, pine) in woodburning stoves and fireplaces. Hardwoods are better because they burn hotter and form less creosote, an oily, black tar that sticks to chimneys and stove pipes. Do not use green or wet woods as the primary wood because they make more creosote and smoke. Never burn painted scrap wood or wood treated with preservatives, because they could release highly toxic pollutants, such as arsenic or lead. Plastics, charcoal, and colored paper such as comics, also produce pollutants. Never burn anything that the stove or fireplace manufacturer does not recommend.

Never use a range, oven, or dryer to heat your home. When you misuse gas appliances in this way, they can produce fatal amounts of carbon monoxide. They can produce high levels of nitrogen dioxide, too.

Never use an unvented combustion heater overnight or in a room where you are sleeping. Carbon monoxide from combustion heaters can reach dangerous levels.

Never ignore a safety device when it shuts off an appliance. It means that something is wrong. Read your appliance instructions to find out what you should do or have a professional check out the problem.

Never ignore the smell of fuel. This usually indicates that the appliance is not operating properly or is leaking fuel. Leaking fuel will not always be detectible by smell. If you suspect that you have a fuel leak have it fixed as soon as possible. In most cases you should shut off the appliance, extinguish any other flames or pilot lights, shut off other appliances in the area, open windows and doors, call for help, and leave the area.

Inspection and Maintenance

Have your combustion appliance regularly inspected and maintained to reduce your exposure to pollutants. Appliances that are not working properly can release harmful and even fatal amounts of pollutants, especially carbon monoxide.

Have chimneys and vents inspected when installing or changing vented heating appliances. Some modifications may be required. For example, if a change was made in your heating system from oil to natural gas, the flue gas produced by the gas system could be hot enough to melt accumulated oil combustion debris in the chimney or vent. This debris could block the vent forcing pollutants into the house. It is important to clean your chimney and vents especially when changing heating systems.

What are the inspection and maintenance procedures?

The best advice is to follow the recommendations of the manufacturer. The same combustion appliance may have different inspection and maintenance requirements, depending upon where you live.

In general, check the flame in the furnace combustion chamber at the beginning of the heating season. Natural gas furnaces should have

Table 13.2. Inspection and Maintenance Schedules

Appliance	Inspection/Frequency	Maintenance/Frequency
Gas Hot Air Heating System	*Air Filters:* Clean/change filter—Monthly As needed; Look at flues for rust and soot—Yearly	Qualified person check/clean chimney, clean/adjust burners, check heat exchanger and operation—Yearly (at start of heating season)
Gas/Oil Water/Steam Heating Systems and Water Heaters	Look at flues for rust and soot—Yearly	Qualified person check/clean chimney, clean combustion chamber, adjust burners, check operation—Yearly (at start of heating season)
Kerosene Space Heaters	Look to see that mantle is properly seated—daily when in use; Look to see that fuel tank is free of water and other contaminants—daily or before refueling	Check and replace wick—Yearly (at start of heating season); Clean Combustion chamber—Yearly (at start of heating season); Drain fuel tank—Yearly (at end of heating season)
Wood/Coal Stoves	Look at flues for rust and soot—Yearly	Qualified person check/clean chimney, check seams and gaskets, check operation—Yearly (at start of heating season)

a blue flame with perhaps only a slight yellow tip. Call your appliance service representative to adjust the burner if there is a lot of yellow in the flame, or call your local utility company for this service. LP units should have a flame with a bright blue center that may have a light yellow tip. Pilot lights on gas water heaters and gas cooking appliances should also have a blue flame. Have a trained service representative adjust the pilot light if it is yellow or orange.

Before each heating season, have flues and chimneys inspected and cleaned before each heating season for leakage and for blockage by creosote or debris. Creosote buildup or leakage could cause black stains on the outside of the chimney or flue. These stains can mean that pollutants are leaking into the house.

Table 13.2 shows how and when to take care of your appliance.

Chapter 14

Formaldehyde in Indoor Air

Formaldehyde is an important industrial chemical used to make other chemicals, building materials, and household products. It is one of the large family of chemical compounds called volatile organic compounds or VOCs. The term volatile means that the compounds vaporize, that is, become a gas, at normal room temperatures. Formaldehyde serves many purposes in products. It is used as a part of:

- the glue or adhesive in pressed wood products (particleboard, hardwood plywood, and medium density fiberboard [MDF]);

- preservatives in some paints, coatings, and cosmetics;

- the coating that provides permanent press quality to fabrics and draperies;

- the finish used to coat paper products; and

- certain insulation materials (urea-formaldehyde foam and fiberglass insulation).

Formaldehyde is released into the air by burning wood, kerosene or natural gas, by automobiles, and by cigarettes. Formaldehyde can off-gas from materials made with it. It is also a naturally occurring substance.

"An Update on Formaldehyde—1997 Revision," a fact sheet produced by the U.S. Consumer Product Safety Commission (CPSC), 1997, CPSC Document #725. This document was deemed current by the CPSC as of February 2003. Available online at http://www.cpsc.gov/cpscpub/pubs/725.html.

115

The U.S. Consumer Safety Commission has produced this information to tell you about formaldehyde found in the indoor air. This chapter tells you where you may come in contact with formaldehyde, how it may affect your health, and how you might reduce your exposure to it.

Why should you be concerned?

Formaldehyde is a colorless, strong-smelling gas. When present in the air at levels above 0.1 ppm (parts in a million parts of air), it can cause watery eyes, burning sensations in the eyes, nose and throat, nausea, coughing, chest tightness, wheezing, skin rashes, and allergic reactions. It has also been observed to cause cancer in scientific studies using laboratory animals and may cause cancer in humans. Typical exposures to humans are much lower; thus any risk of causing cancer is believed to be small at the level at which humans are exposed.

Formaldehyde can affect people differently. Some people are very sensitive to formaldehyde while others may not have any noticeable reaction to the same level.

Persons have developed allergic reactions (allergic skin disease and hives) to formaldehyde through skin contact with solutions of formaldehyde or durable-press clothing containing formaldehyde. Others have developed asthmatic reactions and skin rashes from exposure to formaldehyde.

Formaldehyde is just one of several gases present indoors that may cause illnesses. Many of these gases, as well as colds and flu, cause similar symptoms.

What levels of formaldehyde are normal?

Formaldehyde is normally present at low levels, usually less than 0.03 ppm, in both outdoor and indoor air. The outdoor air in rural areas has lower concentrations while urban areas have higher concentrations. Residences or offices that contain products that release formaldehyde to the air can have formaldehyde levels of greater than 0.03 ppm. Products that may add formaldehyde to the air include particleboard used as flooring underlayment, shelving, furniture and cabinets; MDF in cabinets and furniture; hardwood plywood wall panels, and urea-formaldehyde foam used as insulation. As formaldehyde levels increase, illness or discomfort is more likely to occur and may be more serious.

Efforts have been made by both the government and industry to reduce exposure to formaldehyde. CPSC voted to ban urea-formaldehyde foam insulation in 1992. That ban was over-turned in the courts, but this action greatly reduced the residential use of the insulation product. CPSC, the Department of Housing and Urban Development (HUD) and other federal agencies have historically worked with the pressed wood industry to further reduce the release of the chemical from their products. A 1985 HUD regulation covering the use of pressed wood products in manufactured housing was designed to ensure that indoor levels are below 0.4 ppm. However, it would be unrealistic to expect to completely remove formaldehyde from the air. Some persons who are extremely sensitive to formaldehyde may need to reduce or stop using these products.

What affects formaldehyde levels?

Formaldehyde levels in the indoor air depend mainly on what is releasing the formaldehyde (the source), the temperature, the humidity, and the air exchange rate (the amount of outdoor air entering or leaving the indoor area). Increasing the flow of outdoor air to the inside decreases the formaldehyde levels. Decreasing this flow of outdoor air by sealing the residence or office increases the formaldehyde level in the in door air.

As the temperature rises, more formaldehyde is emitted from the product. The reverse is also true; less formaldehyde is emitted at lower temperature. Humidity also affects the release of formaldehyde from the product. As humidity rises more formaldehyde is released.

The formaldehyde levels in a residence change with the season and from day-to-day and day-to-night. Levels may be high on a hot and humid day and low on a cool, dry day. Understanding these factors is important when you consider measuring the levels of formaldehyde.

Some sources—such as pressed wood products containing urea-formaldehyde glues, urea-formaldehyde foam insulation, durable press fabrics, and draperies—release more formaldehyde when new. As they age, the formaldehyde release decreases.

What are the major sources?

Urea-formaldehyde foam insulation: During the 1970s, many home owners installed this insulation to save energy. Many of these homes had high levels of formaldehyde soon afterwards. Sale of urea-formaldehyde foam insulation has largely stopped. Formaldehyde released from this product decreases rapidly after the first few months and reaches background levels in a few years. Therefore, urea-formaldehyde foam insulation installed 5 to 10 years ago is unlikely to still release formaldehyde.

Durable-press fabrics, draperies, and coated paper products: In the early 1960s, there were several reports of allergic reactions to formaldehyde from durable-press fabrics and coated paper products. Such reports have declined in recent years as industry has taken steps to reduce formaldehyde levels. Draperies made of formaldehyde-treated durable press fabrics may add slightly to indoor formaldehyde levels.

Cosmetics, paints, coatings, and some wet-strength paper products: The amount of formaldehyde present in these products is small and is of slight concern. However, persons sensitive to formaldehyde may have allergic reactions.

Pressed Wood Products: Pressed wood products, especially those containing urea-formaldehyde glues, are a source of formaldehyde. These products include particleboard used in flooring underlayment, shelves, cabinets, and furniture; plywood wall panels, and medium density fiberboard used in drawers, cabinets and furniture. When the surfaces and edges of these products are unlaminated or uncoated they have the potential to release more formaldehyde. Manufacturers have reduced formaldehyde emissions from pressed wood products by 80-90% from the levels of the early 1980's.

Combustion Sources: Burning materials such as wood, kerosene, cigarettes and natural gas, and operating internal combustion engines (e.g. automobiles), produce small quantities of formaldehyde. Combustion sources add small amounts of formaldehyde to indoor air.

Products such as carpets or gypsum board do not contain significant amounts of formaldehyde when new. They may trap formaldehyde emitted from other sources and later release the formaldehyde into the indoor air when the temperature and humidity change.

Do you have formaldehyde-related symptoms?

There are several formaldehyde-related symptoms, such as watery eyes, runny nose, burning sensation in eyes, nose, and throat, headaches, and fatigue. These symptoms may also occur because of the common cold, the flu or other pollutants that may be present in the indoor air. If these symptoms lessen when you are away from home or office but reappear upon your return, they may be caused by indoor pollutants, including formaldehyde. Examine your environment. Have you recently moved into a new or different home or office? Have you recently remodeled or installed new cabinets or furniture? Symptoms may be due to formaldehyde exposure. You should contact your physician and/or state or local health department for help. Your physician can help to determine if the cause of your symptoms is formaldehyde or other pollutants.

Should you measure formaldehyde?

Only trained professionals should measure formaldehyde because they know how to interpret the results. If you become ill, and the illness persists following the purchase of furniture or remodeling with pressed wood products, you might not need to measure formaldehyde. Since these are likely sources, you can take action. You may become ill after painting, sealing, making repairs, and/or applying pest control treatment in your home or office. In such cases, indoor air pollutants other than formaldehyde may be the cause. If the source is not obvious, you should consult a physician to determine whether or not your symptoms might relate to indoor air quality problems. If your physician believes that you may be sensitive to formaldehyde, you may want to make some measurements. As discussed earlier, many factors can affect the level of formaldehyde on a given day in an office or residence. This is why a professional is best suited to make an accurate measurement of the levels.

Do-it-yourself formaldehyde measuring devices are available, however these devices can only provide a ball park figure for the formaldehyde level in the area. If you use such a device, you must carefully follow the instructions.

How do you reduce formaldehyde exposure?

Every day you probably use many products that contain formaldehyde. You may not be able to avoid coming in contact with some formaldehyde in your normal daily routine. If you are sensitive to formaldehyde, you will need to avoid many everyday items to reduce symptoms. For most people, a low-level exposure to formaldehyde (up to 0.1 ppm) does not produce symptoms. People who suspect they are sensitive to formaldehyde should work closely with a knowledgeable physician to make sure that formaldehyde is causing their symptoms. You can avoid exposure to higher levels by:

- Purchasing pressed wood products such as particleboard, MDF, or hardwood plywood for construction or remodeling of homes, or for do-it-yourself projects that are labeled or stamped to be in conformance with American National Standards Institute (ANSI) criteria. Particleboard should be in conformance with ANSI A208.1-1993. For particleboard flooring, look for ANSI grades "PBU", "D2", or "D3" actually stamped on the panel. MDF should be in conformance with ANSI A208.2-1994; and hardwood plywood with ANSI/HPVA HP-1-1994. These standards all specify lower formaldehyde emission levels.

- Purchasing furniture or cabinets that contain a high percentage of panel surfaces and edges that are laminated or coated. Unlaminated or uncoated (raw) panels of pressed wood products will generally emit more formaldehyde than those that are laminated or coated.

- Using alternative products such as wood panel products not made with urea-formaldehyde glues, lumber or metal.

- Avoiding the use of foamed-in-place insulation containing formaldehyde, especially urea-formaldehyde foam insulation.

- Washing durable-press fabrics before use.

How do you reduce existing formaldehyde levels?

The choice of methods to reduce formaldehyde is unique to your situation. People who can help you select appropriate methods are your state or local health department, physician, or professional expert in indoor air problems. Following are some of the methods to reduce indoor levels of formaldehyde.

1. Bring large amounts of fresh air into the home. Increase ventilation by opening doors and windows and installing an exhaust fan(s).

2. Seal the surfaces of the formaldehyde-containing products that are not already laminated or coated. You may use a vapor barrier such as some paints, varnishes, or a layer of vinyl or polyurethane-like materials. Be sure to seal completely, with a

material that does not itself contain formaldehyde. Many paints and coatings will emit other VOCs when curing, so be sure to ventilate the area well during and after treatment.

3. Remove from your home the product that is releasing formaldehyde in the indoor air. When other materials in the area such as carpets, gypsum boards, etc., have absorbed formaldehyde, these products may also start releasing it into the air. Overall levels of formaldehyde can be lower if you increase the ventilation over an extended period.

One method NOT recommended by CPSC is a chemical treatment with strong ammonia (28-29% ammonia in water) which results in a temporary decrease in formaldehyde levels. We strongly discourage such treatment since ammonia in this strength is extremely dangerous to handle. Ammonia may damage the brass fittings of a natural gas system, adding a fire and explosion danger.

Chapter 15

Mold, Moisture, and Indoor Air Quality

Molds can be found almost anywhere; they can grow on virtually any substance, providing moisture is present. There are molds that can grow on and within wood, paper, carpet, and foods. When excessive moisture accumulates in buildings or on building materials, mold growth will often occur, particularly if the moisture problem remains undiscovered or unaddressed. There is no practical way to eliminate all mold and mold spores in the indoor environment; the way to control indoor mold growth is to control moisture.

Molds produce tiny spores to reproduce. Mold spores waft through the indoor and outdoor air continually. When mold spores land on a damp spot indoors, they may begin growing and digesting whatever they are growing on in order to survive.

There are many different kinds of mold. Molds can produce allergens, toxins, and/or irritants. Molds can cause discoloration and odor problems, deteriorate building materials, and lead to health problems such as asthma episodes and allergic reactions in susceptible individuals.

The key to mold control is moisture control. If mold is a problem, clean up the mold and get rid of excess water or moisture. Maintaining the relative humidity between 30%–60% will help control mold.

Excerpted from "IAQ Tools for Schools Kit— IAQ Coordinator's Guide, Appendix H—Mold and Moisture," a guide produced by the U.S. Environmental Protection Agency (EPA), 2000. Available online at http://www.epa.gov/iaq/schools/tfs/guideh.html.

Condensation, Relative Humidity, and Vapor Pressure

Mold growth does not require the presence of standing water, leaks, or floods; mold can grow when the relative humidity of the air is high. Mold can also grow in damp areas such as unvented bathrooms and kitchens, crawl spaces, utility tunnels, gym areas and locker rooms, wet foundations, leaky roof areas, and damp basements. Relative humidity and the factors that govern it are often misunderstood.

Water enters buildings both as a liquid and as a gas (water vapor). Water is introduced intentionally at bathrooms, gym areas, kitchens, art and utility areas, and accidentally by way of leaks and spills. Some of the water evaporates and joins the water vapor that is exhaled by building occupants. Water vapor also moves into the building through the ventilation system, through openings in the building shell, or directly through building materials.

The ability of air to hold water vapor decreases as the air temperature falls. If a unit of air contains half of the water vapor it can hold, it is said to be at least 50% relative humidity (RH). The RH increases as the air cools and approaches saturation. When air contains all of the water vapor it can hold, it is at least 100% RH, and the water vapor condenses, changing from a gas to a liquid. The temperature at which condensation occurs is the dew point.

It is possible to reach 100% RH without changing the air temperature, by increasing the amount of water vapor in the air (the absolute humidity or vapor pressure). It is also possible to reach 100% RH without changing the amount of water vapor in the air, by lowering the air temperature to the dew point.

The highest RH in a room is always next to the coldest surface. This is referred to as the first condensing surface, as it will be the location where condensation happens first, if the relative humidity of the air next to the surface reaches 100%. It is important to understand this when trying to understand why mold is growing on one patch of wall or only along the wall-ceiling joint. It is likely that the surface of the wall is cooler than the room air because there is a gap in the insulation or because the wind is blowing through cracks in the exterior of the building.

Mold and Health Effects

Molds are a major source of indoor allergens. Molds can also trigger asthma. Even when dead or unable to grow, mold can cause health effects such as allergic reactions. The types and severity of health effects associated with exposure to mold depend, in part, on the type of mold present, and the extent of the occupants' exposure and existing sensitivities or allergies. Prompt and effective remediation of moisture problems is essential to minimize potential mold exposures and their potential health effects.

Taking Steps to Reduce Moisture and Mold

Moisture control is the key to mold control. Respond to water damage within 24–48 hours to prevent mold growth.

Mold growth can be reduced if relative humidities near surfaces can be maintained below the dew point. This can be done by:

1. reducing the moisture content (vapor pressure) of the air,

2. increasing air movement at the surface, or

3. increasing the air temperature (either the general space temperature or the temperature at building surfaces).

Either vapor pressure or surface temperature can be the dominant factor in a mold problem. A vapor pressure dominated mold problem may not respond well to increasing temperatures, whereas a surface temperature dominated mold problem may not respond very well to increasing ventilation. Understanding which factor dominates will help in selecting an effective control strategy.

If the relative humidity near the middle of a room is fairly high (e.g., 50% at 70° F), mold or mildew problems in the room are likely to be vapor pressure dominated. If the relative humidity near the middle of a room is fairly low (e.g. 30% at 70° F), mold or mildew problems in the room are likely to be surface temperature dominated.

Vapor Pressure Dominated Mold Growth

Vapor pressure dominated mold growth can be reduced by using one or more of the following strategies:

*   use source control (e.g., direct venting of moisture-generating activities such as showers to the exterior)

*   dilute moisture-laden indoor air with outdoor air at a lower absolute humidity

*   dehumidify the indoor air

Note that dilution is only useful as a control strategy during heating periods, when cold outdoor air contains little total moisture. During cooling periods, outdoor air often contains as much moisture as indoor air.

Consider an old, leaky, poorly insulated school in Maine that has mold and mildew in the coldest corners of one classroom. The indoor relative humidity is low (30%). It is winter and cold air cannot hold much water vapor. Therefore, outdoor air entering through leaks in the building lowers the airborne moisture levels indoors. This is an example of a surface temperature dominated mold problem. In this building, increasing the outdoor air ventilation rate is probably not an effective way to control interior mold and mildew. A better strategy would be to increase surface temperatures by insulating the exterior walls, thereby reducing relative humidity in the corners.

Consider a school locker room that has mold on the ceiling. The locker room exhaust fan is broken, and the relative humidity in the room is 60% at 70° F. This is an example of a vapor pressure dominated mold problem. In this case, increasing the surface temperature is probably not an effective way to correct the mold problem. A better strategy is to repair or replace the exhaust fan.

Surface Temperature Dominated Mold Growth

Surface temperature dominated mold growth can be reduced by increasing the surface temperature using one or more of the following approaches:

- raise the temperature of the air near room surfaces

- raise the thermostat setting

- improve air circulation so that supply air is more effective at heating the room surfaces

- decrease the heat loss from room surfaces

- add insulation

- close cracks in the exterior wall to prevent wind washing (air that enters a wall at one exterior location and exits another exterior location without penetrating into the building)

Mold Clean Up

The key to mold control is moisture control. It is essential to clean up the mold and get rid of excess water or moisture. If the excess water or moisture problem is not fixed, mold will most probably grow again, even if the area was completely cleaned. Clean hard surfaces with water and detergent and dry quickly and completely. Absorbent materials such as ceiling tiles may have to be discarded.

Note that mold can cause health effects such as allergic reactions; remediators should avoid exposing themselves and others to mold.

Wear waterproof gloves during clean up; do not touch mold or moldy items with bare hands. Respiratory protection should be used in most remediation situations to prevent inhalation exposure to mold. Respiratory protection may not be necessary for small remediation jobs with little exposure potential. When in doubt consult a professional, experienced remediator.

Identifying and Correcting Common Mold and Moisture Problems

Exterior Corners and Walls

The interior surfaces of exterior corners and behind furnishings such as chalk boards, file cabinets, and desks next to outside walls are common locations for mold growth in heating climates. They tend to be closer to the outdoor temperature than other parts of the building surface for one or more of the following reasons:

- poor indoor air circulation
- wind washing
- low insulation levels
- greater surface area of heat loss

Sometimes mold growth can be reduced by removing obstructions to airflow (e.g., rearranging furniture). Buildings with forced air heating systems and/or room ceiling fans tend to have fewer mold problems than buildings with less air movement.

Set-Back Thermostats

Set-back thermostats (programmable thermostats) are commonly used to reduce energy consumption during the heating season. Mold growth can occur when temperatures are lowered in buildings with high relative humidity. (Maintaining a room at too low a temperature can have the same effect as a set-back thermostat.) Mold can often be controlled in heating climates by increasing interior temperatures during heating periods. Unfortunately, this also increases energy consumption and reduces relative humidity in the breathing zone, which can create discomfort.

Air-Conditioned Spaces

Mold problems can be as extensive in cooling climates as in heating climates. The same principles apply: either surfaces are too cold, moisture levels are too high or both.

One common example of mold growth in cooling climates can be found in rooms where conditioned cold air blows against the interior surface of an exterior wall. This condition, which may be due to poor duct design, diffuser location, or diffuser performances, creates a cold spot at the interior finish surfaces, possibly allowing moisture to condense.

Possible solutions for this problem include:

- eliminate the cold spots (i.e., elevate the temperature of the surface) by adjusting the diffusers or deflecting the air away from the condensing surface

- increase the room temperature to avoid overcooling. NOTE: During the cooling season, increasing temperature decreases energy consumption, though it could cause comfort problems.

Mold problems can also occur within the wall cavity, when outdoor air comes in contact with the cavity side of the cooled interior surface. It is a particular problem in room decorated with low maintenance interior finishes (e.g., impermeable wall covering such as vinyl wallpaper) which can trap moisture between the interior finish and the gypsum board. Mold growth can be rampant when these interior finishes are coupled with cold spots and exterior moisture.

A possible solution for this problem is to ensure that vapor barriers, facing sealants, and insulation are properly specified, installed and maintained.

Thermal Bridges

Localized cooling of surfaces commonly occurs as a result of thermal bridges—elements of the building structure that are highly conductive of heat (e.g., steel studs in exterior frame walls, uninsulated window lintels, and the edges of concrete floor slabs). Dust particles sometimes mark the locations of thermal bridges, because dust tends to adhere to cold spots.

The use of insulating sheathings significantly reduces the impact of thermal bridges in building envelopes.

Window

In winter, windows are typically the coldest surfaces in a room. The interior surface of a window is often the first condensing surface in a room.

Condensation on window surfaces has historically been controlled by using storm windows or insulated glass (e.g., double-glazed windows or selective surface gas-filled windows) to raise interior surface temperatures. In older building enclosures with less advanced glazing systems, visible condensation on the windows often alerted occupants to the need for ventilation to flush out interior moisture, so they knew to open the windows.

The advent of higher performance glazing systems has led to a greater number of moisture problems in heating climate building enclosures, because the buildings can now be operated at higher interior vapor pressures (moisture levels) without visible surface condensation on windows.

Concealed Condensation

The use of thermal insulation in wall cavities increases interior surface temperatures in heating climates, reducing the likelihood of interior surface mold and condensation. However, the use of thermal insulation without a properly installed air barrier may increase moisture condensation within the wall cavity.

The first condensing surface in a wall cavity in a heating climate is typically the inner surface of the exterior sheathing. Concealed condensation can be controlled by either or both of the following strategies:

- reducing the entry of moisture into the wall cavities (e.g., by controlling entry and/or exit of moisture-laden air)

- raising the temperature of the first condensing surface

- in heating-climate locations: installing exterior insulation (assuming that no significant wind-washing is occurring)

- in cooling-climate locations: installing insulating sheathing to the interior of the wall framing and between the wall framing and the interior gypsum board

Chapter 16

Environmental Tobacco Smoke

Environmental tobacco smoke (ETS) is a mixture of particles that are emitted from the burning end of a cigarette, pipe, or cigar, and smoke exhaled by the smoker. Smoke can contain any of more than 4,000 compounds, including carbon monoxide and formaldehyde. More than 40 of the compounds are known to cause cancer in humans or animals, and many of them are strong irritants. ETS is often referred to as "secondhand smoke" and exposure to ETS is often called "passive smoking."

What Are the Health Effects?

Secondhand smoke has been classified as a Group A carcinogen by the U.S. Environmental Protection Agency (EPA), a rating used only for substances proven to cause cancer in humans. A study conducted in 1992 by the EPA concluded that each year approximately 3,000 lung cancer deaths in nonsmoking adults are attributable to ETS. Exposure to secondhand smoke also causes eye, nose, and throat irritation. It may affect the cardiovascular system and some studies have linked exposure to secondhand smoke with the onset of chest pain. ETS is an even greater health threat to people who already have heart and lung illnesses.

This material is reprinted from "Environmental Tobacco Smoke," a fact sheet produced by the National Safety Council. © 2000. Permission to reprint granted by the National Safety Council, a membership organization dedicated to protecting life and promoting health. For more information visit the website of the National Safety Council at www.nsc.org.

Infants and young children whose parents smoke in their presence are at increased risk of lower respiratory tract infections (pneumonia and bronchitis) and are more likely to have symptoms of respiratory irritation like coughing, wheezing, and excess phlegm. In children under 18 months of age, passive smoking causes between 150,000 and 300,000 lower respiratory tract infections, resulting in 7,500 to 15,000 hospitalizations each year, according to EPA estimates. These children may also have a buildup of fluid in the middle ear, which can lead to ear infections. Slightly reduced lung function may occur in older children who have been exposed to secondhand smoke.

Children with asthma are especially at risk from ETS. The EPA estimates that exposure to ETS increases the number of asthma episodes and the severity of symptoms in 200,000 to 1 million children annually. Secondhand smoke may also cause thousands of non-asthmatic children to develop the disease each year.

What Can Be Done to Reduce Exposure to ETS?

* Do not allow smoking in the home, especially around children. Do not allow babysitters and others who work in the home to smoke in the home or near your children. If someone does smoke at home, increase ventilation in the area where smoking takes place.

* Make sure that any outside group that assists in the care of children, such as schools and daycare facilities, has a smoking policy in force that protects children from exposure to ETS.

* If your workplace does not have a smoking policy that protects nonsmokers from exposure to ETS, try to get it to implement one. See if it will either ban smoking indoors or designate a separately ventilated smoking room that nonsmokers do not have to enter as part of their work responsibilities.

Chapter 17

Air Ducts and Indoor Air Quality

Most people are now aware that indoor air pollution is an issue of growing concern and increased visibility. Many companies are marketing products and services intended to improve the quality of your indoor air. You have probably seen an advertisement, received a coupon in the mail, or been approached directly by a company offering to clean your air ducts as a means of improving your home's indoor air quality. These services typically—but not always—range in cost from $450 to $1,000 per heating and cooling system, depending on the services offered, the size of the system to be cleaned, system accessibility, climatic region, and level of contamination.

Duct cleaning generally refers to the cleaning of various heating and cooling system components of forced air systems, including the supply and return air ducts and registers, grilles and diffusers, heat exchangers heating and cooling coils, condensate drain pans (drip pans), fan motor and fan housing, and the air handling unit housing.

If not properly installed, maintained, and operated, these components may become contaminated with particles of dust, pollen or other debris. If moisture is present, the potential for microbiological growth (e.g., mold) is increased and spores from such growth may be released

"Should You Have the Air Ducts in Your Home Cleaned?" Indoor Environments Division (6609J), Office of Air and Radiation (OAR), EPA-402-K-97-002, October 1997. Available online at http://www.epa.gov/iaq/pubs/airduct.html. Cited February 2003. Despite the older date of this document, the information will be beneficial to those seeking knowledge about the potential benefits and possible problems of air duct cleaning and indoor air quality.

into the home's living space. Some of these contaminants may cause allergic reactions or other symptoms in people if they are exposed to them. If you decide to have your heating and cooling system cleaned, it is important to make sure the service provider agrees to clean all components of the system and is qualified to do so. Failure to clean a component of a contaminated system can result in re-contamination of the entire system, thus negating any potential benefits. Methods of duct cleaning vary, although standards have been established by industry associations concerned with air duct cleaning. Typically, a service provider will use specialized tools to dislodge dirt and other debris in ducts, then vacuum them out with a high-powered vacuum cleaner.

In addition, the service provider may propose applying chemical biocides, designed to kill microbiological contaminants, to the inside of the duct work and to other system components. Some service providers may also suggest applying chemical treatments (sealants or other encapsulants) to seal or cover the inside surfaces of the air ducts and equipment housings because they believe the sealant will control mold growth or prevent the release of dirt particles or fibers from ducts. These practices have yet to be fully researched and you should be fully informed before deciding to permit the use of biocides or sealants in your air ducts. They should only be applied, if at all, after the system has been properly cleaned of all visible dust or debris.

Deciding Whether or Not to Have Your Air Ducts Cleaned

Knowledge about the potential benefits and possible problems of air duct cleaning is limited. Since conditions in every home are different, it is impossible to generalize about whether or not air duct cleaning in your home would be beneficial.

If no one in your household suffers from allergies or unexplained symptoms or illnesses and if, after a visual inspection of the inside of the ducts, you see no indication that your air ducts are contaminated with large deposits of dust or mold (no musty odor or visible mold growth), having your air ducts cleaned is probably unnecessary. It is normal for the return registers to get dusty as dust-laden air is pulled through the grate. This does not indicate that your air ducts are contaminated with heavy deposits of dust or debris; the registers can be easily vacuumed or removed and cleaned.

On the other hand, if family members are experiencing unusual or unexplained symptoms or illnesses that you think might be related to your home environment, you should discuss the situation with your doctor.

You may consider having your air ducts cleaned simply because it seems logical that air ducts will get dirty over time and should occasionally be cleaned. While the debate about the value of periodic duct cleaning continues, no evidence suggests that such cleaning would be detrimental, provided that it is done properly.

On the other hand, if a service provider fails to follow proper duct cleaning procedures, duct cleaning can cause indoor air problems. For example, an inadequate vacuum collection system can release more dust, dirt, and other contaminants than if you had left the ducts alone. A careless or inadequately trained service provider can damage your ducts or heating and cooling system, possibly increasing your heating and air conditioning costs or forcing you to undertake difficult and costly repairs or replacements.

You should consider having the air ducts in your home cleaned if:

- There is substantial visible mold growth inside hard surface (e.g., sheet metal) ducts or on other components of your heating and cooling system. There are several important points to understand concerning mold detection in heating and cooling systems:

  Many sections of your heating and cooling system may not be accessible for a visible inspection, so ask the service provider to show you any mold they say exists.

  You should be aware that although a substance may look like mold, a positive determination of whether it is mold or not can be made only by an expert and may require laboratory analysis for final confirmation. For about $50, some microbiology laboratories can tell you whether a sample sent to them on a clear strip of sticky household tape is mold or simply a substance that resembles it.

  If you have insulated air ducts and the insulation gets wet or moldy it cannot be effectively cleaned and should be removed and replaced.

  If the conditions causing the mold growth in the first place are not corrected, mold growth will recur.

- Ducts are infested with vermin, e.g. (rodents or insects); or

- Ducts are clogged with excessive amounts of dust and debris and/or particles are actually released into the home from your supply registers.

Other Important Considerations

Duct cleaning has never been shown to actually prevent health problems. Neither do studies conclusively demonstrate that particle (e.g., dust) levels in homes increase because of dirty air ducts or go down after cleaning. This is because much of the dirt that may accumulate inside air ducts adheres to duct surfaces and does not necessarily enter the living space. It is important to keep in mind that dirty air ducts are only one of many possible sources of particles that are present in homes. Pollutants that enter the home both from outdoors and indoor activities such as cooking, cleaning, smoking, or just moving around can cause greater exposure to contaminants than dirty air ducts. Moreover, there is no evidence that a light amount of household dust or other particulate matter in air ducts poses any risk to health.

EPA does not recommend that air ducts be cleaned except on an as needed basis because of the continuing uncertainty about the benefits of duct cleaning under most circumstances. If a service provider or advertiser asserts that EPA recommends routine duct cleaning or makes claims about its health benefits, you should notify EPA by writing to the address listed at the end of this guidance. EPA does, however, recommend that if you have a fuel burning furnace, stove, or fireplace, they be inspected for proper functioning and serviced before each heating season to protect against carbon monoxide poisoning. Some research also suggests that cleaning dirty cooling coils, fans and heat exchangers can improve the efficiency of heating and cooling systems. However, little evidence exists to indicate that simply cleaning the duct system will increase your system's efficiency.

If you think duct cleaning might be a good idea for your home, but you are not sure, talk to a professional. The company that services your heating and cooling system may be a good source of advice. You may also want to contact professional duct cleaning service providers and ask them about the services they provide. Remember, they are trying to sell you a service, so ask questions and insist on complete and knowledgeable answers.

Suggestions for Choosing a Duct Cleaning Service Provider

To find companies that provide duct cleaning services, check your Yellow Pages under "duct cleaning" or contact the National Air Duct Cleaners Association (NADCA). Do not assume that all duct cleaning service providers are equally knowledgeable and responsible. Talk to at least three different service providers and get written estimates before deciding whether to have your ducts cleaned. When the service providers come to your home, ask them to show you the contamination that would justify having your ducts cleaned.

Do not hire duct cleaners who make sweeping claims about the health benefits of duct cleaning—such claims are unsubstantiated. Do not hire duct cleaners who recommend duct cleaning as a routine part of your heating and cooling system maintenance. You should also be wary of duct cleaners who claim to be certified by EPA. EPA neither establishes duct cleaning standards nor certifies, endorses, or approves duct cleaning companies.

Do not allow the use of chemical biocides or sealants unless you fully understand the pros and the cons.

Check references to be sure other customers were satisfied and did not experience any problems with their heating and cooling system after cleaning.

Contact your county or city office of consumer affairs or local Better Business Bureau to determine if complaints have been lodged against any of the companies you are considering. Interview potential service providers to ensure:

- they are experienced in duct cleaning and have worked on systems like yours;

- they will use procedures to protect you, your pets, and your home from contamination; and

- they comply with NADCA's air duct cleaning standards and, if your ducts are constructed of fiber glass duct board or insulated internally with fiber glass duct liner, with the North American Insulation Manufacturers Association's (NAIMA) recommendations.

Ask the service provider whether they hold any relevant state licenses. As of 1996, the following states require air duct cleaners to hold special licenses: Arizona, Arkansas, California, Florida, Georgia, Michigan and Texas. Other states may require them as well.

If the service provider charges by the hour, request an estimate of the number of hours or days the job will take, and find out whether there will be interruptions in the work. Make sure the duct cleaner you choose will provide a written agreement outlining the total cost and scope of the job before work begins.

137

What to Expect from an Air Duct Cleaning Service Provider

If you choose to have your ducts cleaned, the service provider should:

- Open access ports or doors to allow the entire system to be cleaned and inspected.

- Inspect the system before cleaning to be sure that there are no asbestos-containing materials (e.g., insulation, register boots, etc.) in the heating and cooling system. Asbestos-containing materials require specialized procedures and should not be disturbed or removed except by specially trained and equipped contractors.

- Use vacuum equipment that exhausts particles outside of the home or use only high-efficiency particle air (HEPA) vacuuming equipment if the vacuum exhausts inside the home.

- Protect carpet and household furnishings during cleaning.

- Use well-controlled brushing of duct surfaces in conjunction with contact vacuum cleaning to dislodge dust and other particles.

- Use only soft-bristled brushes for fiberglass duct board and sheet metal ducts internally lined with fiberglass. (Although flex duct can also be cleaned using soft-bristled brushes, it can be more economical to simply replace accessible flex duct.)

- Take care to protect the duct work, including sealing and re-insulating any access holes the service provider may have made or used so they are airtight.

- Follow NADCA's standards for air duct cleaning and NAIMA's recommended practice for ducts containing fiber glass lining or constructed of fiber glass duct board.

How to Determine If the Duct Cleaner Did a Thorough Job

A thorough visual inspection is the best way to verify the cleanliness of your heating and cooling system. Some service providers use remote photography to document conditions inside ducts. All portions of the system should be visibly clean; you should not be able to detect any debris with the naked eye. Show the Post-Cleaning Consumer Checklist (Table 17.1) to the service provider before the work begins.

After completing the job, ask the service provider to show you each component of your system to verify that the job was performed satisfactorily.

If you answer "No" to any of the questions on the checklist, this may indicate a problem with the job. Ask your service provider to correct any deficiencies until you can answer "yes" to all the questions on the checklist.

Table 17.1. Post-Cleaning Consumer Checklist (*continued on next page*)

General	Yes	No
Did the service provider obtain access to and clean the entire heating and cooling system, including ductwork and all components (drain pans, humidifiers, coils, and fans)?	❏	❏
Has the service provider adequately demonstrated that duct work and plenums are clean? (Plenum is a space in which supply or return air is mixed or moves; can be duct, joist space, attic and crawl spaces, or wall cavity.)	❏	❏
Heating		
Is the heat exchanger surface visibly clean?	❏	❏
Cooling Components		
Are both sides of the cooling coil visibly clean?	❏	❏
If you point a flashlight into the cooling coil, does light shine through the other side? It should if the coil is clean.	❏	❏
Are the coil fins straight and evenly spaced (as opposed to being bent over and smashed together)?	❏	❏
Is the coil drain pan completely clean and draining properly?	❏	❏
Blower		
Are the blower blades clean and free of oil and debris?	❏	❏
Is the blower compartment free of visible dust or debris?	❏	❏
Plenums		
Is the return air plenum free of visible dust or debris?	❏	❏
Do filters fit properly and are they the proper efficiency as recommended by HVAC system manufacturer?	❏	❏
Is the supply air plenum (directly downstream of the air handling unit) free of moisture stains and contaminants?	❏	❏

Table 17.1. Post-Cleaning Consumer Checklist (*continued from previous page*)

	Yes	No
Metal Ducts		
Are interior ductwork surfaces free of visible debris? (Select several sites at random in both the return and supply sides of the system.)	❏	❏
Fiber Glass		
Is all fiber glass material in good condition (i.e., free of tears and abrasions; well adhered to underlying materials)?	❏	❏
Access Doors		
Are newly installed access doors in sheet metal ducts attached with more than just duct tape (e.g., screws, rivets, mastic, etc.)?	❏	❏
With the system running, is air leakage through access doors or covers very slight or non-existent?	❏	❏
Air Vents		
Have all registers, grilles, and diffusers been firmly reattached to the walls, floors, and/or ceilings?	❏	❏
Are the registers, grilles, and diffusers visibly clean?	❏	❏
System Operation		
Does the system function properly in both the heating and cooling modes after cleaning?	❏	❏

How to Prevent Duct Contamination

Whether or not you decide to have the air ducts in your home cleaned, committing to a good preventive maintenance program is essential to minimize duct contamination. To prevent dirt from entering the system:

- Use the highest efficiency air filter recommended by the manufacturer of your heating and cooling system.

- Change filters regularly.

- If your filters become clogged, change them more frequently.

- Be sure you do not have any missing filters and that air cannot bypass filters through gaps around the filter holder.

- When having your heating and cooling system maintained or checked for other reasons, be sure to ask the service provider to clean cooling coils and drain pans.

- During construction or renovation work that produces dust in your home, seal off supply and return registers and do not operate the heating and cooling system until after cleaning up the dust.

- Remove dust and vacuum your home regularly. (Use a high efficiency vacuum (HEPA) cleaner or the highest efficiency filter bags your vacuum cleaner can take. Vacuuming can increase the amount of dust in the air during and after vacuuming as well as in your ducts).

- If your heating system includes in-duct humidification equipment, be sure to operate and maintain the humidifier strictly as recommended by the manufacturer.

To Prevent Ducts from Becoming Wet

Moisture should not be present in ducts. Controlling moisture is the most effective way to prevent biological growth in air ducts.

Moisture can enter the duct system through leaks or if the system has been improperly installed or serviced. Research suggests that condensation (which occurs when a surface temperature is lower than the dew point temperature of the surrounding air) on or near cooling coils of air conditioning units is a major factor in moisture contamination of the system. The presence of condensation or high relative humidity is an important indicator of the potential for mold growth on any type of duct. Controlling moisture can often be difficult, but here are some steps you can take:

- Promptly and properly repair any leaks or water damage.

- Pay particular attention to cooling coils, which are designed to remove water from the air and can be a major source of moisture contamination of the system that can lead to mold growth. Make sure the condensate pan drains properly. The presence of substantial standing water and/or debris indicates a problem requiring immediate attention. Check any insulation near cooling coils for wet spots.

- Make sure ducts are properly sealed and insulated in all non-air-conditioned spaces (e.g., attics and crawl spaces). This will help to prevent moisture due to condensation from entering the system and is important to make the system work as intended. To prevent water condensation, the heating and cooling system must be properly insulated.

Unresolved Issues of Duct Cleaning

Does duct cleaning prevent health problems?

The bottom line is—no one knows. There are examples of ducts that have become badly contaminated with a variety of materials that may pose risks to your health. The duct system can serve as a means to distribute these contaminants throughout a home. In these cases, duct cleaning may make sense. However, a light amount of household dust in your air ducts is normal. Duct cleaning is not considered to be a necessary part of yearly maintenance of your heating and cooling system, which consists of regular cleaning of drain pans and heating and cooling coils, regular filter changes and yearly inspections of heating equipment. Research continues in an effort to evaluate the potential benefits of air duct cleaning.

In the meantime educate yourself about duct cleaning by contacting some or all of the sources of information and asking questions of potential service providers.

Are duct materials other than bare sheet metal ducts more likely to be contaminated with mold and other biological contaminants?

You may be familiar with air ducts that are constructed of sheet metal. However, many modern residential air duct systems are constructed of fiberglass duct board or sheet metal ducts that are lined on the inside with fiberglass duct liner. Since the early 1970's, a significant increase in the use of flexible duct, which generally is internally lined with plastic or some other type of material, has occurred. The use of insulated duct material has increased due to improved temperature control, energy conservation, and reduced condensation. Internal insulation provides better acoustical (noise) control. Flexible duct is very low cost. These products are engineered specifically for use in ducts or as ducts themselves, and are tested in accordance with standards established by Underwriters Laboratories (UL), the American Society for Testing and Materials (ASTM), and the National Fire Protection Association (NFPA).

Many insulated duct systems have operated for years without supporting significant mold growth. Keeping them reasonably clean and dry is generally adequate. However, there is substantial debate about whether porous insulation materials (e.g., fiberglass) are more prone to microbial contamination than bare sheet metal ducts. If enough dirt and moisture are permitted to enter the duct system, there may be no significant difference in the rate or extent of microbial growth in internally lined or bare sheet metal ducts. However, treatment of mold contamination on bare sheet metal is much easier. Cleaning and treatment with an EPA-registered biocide are possible. Once fiberglass duct liner is contaminated with mold, cleaning is not sufficient to prevent re-growth and there are no EPA-registered biocides for the treatment of porous duct materials. EPA, NADCA, and NAIMA all recommend the replacement of wet or moldy fiberglass duct material.

In the meantime experts do agree that moisture should not be present in ducts and if moisture and dirt are present, the potential exists for biological contaminants to grow and be distributed throughout the home. Controlling moisture is the most effective way to prevent biological growth in all types of air ducts.

Correct any water leaks or standing water. Remove standing water under cooling coils of air handling units by making sure that drain pans slope toward the drain and if humidifiers are used, they must be properly maintained.

Air handling units should be constructed so that maintenance personnel have easy, direct access to heat exchange components and drain pans for proper cleaning and maintenance.

Fiberglass, or any other insulation material that is wet or visibly moldy (or if an unacceptable odor is present) should be removed and replaced by a qualified heating and cooling system contractor.

Steam cleaning and other methods involving moisture should not be used on any kind of duct work.

Should chemical biocides be applied to the inside of air ducts?

Air duct cleaning service providers may tell you that they need to apply a chemical biocide to the inside of your ducts to kill bacteria (germs), and fungi (mold) and prevent future biological growth. Some duct cleaning service providers may propose to introduce ozone to kill biological contaminants. Ozone is a highly reactive gas that is regulated in the outside air as a lung irritant. However, there remains considerable controversy over the necessity and wisdom of introducing chemical biocides or ozone into the ductwork.

Among the possible problems with biocide and ozone application in air ducts:

- Little research has been conducted to demonstrate the effectiveness of most biocides and ozone when used inside ducts. Simply spraying or otherwise introducing these materials into the operating duct system may cause much of the material to be transported through the system and released into other areas of your home.

- Some people may react negatively to the biocide or ozone, causing adverse health reactions. Chemical biocides are regulated by EPA under Federal pesticide law. A product must be registered by EPA for a specific use before it can be legally used for that purpose. The specific use(s) must appear on the pesticide (e.g., biocide) label, along with other important information. It is a violation of federal law to use a pesticide product in any manner inconsistent with the label directions.

A small number of products are currently registered by EPA specifically for use on the inside of bare sheet metal air ducts. A number of products are also registered for use as sanitizers on hard surfaces, which could include the interior of bare sheet metal ducts. While many such products may be used legally inside of unlined ducts if all label directions are followed, some of the directions on the label may be inappropriate for use in ducts. For example, if the directions indicate "rinse with water," the added moisture could stimulate mold growth.

All of the products discussed above are registered solely for the purpose of sanitizing the smooth surfaces of unlined (bare) sheet metal ducts. No products are currently registered as biocides for use on fiberglass duct board or fiberglass lined ducts, so it is important to determine if sections of your system contain these materials before permitting the application of any biocide.

In the meantime—before allowing a service provider to use a chemical biocide in your duct work, the service provider should:

- Demonstrate visible evidence of microbial growth in your duct work. Some service providers may attempt to convince you that your air ducts are contaminated by demonstrating that the microorganisms found in your home grow on a settling plate (i.e., petri dish). This is inappropriate. Some microorganisms are always present in the air, and some growth on a settling plate is normal. As noted earlier, only an expert can positively identify a substance as biological growth and lab analysis may be required for final confirmation. Other testing methods are not reliable.

- Explain why biological growth cannot be removed by physical means, such as brushing, and further growth prevented by controlling moisture.

If you decide to permit the use of a biocide, the service provider should:

- Show you the biocide label, which will describe its range of approved uses.

- Apply the biocide only to un-insulated areas of the duct system after proper cleaning, if necessary to reduce the chances for re-growth of mold.

- Always use the product strictly according to its label instructions.

While some low toxicity products may be legally applied while occupants of the home are present, you may wish to consider leaving the premises while the biocide is being applied as an added precaution.

Do sealants prevent the release of dust and dirt particles into the air?

Manufacturers of products marketed to coat and seal duct surfaces claim that these sealants prevent dust and dirt particles inside air ducts from being released into the air. As with biocides, a sealant is often applied by spraying it into the operating duct system. Laboratory tests indicate that materials introduced in this manner tend not to completely coat the duct surface. Application of sealants may also affect the acoustical (noise) and fire-retarding characteristics of fiberglass lined or constructed ducts and may invalidate the manufacturer's warranty.

Questions about the safety, effectiveness and overall desirability of sealants remain. For example, little is known about the potential toxicity of these products under typical use conditions or in the event they catch fire.

In addition, sealants have yet to be evaluated for their resistance to deterioration over time which could add particles to the duct air.

Most organizations concerned with duct cleaning, including EPA, NADCA, NAIMA, and the Sheet Metal and Air Conditioning Contractors' National Association (SMACNA) do not currently recommend the routine use of sealants in any type of duct. Instances when the use of sealants may be appropriate include the repair of damaged fiberglass insulation or when combating fire damage within ducts. Sealants should never be used on wet duct liner, to cover actively growing mold, or to cover debris in the ducts, and should only be applied after cleaning according to NADCA or other appropriate guidelines or standards.

Consumer Checklist

- Learn as much as possible about air duct cleaning before you decide to have your ducts cleaned by reading this guidance and contacting the sources of information provided.

- Consider other possible sources of indoor air pollution first if you suspect an indoor air quality problem exists in your home.

- Have your air ducts cleaned if they are visibly contaminated with substantial mold growth, pests or vermin, or are clogged with substantial deposits of dust or debris.

- Ask the service provider to show you any mold or other biological contamination they say exists. Get laboratory confirmation of mold growth or decide to rely on your own judgment and common sense in evaluating apparent mold growth.

- Get estimates from at least three service providers.

- Check references.

- Ask the service provider whether he/she holds any relevant state licenses. As of 1996, the following states require air duct cleaners to hold special licenses: Arizona, Arkansas, California, Florida, Georgia, Michigan and Texas. Other states may also require licenses.

- Insist that the service provider give you knowledgeable and complete answers to your questions.

- Find out whether your ducts are made of sheet metal, flex duct, or constructed of fiberglass duct board or lined with fiber glass since the methods of cleaning vary depending on duct type. Remember, a combination of these elements may be present.

- Permit the application of biocides in your ducts only if necessary to control mold growth and only after assuring yourself that the product will be applied strictly according to label directions. As a precaution, you and your pets should leave the premises during application.

- Do not permit the use of sealants except under unusual circumstances where other alternatives are not feasible.

- Make sure the service provider follows the National Air Duct Cleaning Association's (NADCA) standards and, if the ducts are constructed of flex duct, duct board, or lined with fiberglass, the guidelines of the North American Insulation Manufacturers Association (NAIMA).

- Commit to a preventive maintenance program of yearly inspections of your heating and cooling system, regular filter changes, and steps to prevent moisture contamination.

Chapter 18

Outdoor Air Quality: The Six Common Air Pollutants

The Clean Air Act established two types of National Ambient Air Quality Standards. "Primary" standards are designed to establish limits to protect public health, including the health of "sensitive" populations such as asthmatics, children, and the elderly. "Secondary" standards set limits to protect public welfare, including protection against decreased visibility and damage to animals, crops, vegetation, and buildings.

For each of these pollutants, EPA tracks two kinds of air pollution trends: air concentrations based on actual measurements of pollutant concentrations in the ambient (outside) air at selected monitoring sites throughout the country, and emissions based on engineering estimates of the total tons of pollutants released into the air each year. Despite the progress made in the last 30 years, millions of people live in counties with monitor data showing unhealthy air for one or more of the six common pollutants.

Text in this chapter is from the "Air Quality Where You Live" series of fact sheets produced by the U.S. Environmental Protection Agency (EPA), 2000: "What are the Six Common Air Pollutants?" "How Ground-Level Ozone Affects the Way We Live and Breathe," "How Particulate Matter Affects the Way We Live and Breathe," "How Carbon Monoxide Affects the Way We Live and Breathe," "How Nitrogen Oxides Affect the Way We Live and Breathe," "How Sulfur Dioxide Affects the Way We Live and Breathe," and "How Lead Affects the Way We Live and Breathe," available online at http://www.epa.gov/air/urbanair.

Exposure to these pollutants is associated with numerous effects on human health, including increased respiratory symptoms, hospitalization for heart or lung diseases, and even premature death.

Ground-Level Ozone

What Is It? Where Does It Come From?

Ozone (O_3) is a gas composed of three oxygen atoms. It is not usually emitted directly into the air, but at ground level is created by a chemical reaction between oxides of nitrogen (NO_x) and volatile organic compounds (VOC) in the presence of heat and sunlight. Ozone has the same chemical structure whether it occurs miles above the earth or at ground level and can be good or bad, depending on its location in the atmosphere. Good ozone occurs naturally in the stratosphere approximately 10 to 30 miles above the earth's surface and forms a layer that protects life on earth from the sun's harmful rays. In the earth's lower atmosphere, ground-level ozone is considered bad.

VOC + NO$_X$ + Heat + Sunlight = Ozone

Motor vehicle exhaust and industrial emissions, gasoline vapors, and chemical solvents are some of the major sources of NO_x and VOC, that help to form ozone. Sunlight and hot weather cause ground-level ozone to form in harmful concentrations in the air. As a result, it is known as a summertime air pollutant. Many urban areas tend to have high levels of bad ozone, but even rural areas are also subject to increased ozone levels because wind carries ozone and pollutants that form it hundreds of miles away from their original sources.

Chief Causes for Concern

Ground-level ozone:

• Triggers a variety of health problems even at very low levels

• May cause permanent lung damage after long-term exposure

• Damages plants and ecosystems

The Summertime Pollutant

Peak ozone levels typically occur during hot, dry, stagnant summertime conditions. The length of the ozone season varies from one area of the United States to another. Southern and Southwestern states may have an ozone season that lasts nearly the entire year.

Ozone Can Be Transported over Long Distances

Ozone and the chemicals that react to form it can be carried hundreds of miles from their origins, causing air pollution over wide regions. Millions of Americans live in areas where ozone levels exceed EPA's health-based air quality standards, primarily in parts of the Northeast, the Lake Michigan area, parts of the Southeast, southeastern Texas, and parts of California.

Ozone and the pollutants that form it can cause air quality problems hundreds of miles away.

Particulate Matter

What Is It? Where Does It Come From?

Particulate matter, or PM, is the term for particles found in the air, including dust, dirt, soot, smoke, and liquid droplets. Particles can be suspended in the air for long periods of time. Some particles are large or dark enough to be seen as soot or smoke. Others are so small that individually they can only be detected with an electron microscope.

Some particles are directly emitted into the air. They come from a variety of sources such as cars, trucks, buses, factories, construction sites, tilled fields, unpaved roads, stone crushing, and burning of wood.

Other particles may be formed in the air from the chemical change of gases. They are indirectly formed when gases from burning fuels react with sunlight and water vapor. These can result from fuel combustion in motor vehicles, at power plants, and in other industrial processes.

Chief Causes for Concern

Particulate Matter:

- is associated with serious health effects.

- is associated with increased hospital admissions and emergency room visits for people with heart and lung disease.

- is associated with work and school absences.

- is the major source of haze that reduces visibility in many parts of the United States, including our National Parks.

- settles on soil and water and harms the environment by changing the nutrient and chemical balance.

- causes erosion and staining of structures including culturally important objects such as monuments and statues.

Health problems for sensitive people can get worse if they are exposed to high levels of PM for several days in a row.

CO

What Is It? Where Does It Come From?

Carbon monoxide, or CO, is a colorless, odorless gas that is formed when carbon in fuel is not burned completely. It is a component of motor vehicle exhaust, which contributes about 56 percent of all CO emissions nationwide. Other non-road engines and vehicles (such as construction equipment and boats) contribute about 22 percent of all CO emissions nationwide. Higher levels of CO generally occur in areas with heavy traffic congestion. In cities, 85 to 95 percent of all CO emissions may come from motor vehicle exhaust. Other sources of CO emissions include industrial processes (such as metals processing and chemical manufacturing), residential wood burning, and natural sources such as forest fires. Woodstoves, gas stoves, cigarette smoke, and unvented gas and kerosene space heaters are sources of CO indoors. The highest levels of CO in the outside air typically occur during the colder months of the year when inversion conditions are more frequent. The air pollution becomes trapped near the ground beneath a layer of warm air.

Chief Causes for Concern

CO:

- is poisonous even to healthy people at high levels in the air.
- can affect people with heart disease.
- can affect the central nervous system.

Motor Vehicle Use Is Increasing

Nationwide, three-quarters of carbon monoxide emissions come from on-road motor vehicles (cars and trucks) and non-road engines (such as boats and construction equipment). Control measures have reduced pollutant emissions per vehicle over the past 20 years, but the number of cars and trucks on the road and the miles they are driven have doubled in the past 20 years. Vehicles are now driven two trillion miles each year in the United States. With more and more cars traveling more and more miles, growth in vehicle travel may eventually offset progress in vehicle emissions controls.

Malfunctions and Tampering Reduce the Effectiveness of Emission Control Systems

Today's sophisticated emission control systems on vehicles are designed to keep pollution to a minimum, but vehicles quickly become polluters when their emission controls do not work correctly or if drivers tamper with them.

NO_x

What Is It? Where Does It Come From?

Nitrogen oxides, or NO_x, is the generic term for a group of highly reactive gases, all of which contain nitrogen and oxygen in varying amounts. Many of the nitrogen oxides are colorless and odorless. However, one common pollutant, nitrogen dioxide (NO_2) along with particles in the air can often be seen as a reddish-brown layer over many urban areas.

Nitrogen oxides form when fuel is burned at high temperatures, as in a combustion process. The primary sources of NO_x are motor vehicles, electric utilities, and other industrial, commercial, and residential sources that burn fuels.

Chief Causes for Concern

NO_x:

- is one of the main ingredients involved in the formation of ground-level ozone, which can trigger serious respiratory problems.

- reacts to form nitrate particles, acid aerosols, as well as NO_2, which also cause respiratory problems.

- contributes to formation of acid rain.

- contributes to nutrient overload that deteriorates water quality.

- contributes to atmospheric particles, that cause visibility impairment most noticeable in national parks.

- reacts to form toxic chemicals.

- contributes to global warming.

NO_X and the pollutants formed from NO_X can be transported over long distances, following the pattern of prevailing winds in the U.S. This means that problems associated with NO_X are not confined to areas where NO_X are emitted. Therefore, controlling NO_X is often most effective if done from a regional perspective, rather than focusing on sources in one local area. NO_X emissions are increasing.

Since 1970, EPA has tracked emissions of the six principal air pollutants—carbon monoxide, lead, nitrogen oxides, particulate matter, sulfur dioxide, and volatile organic compounds. Emissions of all of these pollutants have decreased significantly except for NO_X which has increased approximately 10 percent over this period.

SO_2

What Is It? Where Does It Come From?

Sulfur dioxide, or SO_2, belongs to the family of sulfur oxide gases (SO_X). These gases dissolve easily in water. Sulfur is prevalent in all raw materials, including crude oil, coal, and ore that contains common metals like aluminum, copper, zinc, lead, and iron. SO_X gases are formed when fuel containing sulfur, such as coal and oil, is burned, and when gasoline is extracted from oil, or metals are extracted from ore. SO_2 dissolves in water vapor to form acid, and interacts with other gases and particles in the air to form sulfates and other products that can be harmful to people and their environment.

Over 65% of SO_2 released to the air, or more than 13 million tons per year, comes from electric utilities, especially those that burn coal. Other sources of SO_2 are industrial facilities that derive their products from raw materials like metallic ore, coal, and crude oil, or that burn coal or oil to produce process heat. Examples are petroleum refineries, cement manufacturing, and metal processing facilities. Also, locomotives, large ships, and some non-road diesel equipment currently burn high sulfur fuel and release SO_2 emissions to the air in large quantities.

Chief Causes for Concern

SO_2 contributes to respiratory illness, particularly in children and the elderly, and aggravates existing heart and lung diseases.

SO_2 contributes to the formation of acid rain, which:

- damages trees, crops, historic buildings, and monuments; and
- makes soils, lakes, and streams acidic.

SO_2 contributes to the formation of atmospheric particles that cause visibility impairment, most noticeably in national parks.

SO_2 can be transported over long distances.

SO_2 and the pollutants formed from SO_2, such as sulfate particles, can be transported over long distances and deposited far from the point of origin. This means that problems with SO_2 are not confined to areas where it is emitted.

People with asthma are particularly affected by peak levels of SO_2.

Short-Term Peak Levels

High levels of SO_2 emitted over a short period, such as a day, can be particularly problematic for people with asthma. EPA encourages communities to learn about the types of industries in their communities and to work with local industrial facilities to address pollution control equipment failures or process upsets that could result in peak levels of SO_2.

Lead

What Is It? Where Does It Come From?

Lead is a metal found naturally in the environment as well as in manufactured products. The major sources of lead emissions have historically been motor vehicles (such as cars and trucks) and industrial sources. Due to the phase out of leaded gasoline, metals processing is the major source of lead emissions to the air today. The highest levels of lead in air are generally found near lead smelters. Other stationary sources are waste incinerators, utilities, and lead-acid battery manufacturers.

Chief Causes for Concern

Lead:

- particularly affects young children and infants
- is still found at high levels in urban and industrial areas
- deposits on soil and water and harms animals and fish

Children Are at Greatest Risk

Although overall blood lead levels have decreased since 1976, infants and young children still have the highest blood lead levels. Children and others can be exposed to lead not only through the air, but also through accidentally or intentionally eating soil or paint chips, as well as food or water contaminated with lead.

High levels of lead are still of concern in localized areas.

Urban areas with high levels of traffic, trash incinerators, or other industry, as well as areas near lead smelters, battery plants, or industrial facilities that burn fuel, may still have high lead levels in air. In 1999, ten areas of the country did not meet the national health-based air quality standards for lead.

Chapter 19

Acid Rain

What Is Acid Rain and What Causes It?

Acid rain is a broad term used to describe several ways that acids fall out of the atmosphere. A more precise term is acid deposition, which has two parts: wet and dry.

Wet deposition refers to acidic rain, fog, and snow. As this acidic water flows over and through the ground, it affects a variety of plants and animals. The strength of the effects depend on many factors, including how acidic the water is, the chemistry and buffering capacity of the soils involved, and the types of fish, trees, and other living things that rely on the water.

Dry deposition refers to acidic gases and particles. About half of the acidity in the atmosphere falls back to earth through dry deposition. The wind blows these acidic particles and gases onto buildings, cars, homes, and trees. Dry deposited gases and particles can also be washed from trees and other surfaces by rainstorms. When that happens, the runoff water adds those acids to the acid rain, making the combination more acidic than the falling rain alone.

"Acid Raid," an undated fact sheet from the U.S. Environmental Protection Agency (EPA). Available online at http://www.epa.gov/airmarkets/acidrain/index.html. Cited February 2003; and "What Society Can Do about Acid Deposition," an undated fact sheet from the EPA. Available online at http://www. epa.gov/airmarkets/acidrain/society/index.html. Cited February 2003.

Prevailing winds blow the compounds that cause both wet and dry acid deposition across state and national borders, and sometimes over hundreds of miles.

Scientists discovered, and have confirmed, that sulfur dioxide (SO_2) and nitrogen oxides (NO_x) are the primary causes of acid rain. In the U.S., about 2/3 of all SO_2 and 1/4 of all NO_x comes from electric power generation that relies on burning fossil fuels like coal.

Acid rain occurs when these gases react in the atmosphere with water, oxygen, and other chemicals to form various acidic compounds. Sunlight increases the rate of most of these reactions. The result is a mild solution of sulfuric acid and nitric acid.

How Do We Measure Acid Rain?

Acid rain is measured using a scale called pH. The lower a substance's pH, the more acidic it is.

Pure water has a pH of 7.0. Normal rain is slightly acidic because carbon dioxide dissolves into it, so it has a pH of about 5.5. As of the year 2000, the most acidic rain falling in the U.S. has a pH of about 4.3.

Acid rain's pH, and the chemicals that cause acid rain, are monitored by two networks, both supported by EPA. The National Atmospheric Deposition Program measures wet deposition, and its website features maps of rainfall pH and other important precipitation chemistry measurements. The Clean Air Status and Trends Network (CASTNET) measures dry deposition. Its website features information about the data it collects, the measuring sites, and the kinds of equipment it uses.

What Are Acid Rain's Effects?

Acid deposition has a variety of effects, including damage to forests and soils, fish and other living things, materials, and human health. Acid rain also reduces how far and how clearly we can see through the air, an effect called visibility reduction.

What Society Can Do about Acid Deposition

There are several ways to reduce acid deposition, more properly called acid deposition, ranging from societal changes to individual action.

Understand Acid Deposition's Causes and Effects

To understand acid deposition's causes and effects and track changes in the environment, scientists from EPA, state governments, and academic study acidification processes. They collect air and water samples and measure them for various characteristics like pH and chemical composition, and they research the effects of acid deposition on human-made materials such as marble and bronze. Finally, scientists work to understand the effects of sulfur dioxide (SO_2) and nitrogen oxides (NO_x)—the pollutants that cause acid deposition and fine particles—on human health.

To solve the acid rain problem, people need to understand how acid rain causes damage to the environment. They also need to understand what changes could be made to the air pollution sources that cause the problem. The answers to these questions help leaders make better decisions about how to control air pollution and therefore how to reduce—or even eliminate—acid rain. Since there are many solutions to the acid rain problem, leaders have a choice of which options or combination of options are best.

Clean Up Smokestacks and Exhaust Pipes

Almost all of the electricity that powers modern life comes from burning fossil fuels like coal, natural gas, and oil. Acid deposition is caused by two pollutants that are released into the atmosphere, or emitted, when these fuels are burned: sulfur dioxide (SO_2) and nitrogen oxides (NO_x).

Coal accounts for most U.S. sulfur dioxide (SO_2) emissions and a large portion of NO_x emissions. Sulfur is present in coal as an impurity, and it reacts with air when the coal is burned to form SO_2. In contrast, NO_x is formed when any fossil fuel is burned.

There are several options for reducing SO_2 emissions, including using coal containing less sulfur, washing the coal, and using devices called scrubbers to chemically remove the SO_2 from the gases leaving the smokestack. Power plants can also switch fuels; for example burning natural gas creates much less SO_2 than burning coal. Certain approaches will also have additional benefits of reducing other pollutants such as mercury and carbon dioxide. Understanding these co-benefits has become important in seeking cost-effective air pollution reduction strategies. Finally, power plants can use technologies that don't burn fossil fuels. Each of these options has its own costs and benefits, however; there is no single universal solution.

Similar to scrubbers on power plants, catalytic converters reduce NO_x emissions from cars. These devices have been required for over twenty years in the U.S., and it is important to keep them working properly and tailpipe restrictions have been tightened recently. EPA has also made, and continues to make, changes to gasoline that allows it to burn cleaner.

Use Alternative Energy Sources

There are other sources of electricity besides fossil fuels. They include: nuclear power, hydropower, wind energy, geothermal energy, and solar energy. Of these, nuclear and hydropower are used most widely; wind, solar, and geothermal energy have not yet been harnessed on a large scale in this country.

There are also alternative energies available to power automobiles, including natural gas powered vehicles, battery-powered cars, fuel cells, and combinations of alternative and gasoline powered vehicles.

All sources of energy have environmental costs as well as benefits. Some types of energy are more expensive to produce than others, which means that not all Americans can afford all types of energy. Nuclear power, hydropower, and coal are the cheapest forms today, but changes in technologies and environmental regulations may shift that in the future. All of these factors must be weighed when deciding which energy source to use today and which to invest in for tomorrow.

Restore a Damaged Environment

Acid deposition penetrates deeply into the fabric of an ecosystem, changing the chemistry of the soil as well as the chemistry of the streams and narrowing, sometimes to nothing, the space where certain plants and animals can survive. Because there are so many changes, it takes many years for ecosystems to recover from acid deposition, even after emissions are reduced and the rain becomes normal again. For example, while the visibility might improve within days, and small or episodic chemical changes in streams improve within months, chronically acidified lakes, streams, forests, and soils can take years to decades or even centuries (in the case of soils) to heal.

However, there are some things that people do to bring back lakes and streams more quickly. Limestone or lime (a naturally-occurring basic compound) can be added to acidic lakes to cancel out the acidity. This process, called liming, has been used extensively in Norway and Sweden but is not used very often in the United States. Liming tends to be expensive, has to be done repeatedly to keep the water from returning to its acidic condition, and is considered a short-term remedy in only specific areas rather than an effort to reduce or prevent pollution. Furthermore, it does not solve the broader problems of changes in soil chemistry and forest health in the watershed, and does nothing to address visibility reductions, materials damage, and risk to human health. However, liming does often permit fish to remain in a lake, so it allows the native population to survive in place until emissions reductions reduce the amount of acid deposition in the area.

Look to the Future

As emissions from the largest known sources of acid deposition—power plants and automobiles—are reduced, EPA scientists and their colleagues must assess the reductions to make sure they are achieving the results Congress anticipated. If these assessments show that acid deposition is still harming the environment, Congress may begin to consider additional ways to reduce emissions that cause acid deposition. They may consider additional emissions reductions from sources that have already been controlled, or methods to reduce emissions from other sources. They may also invest in energy efficiency and alternative energy. The cutting edge of protecting the environment from acid deposition will continue to develop and implement cost-effective mechanisms to cut emissions and reduce their impact on the environment.

Take Action as Individuals

It may seem like there is not much that one individual can do to stop acid deposition. However, like many environmental problems, acid deposition is caused by the cumulative actions of millions of individual people. Therefore, each individual can also reduce their contribution to the problem and become part of the solution. One of the first steps is to understand the problem and its solutions.

Individuals can contribute directly by conserving energy, since energy production causes the largest portion of the acid deposition problem. For example, you can:

- Turn off lights, computers, and other appliances when you're not using them

- Use energy efficient appliances: lighting, air conditioners, heaters, refrigerators, washing machines, etc.

- Only use electric appliances when you need them.

- Keep your thermostat at 68° F in the winter and 72° F in the summer. You can turn it even lower in the winter and higher in the summer when you are away from home.

- Insulate your home as best you can.

- Carpool, use public transportation, or better yet, walk or bicycle whenever possible.

- Buy vehicles with low NO_x emissions, and maintain all vehicles well.

- Be well-informed.

Chapter 20

Ozone

What Ozone Is

Ozone is unstable and irritating: As when a third person breaks in to dance with a happy pair. Ozone is a special form of oxygen. Like ordinary oxygen, ozone is one of the many gases in the air we breathe. Like oxygen, ozone is made up of oxygen molecules. But, while the molecules of ordinary oxygen are made up of two chemically linked oxygen atoms, the molecules of ozone are made of three such atoms. With its third atom of oxygen, ozone is not very stable—that is, it ordinarily doesn't last very long.

A little ozone occurs naturally. An energy source such as lightning can produce it—temporarily breaking up pairs of oxygen atoms and reforming them as chemically linked clusters of three oxygen atoms: ozone. People, other animals and plants tolerate such naturally occurring, short-lived ozone pretty well. But when ozone builds up—generally as a result of our use of fossil fuels—it reacts very strongly with animal and plant tissues, and even damages tough materials such as rubber, plastics and outdoor paints.

You've probably seen hydrogen peroxide fizz—and perhaps felt it burn your gums or skin tissues. Like ozone, hydrogen peroxide is closely related to a very stable molecule: water, or H^2O. With an added oxygen atom, it changes to H_2O_2, becoming very reactive.

Excerpted from "Ozone Alerts," a fact sheet produced by the National Institute of Environmental Health Sciences (NIEHS), 1999. Available online at http://www.niehs.nih.gov/oc/factsheets/ozone/phome.htm.

The fizz and burn of hydrogen peroxide on a scratch or wound illustrate how, at high concentrations, ozone's own strong reactivity can irritate and damage the sensitive tissues of your eyes, lungs, nose, sinuses and throat, causing burning eyes, shortness of breath, chest tightness, wheezing, coughing and nausea.

The sustained, higher levels of ozone that cause these effects usually begin with human activity. That is, when we use electricity for our lights, computer and TV, when we heat our houses and run our cars and SUVs, or even when we roast chestnuts on an open fire or charcoal a steak, these activities often require the burning of fossil fuels—hydrocarbons such as gasoline, heating oil, firewood, charcoal and the coal for power plants. This combustion releases oxides of nitrogen, which are gaseous combinations of oxygen and nitrogen, nitrogen being another common gas in our atmosphere. One of these combinations is nitrogen dioxide (NO_2). When NO_2 absorbs energy from sunlight, it breaks down to nitric oxide (NO) and a free oxygen atom.

The free oxygen atom then barges into the oxygen pair to form the linked triplet of ozone (O_3).

How It Hurts You

When ozone accumulates, it hurts people, pets, and crops. Normally, ozone converts back to oxygen. However, airborne hydrocarbons (from motor vehicles, industrial emissions and other kinds of incomplete combustion and solvent use) can disrupt this conversion, allowing the ozone to accumulate. Because sunlight and heat play roles in the smog process, ozone concentrations most often rise in the warmer months of the year and peak in the warmer hours of the day.

While winds might dissipate the ozone, temperature inversions frequently occurring during warm weather over many cities can hold down and stagnate the lower atmosphere, allowing ozone to build up. And there you have it: grey, thick, photochemical smog— urban smog.

Thus, the centers of ozone pollution are the great centers and suburbs of humankind's activity: Los Angeles, Houston, Atlanta, New York, Boston and other large metropolitan areas. (That's why in some cities in developing countries, people are somewhat proud of smog— as a sign of industrialization's progress.)

An Inversion. You hear about it on TV weather a lot: Normally, warm air rises until it cools at lower altitudes, thus moving and mixing the air. A temperature inversion occurs when the upper air is warmer and prevents the lower air from rising, trapping it in place.

In rural areas, less ozone is likely to accumulate. There are fewer gasoline automobiles, homes and factories. In addition, moisture in rural soil and trees absorbs some of the radiant energy from the sun, keeping these areas cooler than nearby cities. But rural areas do not escape the effects of ozone entirely. Trees themselves generate some hydrocarbons and add to ozone levels. Many power plants that burn fossil fuels are in rural areas, increasing the concentrations of oxides of nitrogen in rural air. According to the weatherman, the National Oceanic and Atmospheric Administration, rural sections of the East and South have among the highest summer ozone readings in North America partly as a result of spillover from cities and suburbs.

A study of hikers on the White Mountain in New Hampshire in the NIEHS *Journal Environmental Health Perspectives* for February 1998 showed lung function rose and fell with ozone levels, even though they remained within the range common in urban parts of the United States.

Crops suffer as well, with up to $3 billion in agricultural losses a year in the United States. The forests that we harvest for paper and building materials are also susceptible to ozone-induced damage. In China, heavy regional haze may cut food production 10-30 percent, according to one estimate, contributing to food scarcities and hunger.

How Ozone Disturbs Your Body

Inhaled ozone travels down the windpipe and enters the lungs through the large bronchial tubes, which branch into smaller airways, or bronchioles. At the end of the bronchioles are tiny air sacs called alveoli, which fill up and expand like little balloons to put oxygen into the bloodstream. Ozone primarily injures these key oxygen exchangers, the alveoli, along with the bronchioles. Animals also suffer from ozone. Studies demonstrate how ozone exposure injures their lung cells and causes unusual changes in lung tissue. Other studies have shown that ozone can make people more susceptible to bacterial pneumonia, a potential killer.

People with existing lung diseases—asthma, bronchitis, or emphysema—are particularly vulnerable to the respiratory effects of ozone. There are also particularly sensitive individuals.

New Research Results

A third group that may be particularly susceptible to ozone is made up—ironically—of healthy, not-particularly-sensitive people who exercise a lot outdoors. Studies show that adults exercising vigorously react more to ozone exposure than do adults at rest. People working or exercising increase their breathing rate, so that they inhale more ozone and thus a higher dose reaches the target tissues of the bronchioles and alveoli.

Other tests have shown:

- Ozone affects a person's vital lung capacity—the volume of air that can be expelled from fully inflated lungs. In controlled tests, a 5 to 10 percent reduction occurred in volunteers engaged in moderate exercise for 6.5 hours at just 80 ppb. In the real world, active kids at camp showed reduced vital lung function when ozone was higher than normal.

- Athletic ability, as measured by performance on stationary bikes or treadmills, has been shown to be poorer at 180 ppb than among controls performing in normal air.

- Ozone concentrations can make the small bands of muscles that help control breathing more sensitive to dry air, cold or dust, so they contract, narrowing the airways and making breathing more difficult.

- In five cities studied by researchers in Massachusetts, hospital admissions for pneumonia and flu were highest in the cities with higher maximum ozone levels and particulate levels.

A Gene for Ozone Sensitivity, Maybe a Treatment—and Studies That Don't Find Ozone to Be Carcinogenic

In studies funded by the National Institute of Environmental Health Sciences:

- At the Johns Hopkins University in Baltimore, researchers have identified a gene that may play a role in ozone sensitivity, and

- Scientists at Rutgers University in New Jersey have found they can prevent some ozone-related lung damage by pretreating cells with an amino acid called taurine that may develop into a treatment for patients.

Other NIEHS-supported studies include the Harvard University Six-Cities Study—expanded to include 24 locations—which has generated one of the largest known databases on the health effects of outdoor and indoor air pollutants.

166

Because ozone is so reactive, so irritating, you might wonder if it causes cancer. There's some generally good news on that score: The National Toxicology Program, headquartered at NIEHS, found that rats exposed to ozone for from two years to 30 months did not have a significant increase in tumors—nor did ozone add to the risk of rats exposed to a known carcinogen in tobacco smoke. Only at the high exposure of 1 part per million did a marginal increase in lung tumors appear, and that could be coincidental.

Ozone Has Proved Hard to Reduce

Some emissions have been greatly reduced under the Clean Air Act of 1970 (with amendments in 1977 and 1990). Today's air is noticeably cleaner than a few decades ago. But ozone, which results from a reaction between emissions and other substances, has proved harder to reduce. A report of the National Academy of Sciences a few years ago put it pretty bluntly: State and federal restrictions, along with industry practices, had largely failed to decrease ozone exposures. As the century ended there were still 32 nonattainment areas containing 40 cities in which people are exposed to ozone in excess of the air-quality standards set to protect people's health. A nonattainment area may involve three urban, highly populated states, such as New York, New Jersey and Connecticut, so many people are exposed to unacceptably high levels of ozone.

Stratospheric Research Leads to Nobel Prize—But Will the Shield Recover Soon?

In the stratosphere, the news is bad, but probably would be worse except for an eccentric Dutchman and two Americans on a mission.

Even small changes in the ozone layer in the stratosphere have been linked to an increase in skin cancer. Further deterioration could be even more harmful. Indeed, without the ozone layer's filter, life on earth as we know it could not exist.

In the 1980s, an ozone hole was found to be forming every spring over Antarctica, where cold, stratospheric temperatures promote the chemical reactions that destroy ozone. Scientists are watching for UV damage to penguins, whales and the vital food chain of fish and other sea creatures, including the microscopic algae (phytoplankton) that are the base food for the undersea food chain.

The Arctic has no land mass and is warmer than Antarctica, but an ozone hole now appears over the North Pole as well. However, prospects for life on earth are brighter today than they undoubtedly would have been if there had been no Paul Crutzen, a Dutchman who taught himself chemistry. He dresses eccentrically, showing up for a formal-dress lecture in sandals and open shirt and talking from scribbled notes— yet, reported the *New York Times*, mesmerizing his audience. In 1970, Dr. Crutzen showed that the ozone layer is created naturally by the action of sunlight on oxygen—and can be destroyed by compounds called chlorofluorocarbons (CFCs).

This helped lead Mexico-born Mario Molina and F. Sherwood Rowland, both U.S. citizens working at the University of California at Irvine, to discover soon afterward that chlorofluorocarbon gasses from earthly air conditioners and spray cans could waft intact to the stratosphere, where they might persist a hundred years, gradually being broken down by the sun's UV rays into free chlorine atoms.

Drs. Molina and Rowland showed that each chlorine atom could then destroy thousands of ozone molecules in a long chain reaction.

Much of the world, but perhaps not quite enough of it, was shaken by the 1974 prediction by Molina and Rowland that if humans continued to make and emit CFCs, the ozone layer would be weakened. To the consternation of the industries making and using CFCs, the two scientists became salesmen on behalf of ozone protection. Gradually, confirmatory data accumulated and, 11 years later, in 1985, an actual hole in the ozone layer was reported by an English scientist.

That wake-up call was acted upon quickly, as political actions go, in the 1987 Montreal Protocol, which called for the international phasing out of CFC-containing products, as well as in the U.S. Clean Air Act Amendments of 1990. These were major steps toward protecting the ozone shield from further damage by eliminating use of these ozone-depleting chemicals.

In awarding the Nobel Prize in Chemistry to Molina, Rowland and Crutzen in 1995, the Royal Swedish Academy of Sciences said they had contributed to the world's salvation from a global environmental problem that could have catastrophic consequences.

But phasing out the use of ozone-depleting chemicals has been no quick fix. It may slow the destruction of the ozone layer and eventually halt it, perhaps allowing it to rebuild. But a NASA satellite showed the hole in the shield over the Antarctica (South Pole) reached 10.5 million square miles on September 19, 1998—bigger than ever.

No one can predict the future with certainty, but over the 21st Century, the shield may slowly recover.

You Can Help

After that glorious chemistry, what's left to say, but: What can I do?

In terms of ozone concentrations in the lower atmosphere, you can:

- *Run Early or Late.* Protect yourself in warm weather, when ozone concentrates, by exercising in non-congested areas, in the mornings, before ozone levels rise with daily temperatures, or in the evenings, after they've declined.

- *Keep Car Tuned, Tires Inflated.* Protect your environment by keeping your car in tune and your tires inflated to the recommended pressure, and by using your car sparingly, finding alternatives.

- *Cap Chemicals.* Keep household cleaners, solvents and other home and garden chemicals tightly sealed, to reduce the evaporation of volatile organic compounds, which contribute to the hydrocarbon content of the atmosphere.

- *Limit Burning.* Whether your locality permits it or not, avoid burning trash and building inefficient fires, such as smoky grills and fireplaces—especially if your area is experiencing alerts.

- *Conserve Power.* Join in your electric utility's conservation programs, such as periodic air conditioning cut-backs that also reduce your bills. Support local ordinances and regulations related to conservation and to burning and smoke restrictions, so that you and your neighbors can breathe easier.

In terms of the stratosphere, you can:

- *Repair Leaky AC.* Make sure that old-style refrigerants used in your auto are not released into the atmosphere but are recovered in a government-approved program, as required by law. Repair leaky units before refilling them.

- *Dispose of Fridge or AC Carefully.* Check with your local authorities about the proper disposal of old refrigerators and air conditioners.

- *Protect Skin.* Prevent sunburn and reduce your risk of skin cancer, malignant melanomas and cataracts by protecting yourself with a wide-brim hat, tight-weave clothing, sunglasses and a sunscreen of SPF 15 to 30.

169

The story of ozone illustrates what we at the National Institute of Environmental Health Sciences say: Your Environment Is Your Health.

Likewise, the research on ozone-like previous research NIEHS has carried out and supported on asbestos and lead and industrial chemicals, and on the water we drink—illustrates that good environmental health research is the basis for intelligent action—and for preventive health measures that can save health, lives and dollars.

Saving Your Money on Ozone Air Cleaners

Save your money—resist ozone air fresheners. Having just read a bit about ozone, you might think it darn odd that someone might want

Table 20.1. Ozone Alert Values—Ground Level Air Quality Alerts

Too much ozone at ground level can make your eyes smart, can reduce your lung capacity and, in extreme cases, can make it hard to breathe. Too much ozone at ground level can make even a very fit person, an athlete-in-training, pretty sick.

Local broadcast and newspaper air quality alerts generally correspond to federal ozone standards:

Ozone Index Value	Precaution
0-50 (good-GREEN)	Best for outdoor activity.
50-100 (moderate-YELLOW)	Unusually sensitive people should consider limiting prolonged outdoor exertion.
101-150 (unhealthy-ORANGE)	Active children and adults, and people with respiratory disease such as asthma, should limit pro longed outdoor exertion.
151-200 (unhealthy-RED)	Exercise early/late; indoors when possible. Every-one, especially children, should avoid (if sensitive) or limit prolonged outdoor exertion.
Above 200 (very unhealthy—PURPLE)	Active children and adults, and people with respiratory disease such as asthma should avoid all out-door exertion. Everyone else should limit outdoor exertion.

Note: When ozone begins to rise, fires, outdoor grilling and individual auto use should be restricted.

to breathe more of it—or want you to. But, despite Federal Trade Commission and state actions against their claims, there remain people who want to take some money from you in exchange for an air cleaner or air freshener that claims to work by generating ozone.

You can read a long report at http://www.epa.gov/iaq/pubs/ozone gen.html on why this is a silly and potentially harmful idea. The bottom line is, to generate enough ozone to be potentially effective, the ozone equipment would have to produce dangerous amounts of ozone. Contrary to suggestions from some sales people, no federal agency approves, much less recommends, ozone generators for use in occupied spaces.

There are other kinds of air cleaners you can buy. Some use high efficiency particle arrestance (HEPA) filters or charcoal to work safely, according to a California consumer bulletin in 1998. But as for the cleaners using ozone: The bulletin states that air cleaners that rely on ozone generation just don't destroy enough microbes, remove enough odor sources or reduce indoor pollutants enough to provide health benefits—and may contribute to eye and nose irritation or other respiratory health problems and can cause damage to building materials and electronic devices.

Table 20.2. Ozone Alert Values—Ultraviolet (UV) Alerts

To help avoid painful sunburn and blisters and such long-term problems as skin cancer and sight-dulling cataracts, many weather reports now include information on the UV Index. Using two National Oceanic and Atmospheric Administration-operated satellites, the National Weather Service and the Environmental Protection Agency forecast the UV risk (or Index Value) based in part on the wavelengths of the UV radiation (some being more harmful than others) and on whether clear skies or cloudy are expected. They then suggest preventive actions:

UV Index Value	Precaution
0-2 (minimal)	Wear hat or cap.
3-4 (low)	Hat and sunscreen of SPF 15 or more.
5-6 (moderate)	Hat, sunscreen of 15+, stay in shady areas.
7-9 (high)	As above, plus stay indoors 10 a.m. to 4 p.m.

To reduce the risk of cataracts and other eye damage, sunglasses are advised for UV values of 5 (moderate) or higher. Good sunglasses are also advised at the beach, on the water, or on snow, at all times, even when the index is minimal.

So You Want to Be Ozone-Healthy?—A Quiz

1. Ozone at ground level reduces your:

   a. waist,

   b. lung capacity and athletic performance,

   c. IQ,

   d. all of the above.

2. Ozone is made up of how many atoms of oxygen?

   a. three, as in O_3,

   b. two, as in O_2,

   c. three, as in H_2O,

   d. four, as in O_4?

3. When ground-level ozone is high, you get smog and sometimes:

   a. burning eyes,

   b. shortness of breath,

   c. irritation of the nose and throat,

   d. all of the above.

4. Sustained, high levels of ground-level ozone result from human activities such as:

   a. burning fuels,

   b. spilling gasoline,

   c. roasting chestnuts and steaks on an open fire,

   d. all of the above.

5. Combustion produces, among other oxides of nitrogen, nitrogen dioxide (NO_2). One of the oxygen atoms is freed to form the linked triplet of ozone, O_3 when:

   a. NO_2 absorbs energy from sunlight,

   b. NO_2 tires,

   c. NO_2 is inhaled,

   d. all of the above.

6. Without a protective ozone layer in the stratosphere, life as we know it could not exist. But in the 1980s:

   a. an ozone hole appeared over the U.S.,

b. too much ozone accumulated and the sun was dimmed,

c. an ozone hole was found to be forming every spring over the South Pole,

d. ozone-polluted plankton was shown to be making penguins sick.

7. Chlorofluorocarbon gasses were shown to waft up to the stratosphere, from earthly uses in air conditioners and spray cans, and be broken down by the sun's ultraviolet rays into ozone-destroying:

a. hair gel,

b. coolants,

c. free chlorine atoms,

d. calcium-bound fluorosis.

8. Because of political action to reduce chlorofluorocarbons, the ozone shield:

a. has been reformed,

b. may be fine by 2010,

c. may recover over the 21st Century,

d. can't get better.

9. To reduce ground-level ozone, we can:

a. wear sunscreen with an SPF of 15 or more,

b. stay indoors in mid-day,

c. avoid genetically modified foods, drugs and cosmetics,

d. cap chemicals, limit burning and conserve power.

10. In terms of the stratosphere, you can:

a. keep tires low,

b. burn trash,

c. properly dispose of old refrigerators, air conditioners and their coolants, as required by law,

d. watch for air quality alerts.

Answers

1b, 2a, 3d, 4d, but roasting chestnuts and grilling steaks at least smell awfully good; 5a, 6c, and then, later, a North Pole, or Arctic, hole appeared; 7c, fluorosis being a darkening of your teeth from excess fluorides; 8c, at least that's the hope; 9d, though it is good to wear sunscreen for protection against the sun's UV rays because of the damaged ozone shield; 10c, you should also watch for air quality alerts, but these apply to ground-level ozone.

If you got less than eight right, don't bother applying to the major TV quiz shows. If you got less than six, you should have read the chapter first.

Chapter 21

Understanding the Air Quality Index

Increasingly, radio, TV, and newspapers are providing information like this to local communities. But what does it mean to you if you plan to be outdoors that day, or if you have children who play outdoors? What if you are retired, or if you have asthma? This chapter will help you understand what this information means to you and your family and what you can do to protect your health.

Local air quality affects how we live and breathe. Like the weather, it can change from day to day or even hour to hour. The U.S. Environmental Protection Agency (EPA) and others are working to make information about outdoor air quality as available to the public as information about the weather. A key tool in this effort is the Air Quality Index, or AQI. EPA and local officials use the AQI to provide the public with timely and easy-to-understand information on local air quality and whether air pollution levels pose a health concern.

This chapter tells you about the AQI and how it is used to provide air quality information. It also tells you about the possible health effects of major air pollutants at various levels and suggests actions you can take to protect your health when pollutants in your area reach unhealthy concentrations.

What Is the AQI?

The AQI is an index for reporting daily air quality. It tells you how clean or polluted your air is, and what associated health concerns you

"Air Quality Index," a fact sheet produced by the U.S. Environmental Protection Agency (EPA), EPA-454/R-00-005, 2000.

175

should be aware of. The AQI focuses on health effects that can happen within a few hours or days after breathing polluted air. EPA uses the AQI for five major air pollutants regulated by the Clean Air Act: ground-level ozone, particulate matter, carbon monoxide, sulfur dioxide, and nitrogen dioxide. For each of these pollutants, EPA has established national air quality standards to protect against harmful health effects.

How Does the AQI Work?

You can think of the AQI as a yardstick that runs from 0 to 500. The higher the AQI value, the greater the level of air pollution and the greater the health danger. For example, an AQI value of 50 represents good air quality and little potential to affect public health, while an AQI value over 300 represents hazardous air quality.

An AQI value of 100 generally corresponds to the national air quality standard for the pollutant, which is the level EPA has set to protect public health. So, AQI values below 100 are generally thought of as satisfactory. When AQI values are above 100, air quality is considered to be unhealthy—at first for certain sensitive groups of people, then for everyone as AQI values get higher.

Understanding the AQI

The purpose of the AQI is to help you understand what local air quality means to your health. To make the AQI as easy to understand as possible, EPA has divided the AQI scale into six categories as shown in Table 21.1.

Each category corresponds to a different level of health concern. For example, when the AQI for a pollutant is between 51 and 100, the health concern is *Moderate*. Following are the six levels of health concern and what they mean:

- *Good:* The AQI value for your community is between 0 and 50. Air quality is considered satisfactory and air pollution poses little or no risk.

- *Moderate:* The AQI for your community is between 51 and 100. Air quality is acceptable; however, for some pollutants there may be a moderate health concern for a very small number of individuals. For example, people who are unusually sensitive to ozone may experience respiratory symptoms.

- *Unhealthy for Sensitive Groups:* Certain groups of people are particularly sensitive to the harmful effects of certain air pollutants.

This means they are likely to be affected at lower levels than the general public. For example, children and adults who are active outdoors and people with respiratory disease are at greater risk from exposure to ozone, while people with heart disease are at greater risk from carbon monoxide. Some people may be sensitive to more than one pollutant. When AQI values are between 101 and 150, members of sensitive groups may experience health effects. The general public is not likely to be affected when the AQI is in this range.

- *Unhealthy:* AQI values are between 151 and 200. Everyone may begin to experience health effects. Members of sensitive groups may experience more serious health effects.

- *Very Unhealthy:* AQI values between 201 and 300 trigger a health alert, meaning everyone may experience more serious health effects.

- *Hazardous:* AQI values over 300 trigger health warnings of emergency conditions. The entire population is more likely to be affected.

AQI Colors

EPA has assigned a specific color to each AQI category to make it easier for people to understand quickly the significance of air pollution levels in their communities. For example, the color orange means

Table 21.1. Air Quality Index Scale

Air Quality Index (AQI) Values	Levels of Health Concern	Colors
When the AQI is in this range:	*...air quality conditions are:*	*...as symbolized by this color:*
0 to 50	Good	Green
51 to 100	Moderate	Yellow
101 to 150	Unhealthy for Sensitive Groups	Orange
151 to 200	Unhealthy	Red
201 to 300	Very Unhealthy	Purple
301 to 500	Hazardous	Maroon

that conditions are unhealthy for sensitive groups; the color red means that conditions may be unhealthy for everyone, and so on. You may see these colors when the AQI is reported in the newspaper or on television, or on your state or local air pollution agency's web site. The colors can help you rapidly determine whether air pollutants are reaching unhealthy levels in your area.

How Is a Community's AQI Calculated?

Air quality is measured by networks of monitors that record the concentrations of the major pollutants at more than a thousand locations across the country each day. These raw measurements are then converted into AQI values using standard formulas developed by EPA. An AQI value is calculated for each of the individual pollutants in an area (ground-level ozone, particulate matter, carbon monoxide, sulfur dioxide, and nitrogen dioxide). Finally, the highest of the AQI values for the individual pollutants becomes the AQI value for that day. For example, if on July 12 a certain area had AQI values of 90 for ozone and 88 for sulfur dioxide, the AQI value would be 90 for the pollutant ozone on that day.

When and How Is the AQI Reported to the Public?

In large metropolitan areas (more than 350,000 people), state and local agencies are required to report the AQI to the public daily. When the AQI is above 100, they must also report which groups (e.g., children, people with asthma or heart disease) may be sensitive to the specific pollutant. If two or more pollutants have AQI values above 100 on a given day, agencies will report all the groups that are sensitive to those pollutants. Although it is not required, many smaller communities also report the AQI as a public health service.

Many metropolitan areas also report an AQI forecast that allows local residents to plan their activities to protect their health.

The AQI is a national index, so the values and colors used to show local air quality and the associated level of health concern will be the same everywhere you go in the U.S. Look for the AQI to be reported in your local newspaper, on television and radio, on the Internet, and on state and local telephone hotlines.

What Are Typical AQI Values in Most Communities?

In many U.S. communities, AQI values are mostly below 100, with values greater than 100 occurring several times a year. Several metropolitan areas in the United States have more severe air pollution problems, and the AQI in these areas may often exceed 100. AQI values higher than 200 are very infrequent, and AQI values above 300 are extremely rare.

AQI values can vary significantly from one season to another. In winter, for example, carbon monoxide is likely to be the pollutant with the highest AQI values in some areas, because cold weather makes it difficult for car emission control systems to operate effectively. In summer, ozone is the most significant air pollutant in many communities, since it forms in the presence of heat and sunlight.

AQI values also can vary depending on the time of day. For example, ozone levels often peak in the afternoon, while carbon monoxide is usually a problem during morning or evening rush hours.

How Can I Avoid Being Exposed to Harmful Air Pollutants?

The information in Table 21.2 tells you where each pollutant comes from, what health effects may occur for each pollutant, and what you can do to protect your health.

What Is Ozone?

Ozone is an odorless, colorless gas composed of three atoms of oxygen. Ozone occurs both in the Earth's upper atmosphere and at ground level. Ozone can be good or bad, depending on where it is found:

Good Ozone. Ozone occurs naturally in the Earth's upper atmosphere—10 to 30 miles above the Earth's surface—where it forms a protective layer that shields us from the sun's harmful ultraviolet rays. This beneficial ozone is gradually being destroyed by manmade chemicals. An area where ozone has been significantly depleted—for example, over the North or South pole—is sometimes called a hole in the ozone.

Bad Ozone. In the Earth's lower atmosphere, near ground level, ozone is formed when pollutants emitted by cars, power plants, industrial boilers, refineries, chemical plants, and other sources react chemically in the presence of sunlight. Ozone at ground level is a harmful pollutant. Ozone pollution is a concern during the summer months, when the weather conditions needed to form it—lots of sun, hot temperatures—normally occur.

What Are the Health Effects and Who Is Most at Risk?

Roughly one out of every three people in the United States is at a higher risk of experiencing ozone-related health effects. Sensitive people include children and adults who are active outdoors, people with respiratory disease, such as asthma, and people with unusual sensitivity to ozone.

- One group at high risk from ozone exposure is active children because this group often spends a large part of the summer playing outdoors. However, people of all ages who are active outdoors are at increased risk because, during physical activity, ozone penetrates deeper into the parts of the lungs that are more vulnerable to injury.

Table 21.2. Air Quality Index (AQI): Ozone

Index Values	Levels of Health Concern	Cautionary Statements
0-50	Good	None
51-100*	Moderate	Unusually sensitive people should consider limiting prolonged outdoor exertion.
101-150	Unhealthy for Sensitive Groups	Active children and adults, and people with respiratory disease, such as asthma, should limit prolonged outdoor exertion.
151-200	Unhealthy	Active children and adults, and people with respiratory disease, such as asthma, should avoid prolonged outdoor exertion; everyone else, especially children, should limit prolonged outdoor exertion.
202-300	Very Unhealthy	Active children and adults, and people with respiratory disease, such as asthma, should avoid all outdoor exertion; everyone else, especially children, should limit outdoor exertion.
301-500	Hazardous	Everyone should avoid all outdoor exertion.

* Generally, an AQI of 100 for ozone corresponds to an ozone level of 0.08 parts per million (averaged over 8 hours).

- People with respiratory diseases that make their lungs more vulnerable to ozone may experience health effects earlier and at lower ozone levels than less sensitive individuals.

- Though scientists don't yet know why, some healthy people experience health effects at more moderate levels of outdoor exertion or at lower ozone levels than the average person.

- Ozone can irritate the respiratory system, causing coughing, throat irritation, and/or an uncomfortable sensation in the chest.

- Ozone can reduce lung function and make it more difficult to breathe deeply and vigorously. Breathing may become more rapid and shallow than normal. This reduction in lung function may limit a person's ability to engage in vigorous outdoor activities.

- Ozone can aggravate asthma. When ozone levels are high more people with asthma have attacks that require a doctor's attention or the use of additional medication. One reason this happens is that ozone makes people more sensitive to allergens, the most common triggers of asthma attacks.

- Ozone can increase susceptibility to respiratory infections.

- Ozone can inflame and damage the lining of the lungs. Within a few days, the damaged cells are shed and replaced—much like the skin peels after a sunburn. Animal studies suggest that if this type of inflammation happens repeatedly over a long time period (months, years, a lifetime), lung tissue may become permanently scarred, resulting in less lung elasticity, permanent loss of lung function, and a lower quality of life.

What Is Particulate Matter?

The term particulate matter (PM) includes both solid particles and liquid droplets found in air. Many manmade and natural sources emit PM directly or emit other pollutants that react in the atmosphere to form PM. These solid and liquid particles come in a wide range of sizes. Particles less than 10 micrometers in diameter tend to pose the greatest health concern because they can be inhaled into and accumulate in the respiratory system. Particles less than 2.5 micrometers in diameter are referred to as fine particles. Sources of fine particles include all types of combustion (motor vehicles, power plants, wood burning, etc.) and some industrial processes. Particles with diameters

Table 21.3. Air Quality Index (AQI): Particulate Matter (PM)

Index Values	Levels of Health Concern	Cautionary Statements* $PM_{2.5}$	Cautionary Statements* PM_{10}
0-50	Good	None	None
51-100**	Moderate	None	None
101-150	Unhealthy for Sensitive Groups	People with respiratory or heart disease, the elderly, and children should limit prolonged exertion.	People with respiratory disease, such as asthma, should limit outdoor exertion.
151-200	Unhealthy	People with respiratory or heart disease, the elderly, and children should avoid prolonged exertion; everyone else should limit prolonged exertion.	People with respiratory disease, such as asthma, should avoid outdoor exertion; everyone else, especially the elderly and children, should limit prolonged outdoor exertion.
201-300	Very Unhealthy	People with respiratory or heart disease, the elderly, and children should avoid any outdoor activity; everyone else should avoid prolonged exertion.	People with respiratory disease, such as asthma, should avoid any outdoor activity; everyone else, especially the elderly and children, should limit outdoor exertion.
301-500	Hazardous	Everyone should avoid any outdoor exertion; people with respiratory or heart disease, the elderly, and children should remain indoors.	Everyone should avoid any outdoor exertion; people with respiratory disease, such as asthma, should remain indoors.

*   PM has two sets of cautionary statements, which correspond to the two sizes of PM that are measured:
- Particles up to 2.5 micrometers in diameter ($PM_{2.5}$)
- Particles up to 10 micrometers in diameter (PM_{10})

**
- An AQI of 100 for $PM_{2.5}$ corresponds to a $PM_{2.5}$ level of 40 micrograms per cubic meter (averaged over 24 hours).
- An AQI of 100 for PM_{10} corresponds to a PM_{10} level of 150 micrograms per cubic meter (averaged over 24 hours).

between 2.5 and 10 micrometers are referred to as coarse. Sources of coarse particles include crushing or grinding operations, and dust from paved or unpaved roads.

What Are the Health Effects and Who Is Most at Risk?

Both fine and coarse particles can accumulate in the respiratory system and are associated with numerous health effects. Coarse particles can aggravate respiratory conditions such as asthma. Exposure to fine particles is associated with several serious health effects, including premature death. Adverse health effects have been associated with exposures to PM over both short periods (such as a day) and longer periods (a year or more).

- When exposed to PM, people with existing heart or lung diseases—such as asthma, chronic obstructive pulmonary disease, congestive heart disease, or ischemic heart disease are at increased risk of premature death or admission to hospitals or emergency rooms.

- The elderly also are sensitive to PM exposure. They are at increased risk of admission to hospitals or emergency rooms and premature death from heart or lung diseases.

- When exposed to PM, children and people with existing lung disease may not be able to breathe as deeply or vigorously as they normally would, and they may experience symptoms such as coughing and shortness of breath.

- PM can increase susceptibility to respiratory infections and can aggravate existing respiratory diseases, such as asthma and chronic bronchitis, causing more use of medication and more doctor visits.

What Is Carbon Monoxide?

Carbon monoxide (CO) is an odorless, colorless gas. It forms when the carbon in fuels does not completely burn. Vehicle exhaust contributes roughly 60 percent of all carbon monoxide emissions nationwide, and up to 95 percent in cities. Other sources include fuel combustion in industrial processes and natural sources such as wildfires. Carbon monoxide concentrations typically are highest during cold weather, because cold temperatures make combustion less complete and cause inversions that trap pollutants low to the ground.

What Are the Health Effects and Who Is Most at Risk?

Carbon monoxide enters the bloodstream through the lungs and binds chemically to hemoglobin, the substance in blood that carries oxygen to cells. In this way, carbon monoxide reduces the amount of oxygen reaching the body's organs and tissues.

- People with cardiovascular disease, such as angina, are most at risk from carbon monoxide. These individuals may experience chest pain and more cardiovascular symptoms if they are exposed to carbon monoxide, particularly while exercising.

- People with marginal or compromised cardiovascular and respiratory systems (for example, individuals with congestive heart failure, cerebrovascular disease, anemia, chronic obstructive lung disease), and possibly fetuses and young infants, may also be at greater risk from carbon monoxide pollution.

Table 21.4. Air Quality Index (AQI): Carbon Monoxide (CO)

Index Values	Levels of Health Concern	Cautionary Statements
0-50	Good	None
51-100*	Moderate	None
101-150	Unhealthy for Sensitive Groups	People with cardiovascular disease, such as angina, should limit heavy exertion and avoid sources of CO, such as heavy traffic.
151-200	Unhealthy	People with cardiovascular disease, such as angina, should limit moderate exertion and avoid sources of CO, such as heavy traffic.
201-300	Very Unhealthy	People with cardiovascular disease, such as angina, should avoid exertion and sources of CO, such as heavy traffic.
301-500	Hazardous	People with cardiovascular disease, such as angina, should avoid exertion and sources of CO, such as heavy traffic; everyone else should limit heavy exertion.

*An AQI of 100 for carbon monoxide corresponds to a CO level of 9 parts per million (averaged over 8 hours).

- In healthy individuals, exposure to higher levels of carbon monoxide can affect mental alertness and vision.

What Is Sulfur Dioxide?

Sulfur dioxide (SO_2), a colorless, reactive gas, is produced during the burning of sulfur-containing fuels such as coal and oil, during metal smelting, and by other industrial processes. Major sources include power plants and industrial boilers. Generally, the highest concentrations of sulfur dioxide are found near large industrial sources.

What Are the Health Effects and Who Is Most at Risk?

- Children and adults with asthma who are active outdoors are most vulnerable to the health effects of sulfur dioxide. The primary effect they experience, even with brief exposure, is a narrowing of the airways (called bronchoconstriction), which may cause symptoms such as wheezing, chest tightness, and shortness of breath. Symptoms increase as sulfur dioxide concentrations

Table 21.5. Air Quality Index (AQI): Sulfur Dioxide (SO_2)

Index Values	Levels of Health Concern	Cautionary Statements
0-50	Good	None
51-100*	Moderate	None
101-150	Unhealthy for Sensitive Groups	People with asthma should consider limiting outdoor exertion.
151-200	Unhealthy	Children, asthmatics, and people with heart or lung disease should limit outdoor exertion.
201-300	Very Unhealthy	Children, asthmatics, and people with heart or lung disease should avoid outdoor exertion; everyone else should limit outdoor exertion.
301-500	Hazardous	Children, asthmatics, and people with heart or lung disease should remain indoors; everyone else should avoid outdoor exertion.

*An AQI of 100 for sulfur dioxide corresponds to an SO_2 level of 0.14 parts per million (averaged over 24 hours).

and/or breathing rates increase. When exposure ceases, lung function typically returns to normal within an hour.

- At very high levels, sulfur dioxide may cause wheezing, chest tightness, and shortness of breath in people who do not have asthma.

- Long-term exposure to both sulfur dioxide and fine particles can cause respiratory illness, alter the lung's defense mechanisms, and aggravate existing cardiovascular disease. People who may be most susceptible to these effects include individuals with cardiovascular disease or chronic lung disease, as well as children and the elderly.

What Is Nitrogen Dioxide?

Nitrogen dioxide (NO_2) is a reddish brown, highly reactive gas formed when another pollutant (nitric oxide) combines with oxygen in the atmosphere. Once it has formed, nitrogen dioxide reacts with

Table. 21.6. Air Quality Index (AQI): Nitrogen Dioxide (NO_2)

Index Values	Levels of Health Concern	Cautionary Statements
0-50	Good	None
51-100	Moderate	None
101-150	Unhealthy for Sensitive Groups	None
151-200	Unhealthy	None
201*-300	Very Unhealthy	Children and people with respiratory disease, such as asthma, should limit heavy outdoor exertion.
301-500	Hazardous	Children and people with respiratory disease, such as asthma, should limit moderate or heavy outdoor exertion.

*Short-term health effects for nitrogen dioxide do not occur until AQI values are above 200; therefore, the AQI is not calculated below 201 for NO_2. An AQI of 201 for NO_2 corresponds to an NO_2 level of 0.65 parts per million (averaged over 24 hours).

other pollutants (volatile organic compounds). Eventually these reactions result in the formation of ground-level ozone. Major sources include automobiles and power plants.

What Are the Health Effects and Who Is Most at Risk?

- In children and adults with respiratory disease, such as asthma, nitrogen dioxide can cause respiratory symptoms such as coughing, wheezing, and shortness of breath. Even short exposures to nitrogen dioxide affect lung function.

- In children, short-term exposure can increase the risk of respiratory illness.

- Animal studies suggest that long-term exposure to nitrogen dioxide may increase susceptibility to respiratory infection and may cause permanent structural changes in the lungs.

Part Three

Waterborne Hazards

Chapter 22

Drinking Water and Your Health

The United States has one of the safest water supplies in the world. However, national statistics don't tell you specifically about the quality and safety of the water coming out of your tap. That's because drinking water quality varies from place to place, depending on the condition of the source water from which it is drawn and the treatment it receives.

Now you have a new way to find information about your drinking water, if it comes from a public water supplier (EPA doesn't regulate private wells, but recommends that well owners have their water tested annually). Beginning in 1999, every community water supplier must provide an annual report (sometimes called a consumer confidence report) to its customers. The report provides information on your local drinking water quality, including the water's source, the contaminants found in the water, and how consumers can get involved in protecting drinking water. If you have been looking for specific information about your drinking water, this annual report will provide you with the information you need to begin your investigation.

These annual reports will by necessity be short documents. You may want more information, or have more questions. One place you can go is to your water supplier, who is best equipped to answer questions about your specific water supply.

"Drinking Water and Health: What You Need to Know!" a brochure produced by the Environmental Protection Agency (EPA), EPA 816-K-99-001,1999. Available online at http://www.epa.gov/safewater/dwh/dw-health.pdf.

What contaminants may be found in drinking water?

There is no such thing as naturally pure water. In nature, all water contains some impurities. As water flows in streams, sits in lakes, and filters through layers of soil and rock in the ground, it dissolves or absorbs the substances that it touches. Some of these substances are harmless. In fact, some people prefer mineral water precisely because minerals give it an appealing taste. However, at certain levels, minerals, just like man-made chemicals, are considered contaminants that can make water unpalatable or even unsafe.

Some contaminants come from erosion of natural rock formations. Other contaminants are substances discharged from factories, applied to farmlands, or used by consumers in their homes and yards. Sources of contaminants might be in your neighborhood or might be many miles away. Your local water quality report tells which contaminants are in your drinking water, the levels at which they were found, and the actual or likely source of each contaminant.

Some ground water systems have established wellhead protection programs to prevent substances from contaminating their wells. Similarly, some surface water systems protect the watershed around their reservoir to prevent contamination. Right now, states and water suppliers are working systematically to assess every source of drinking water and to identify potential sources of contaminants. This process will help communities to protect their drinking water supplies from contamination, and a summary of the results will be in future water quality reports.

Where does drinking water come from?

A clean, constant supply of drinking water is essential to every community. People in large cities frequently drink water that comes from surface water sources, such as lakes, rivers, and reservoirs. Sometimes these sources are close to the community. Other times, drinking water suppliers get their water from sources many miles away. In either case, when you think about where your drinking water comes from, it's important to consider not just the part of the river or lake that you can see, but the entire watershed. The watershed is the land area over which water flows into the river, lake, or reservoir.

In rural areas, people are more likely to drink ground water that was pumped from a well. These wells tap into aquifers—the natural reservoirs under the earth's surface—that may be only a few miles wide, or may span the borders of many states. As with surface water, it is important to remember that activities many miles away from you may affect the quality of ground water.

Your annual drinking water quality report will tell you where your water supplier gets your water.

How is drinking water treated?

When a water supplier takes untreated water from a river or reservoir, the water often contains dirt and tiny pieces of leaves and other organic matter, as well as trace amounts of certain contaminants. When it gets to the treatment plant, water suppliers often add chemicals called coagulants to the water. These act on the water as it flows very slowly through tanks so that the dirt and other contaminants form clumps that settle to the bottom. Usually, this water then flows through a filter for removal of the smallest contaminants like viruses and *Giardia.*

Most ground water is naturally filtered as it passes through layers of the earth into underground reservoirs known as aquifers. Water that suppliers pump from wells generally contains less organic material than surface water and may not need to go through any or all of the treatments described in the previous paragraph. The quality of the water will depend on local conditions.

The most common drinking water treatment, considered by many to be one of the most important scientific advances of the 20th century, is disinfection. Most water suppliers add chlorine or another disinfectant to kill bacteria and other germs.

Water suppliers use other treatments as needed, according to the quality of their source water. For example, systems whose water is contaminated with organic chemicals can treat their water with activated carbon, which adsorbs or attracts the chemicals dissolved in the water.

What if I have special health needs?

People who have HIV/AIDS, are undergoing chemotherapy, take steroids, or for another reason have a weakened immune system may be more susceptible to microbial contaminants, including *Cryptosporidium*, in drinking water. If you or someone you know fall into one of these categories, talk to your health care provider to find out if you need to take special precautions, such as boiling your water.

Young children are particularly susceptible to the effects of high levels of certain contaminants, including nitrate and lead. To avoid exposure to lead, use water from the cold tap for making baby formula, drinking, and cooking, and let the water run for a minute or more if the water hasn't been turned on for six or more hours. If your water supplier alerts you that your water does not meet EPA's standard for nitrates and you have children less than six months old, consult your health care provider. You may want to find an alternate source of water that contains lower levels of nitrates for your child.

What are the health effects of contaminants in drinking water?

EPA has set standards for more than 80 contaminants that may occur in drinking water and pose a risk to human health. EPA sets these standards to protect the health of everybody, including vulnerable groups like children. The contaminants fall into two groups according to the health effects that they cause. Your local water supplier will alert you through the local media, direct mail, or other means if there is a potential acute or chronic health effect from compounds in the drinking water. You may want to contact them for additional information specific to your area.

Acute effects occur within hours or days of the time that a person consumes a contaminant. People can suffer acute health effects from almost any contaminant if they are exposed to extraordinarily high levels (as in the case of a spill). In drinking water, microbes, such as bacteria and viruses, are the contaminants with the greatest chance of reaching levels high enough to cause acute health effects. Most people's bodies can fight off these microbial contaminants the way they fight off germs, and these acute contaminants typically don't have permanent effects. Nonetheless, when high enough levels occur, they can make people ill, and can be dangerous or deadly for a person whose immune system is already weak due to HIV/AIDS, chemotherapy, steroid use, or another reason.

Chronic effects occur after people consume a contaminant at levels over EPA's safety standards for many years. The drinking water contaminants that can have chronic effects are chemicals (such as disinfection by-products, solvents, and pesticides), radionuclides (such as radium), and minerals (such as arsenic). Examples of these chronic effects include cancer, liver or kidney problems, or reproductive difficulties.

Who is responsible for drinking water quality?

The Safe Drinking Water Act gives the Environmental Protection Agency (EPA) the responsibility for setting national drinking water standards that protect the health of the 250 million people who get their water from public water systems. Other people get their water from private wells which are not subject to federal regulations. Since 1974, EPA has set national standards for over 80 contaminants that may occur in drinking water.

While EPA and state governments set and enforce standards, local governments and private water suppliers have direct responsibility for the quality of the water that flows to your tap. Water systems test and treat their water, maintain the distribution systems that deliver water to consumers, and report on their water quality to the state. States and EPA provide technical assistance to water suppliers and can take legal action against systems that fail to provide water that meets state and EPA standards.

What is a violation of a drinking water standard?

Drinking water suppliers are required to monitor and test their water many times, for many things, before sending it to consumers. These tests determine whether and how the water needs to be treated, as well as the effectiveness of the treatment process. If a water system consistently sends to consumers water that contains a contaminant at a level higher than EPA or state health standards or if the system fails to monitor for a contaminant, the system is violating regulations, and is subject to fines and other penalties. When a water system violates a drinking water regulation, it must notify the people who drink its water about the violation, what it means, and how they should respond. In cases where the water presents an immediate health threat, such as when people need to boil water before drinking it, the system must use television, radio, and newspapers to get the word out as quickly as possible. Other notices may be sent by mail, or delivered with the water bill. Each water suppliers' annual water quality report must include a summary of all the violations that occurred during the previous year.

How can I help protect drinking water?

Using the new information that is now available about drinking water, citizens can both be aware of the challenges of keeping drinking water safe and take an active role in protecting drinking water. There are lots of ways that individuals can get involved. Some people will help clean up the watershed that is the source of their community's water. Other people might get involved in wellhead protection activities to prevent the contamination of the ground water source that provides water to their community. These people will be able to make use of the information that states and water systems are gathering as they assess their sources of water.

Other people will want to attend public meetings to ensure that the community's need for safe drinking water is considered in making decisions about land use. You may wish to participate as your state and water system make funding decisions. And all consumers can do their part to conserve water and to dispose properly of household chemicals.

Chapter 23

Drinking Water Standards

Setting Standards for Safe Drinking Water

The Safe Drinking Water Act (SDWA), passed in 1974 and amended in 1986 and 1996, gives the Environmental Protection Agency (EPA) the authority to set drinking water standards. This chapter describes how EPA establishes these standards.

What are drinking water standards?

Drinking water standards are regulations that EPA sets to control the level of contaminants in the nation's drinking water. These standards are part of the Safe Drinking Water Act's multiple barrier approach to drinking water protection, which includes assessing and protecting drinking water sources; protecting wells and collection systems; making sure water is treated by qualified operators; ensuring the integrity of distribution systems; and making information available to the public on the quality of their drinking water. With the involvement of EPA, states, tribes, drinking water utilities, communities and citizens, these multiple barriers ensure that tap water in the United States and territories is safe to drink. In most cases, EPA

Excerpted from "Setting Standards for Safe Drinking Water," a fact sheet produced by the U.S. Environmental Protection Agency (EPA), 2000, available online at http://www.epa.gpv/safewater/standard/setting.html. Cited February 2003; and "Current Drinking Water Standards," a fact sheet produced by the EPA, EPA 816-F-02-013, 2002, available online at http://www.epa.gov/safewater/mcl.html.

Table 23.1. National Drinking Water Regulations for Microorganisms

Microorganisms	MCLG[1] (mg/L)[2]	MCL or TT[1] (mg/L)[2]	Potential Health Effects from Ingestion of Water	Sources of Contaminant in Drinking Water
Cryptosporidium	zero	TT[3]	Gastrointestinal illness (e.g., diarrhea, vomiting, cramps)	Human and fecal animal waste
Giardia lamblia	zero	TT[3]	Gastrointestinal illness (e.g., diarrhea, vomiting, cramps)	Human and animal fecal waste
Heterotrophic plate count	n/a	TT[3]	HPC has no health effects; it is an analytic method used to measure the variety of bacteria that are common in water. The lower the concentration of bacteria in drinking water, the better maintained the water system is.	HPC measures a range of bacteria that are naturally present in the environment
Legionella zero	zero	TT[3]	Legionnaire's Disease, a type of pneumonia	Found naturally in water; multiplies in heating systems
Total Coliforms (including fecal coliform and *E. Coli)*	zero	5.0%[4]	Not a health threat in itself; it is used to indicate whether other potentially harmful bacteria may be present[5]	Coliforms are naturally present in the environment; as well as feces; fecal coliforms and *E. coli* only come from human and animal fecal waste.
Turbidity	n/a	TT[3]	Turbidity is a measure of the cloudiness of water. It is used to indicate water quality and filtration effectiveness (e.g., whether disease-causing organisms are present). Higher turbidity levels are often associated with higher levels of disease-causing microorganisms such as viruses, parasites and some bacteria. These organisms can cause symptoms such as nausea, cramps, diarrhea, and associated headaches.	Soil runoff
Viruses (enteric)	zero	TT[3]	Gastrointestinal illness (e.g., diarrhea, vomiting, cramps)	Human and animal fecal waste

delegates responsibility for implementing drinking water standards to states and tribes.

There are two categories of drinking water standards:

- A *National Primary Drinking Water Regulation* (NPDWR or primary standard) is a legally-enforceable standard that applies to public water systems. Primary standards protect drinking water quality by limiting the levels of specific contaminants that can adversely affect public health and are known or anticipated to occur in water. They take the form of Maximum Contaminant Levels or Treatment Techniques.

- A *National Secondary Drinking Water Regulation* (NSDWR or secondary standard) is a non-enforceable guideline regarding contaminants that may cause cosmetic effects (such as skin or tooth discoloration) or aesthetic effects (such as taste, odor, or color) in drinking water. EPA recommends secondary standards to water systems but does not require systems to comply. However, states may choose to adopt them as enforceable standards.

Who must comply with drinking water standards?

Drinking water standards apply to public water systems (PWSs), which provide water for human consumption through at least 15 service connections, or regularly serve at least 25 individuals. Public water systems include municipal water companies, homeowner associations, schools, businesses, campgrounds and shopping malls.

Who is involved in the standard setting process?

EPA considers input from many individuals and groups throughout the rulemaking process. One of the formal means by which EPA solicits the assistance of its stakeholders is the National Drinking Water Advisory Council (NDWAC). The 15-member committee was created by the Safe Drinking Water Act. It is comprised of five members of the general public, five representatives of state and local agencies concerned with water hygiene and public water supply, and five representations of private organizations and groups demonstrating an active interest in water hygiene and public water supply, including two members who are associated with small rural public water systems. NDWAC advises EPA's Administrator o n all of the agency's activities relating to drinking water.

In addition to the NDWAC, representatives from water utilities, environmental groups, public interest groups, states, tribes and the general public are encouraged to take an active role in shaping the regulations, by participating in public meetings and commenting on proposed rules. Special meetings are also held to obtain input from minority and low-income communities, as well as representatives of small businesses.

Current Drinking Water Standards

National Primary Drinking Water Regulations (NPDWRs or primary standards) are legally enforceable standards that apply to public water systems. Primary standards protect public health by limiting the levels of contaminants in drinking water. The following tables show the divisions of these contaminants.

Table 23.2. National Drinking Water Regulations for Disinfection Byproducts

Disinfection Byproducts	MCLG[1] (mg/L)[2]	MCL or TT[1] (mg/L)[2]	Potential Health Effects from Ingestion of Water	Sources of Contaminant in Drinking Water
Bromate	zero	0.010	Increased risk of cancer	Byproduct of drinking water disinfection
Chlorite	0.8	1.0	Anemia; infants and young children: nervous system effects	Byproduct of drinking water disinfection
Haloacetic acids (HAA5)	n/a[6]	0.060	Increased risk of cancer	Byproduct of drinking water disinfection
Total Trihalomethanes (TTHMs)	none[7] n/a[6]	0.10 0.080	Liver, kidney or central nervous system problems; increased risk of cancer	Byproduct of drinking water disinfection

Table 23.3. National Drinking Water Regulations for Disinfectants

Disinfectants	MRDL[1] (mg/L)[2]	MRDL[1] (mg/L)[2]	Potential Health Effects from Ingestion of Water	Sources of Contaminant in Drinking Water
Chloramines (as Cl_2)	MRDLG= 4[1]	MRDL= 4.0[1]	Eye/nose irritation; stomach discomfort, anemia	Water additive used to control microbes
Chlorine (as Cl_2)	MRDLG= 4[1]	MRDL= 4.0[1]	Eye/nose irritation; stomach discomfort	Water additive used to control microbes
Chlorine dioxide (as ClO_2)	MRDLG= 0.8[1]	MRDL= 0.8[1]	Anemia; infants and young children: nervous system effects	Water additive used to control microbes

Table 23.4. National Drinking Water Regulations for Inorganic Chemicals (continued on next page)

Inorganic Chemicals	MCLG[1] (mg/L)[2]	MCL or TT[1] (mg/L)[2]	Potential Health Effects from Ingestion of Water	Sources of Contaminant in Drinking Water
Antimony	0.006	0.006	Increase in blood cholesterol; decrease in blood sugar	Discharge from petroleum refineries; fire retardants; ceramics; electronics; solder
Arsenic	0[7]	0.010 as of 01/23/06	Skin damage or problems with circulatory systems, and may have increased risk of getting cancer	Erosion of natural deposits; runoff rom orchards, runoff from glass and electronics production wastes
Asbestos (fiber >10 micrometers)	7 million fibers per liter	7 MFL	Increased risk of developing benign intestinal polyps	Decay of asbestos cement in water mains; erosion of natural deposits
Barium	2	2	Increase in blood pressure	Discharge of drilling wastes; discharge from metal refineries;erosion of natural deposits

Table 23.4. (continued) National Drinking Water Regulations for Inorganic Chemicals (*continued on next page*)

Inorganic Chemicals	MCLG[1] (mg/L)[2]	MCL or TT[1] (mg/L)[2]	Potential Health Effects from Ingestion of Water	Sources of Contaminant in Drinking Water
Beryllium	0.004	0.004	Intestinal lesions	Discharge from metal refineries and coal-burning factories; discharge from electrical, aerospace, and defense industries
Cadmium	0.005	0.005	Kidney damage	Corrosion of galvanized pipes; erosion of natural deposits; discharge from metal refineries; runoff from waste batteries and paints
Chromium (total)	0.1	0.1	Allergic dermatitis	Discharge from steel and pulp mills; erosion of natural deposits
Copper	1.3	TT[8]; Action Level= 1.3	Short term exposure: Gastrointestinal distress; Long term exposure: Liver or kidney damage; People with Wilson's Disease should consult their personal doctor if the amount of copper in their water exceeds the action level	Corrosion of house hold plumbing systems; erosion of natural deposits
Cyanide (as free cyanide)	0.2	0.2	Nerve damage or thyroid problems	Discharge from steel/metal factories; discharge from plastic and fertilizer factories
Fluoride	4.0	4.0	Bone disease (pain and tenderness of the bones); Children may get mottled teeth	Water additive which promotes strong teeth; erosion of natural deposits; discharge from fertilizer and aluminum factories

Table 23.4. (continued) National Drinking Water Regulations for Inorganic Chemicals

Inorganic Chemicals	MCLG[1] (mg/L)[2]	MCL or TT[1] (mg/L)[2]	Potential Health Effects from Ingestion of Water	Sources of Contaminant in Drinking Water
Lead	zero	TT[8]; Action Level= 0.015	Infants and children: Delays in physical or mental development; children could show slight deficits in attention span and learning abilities; Adults: Kidney problems; high blood pressure	Corrosion of house hold plumbing systems; erosion of natural deposits
Mercury (inorganic)	0.002	0.002	Kidney damage	Erosion of natural deposits; discharge from refineries and factories; runoff from landfills and croplands
Nitrate (measured as Nitrogen)	10	10	Infants below the age of six months who drink water containing nitrate in excess of the MCL could become seriously ill and, if untreated, may die. Symptoms include shortness of breath and blue-baby syndrome.	Runoff from fertilizer use; leaching from septic tanks, sewage; erosion of natural deposits
Nitrite (measured as Nitrogen)	1	1	Infants below the age of six months who drink water containing nitrite in excess of the MCL could become seriously ill and, if untreated, may die. Symptoms include shortness of breath and blue-baby syndrome.	Runoff from fertilizer use; leaching from septic tanks, sewage; erosion of natural deposits
Selenium	0.05	0.05	Hair or fingernail loss; numbness in fingers or toes; circulatory problems	Discharge from peroleum refineries; erosion of natural deposits; discharge from mines
Thallium	0.0005	0.002	Hair loss; changes in blood; kidney, intestine, or liver problems	Leaching from ore-processing sites; discharge from electronics, glass, and drug factories

Table 23.5. National Drinking Water Regulations for Organic Chemicals (continued on next page)

Organic Chemicals	MCLG[1] (mg/L)[2]	MCL or TT[1] (mg/L)[2]	Potential Health Effects from Ingestion of Water	Sources of Contaminant in Drinking Water
Acrylamide	zero	TT[9]	Nervous system or blood problems; increased risk of cancer	Added to water during sewage/wastewater treatment
Alachlor	zero	0.002	Eye, liver, kidney or spleen problems; anemia; increased risk of cancer	Runoff from herbicide used on row crops
Atrazine	0.003	0.003	Cardiovascular system or reproductive problems	Runoff from herbicide used on row crops
Benzene	zero	0.005	Anemia; decrease in blood platelets; increased risk ofcancer	Discharge from factories; leaching from gas storage tanks and landfills
Benzo(a)pyrene (PAHs)	zero	0.0002	Reproductive difficulties; increased risk of cancer	Leaching from linings of water storage tanks and distribution lines
Carbofuran	0.04	0.04	Problems with blood, nervous system, or reproductive system	Leaching of soil fumigant used on rice and alfalfa
Carbon tetrachloride	zero	0.005	Liver problems; increased risk of cancer	Discharge from chemical plants and other industrial activities
Chlordane	zero	0.002	Liver or nervous system problems; increased risk of cancer	Residue of banned termiticide
Chlorobenzene	0.1	0.1	Liver or kidney problems	Discharge from chemical and agricultural chemical factories
2,4-D	0.07	0.07	Kidney, liver, or adrenal gland problems	Runoff from herbicide used on row crops
Dalapon	0.2	0.2	Minor kidney changes	Runoff from herbicide used on rights of way
1,2-Dibromo-3-chloropropane (DBCP)	zero	0.0002	Reproductive difficulties; increased risk of cancer	Runoff/leaching from soil fumigant used on soybeans, cotton, pineapples, and orchards
o-Dichlorobenzene	0.6	0.6	Liver, kidney, or circulatory system problems	Discharge from industrial chemical factories

Table 23.5. (continued) National Drinking Water Regulations for Organic Chemicals (continued on next page)

Organic Chemicals	MCLG[1] (mg/L)[2]	MCL or TT[1] (mg/L)[2]	Potential Health Effects from Ingestion of Water	Sources of Contaminant in Drinking Water
p-Dichloro-benzene	0.075	0.075	Anemia; liver, kidney or spleen damage; changes in blood	Discharge from industrial chemical factories
1,2-Dichloro-ethane	zero	0.005	Increased risk of cancer	Discharge from industrial chemical factories
1,1-Dichloro-ethylene	0.007	0.007	Liver problems	Discharge from industrial chemical factories
cis-1,2-Dichloro-ethylene	0.07	0.07	Liver problems	Discharge from industrial chemical factories
trans-1,2-Dichloro-ethylene	0.1	0.1	Liver problems	Discharge from industrial chemical factories
Dichloromethane	zero	0.005	Liver problems; increased risk of cancer	Discharge from drug and chemical factories
1,2-Dichloro-propane	zero	0.005	Increased risk of cancer	Discharge from industrial chemical factories
Di(2-ethylhexyl) adipate	0.4	0.4	General toxic effects or reproductive difficulties	Discharge from chemical factories
Di(2-ethylhexyl) phthalate	zero	0.006	Reproductive difficulties; liver problems; increased risk of cancer	Discharge from rubber and chemical factories
Dinoseb	0.007	0.007	Reproductive difficulties	Runoff from herbicide used on soybeans and vegetables
Dioxin (2,3,7,8-TCDD)	zero	0.00000003	Reproductive difficulties; increased risk of cancer	Emissions from waste incineration and other combustion; discharge from chemical factories
Diquat	0.02	0.02	Cataracts	Runoff from herbicide use
Endothall	0.1	0.1	Stomach and intestinal problems	Runoff from herbicide use
Endrin	0.002	0.002	Liver problems	Residue of banned insecticide
Epichlorohydrin	zero	TT[9]	Increased cancer risk, and over a long period of time, stomach problems	Discharge from industrial chemical factories; an impurity of some water treatment chemicals
Ethylbenzene	0.7	0.7	Liver or kidneys problems	Discharge from petroleum refineries

Table 23.5. (continued) National Drinking Water Regulations for Organic Chemicals (continued on next page)

Organic Chemicals	MCLG[1] (mg/L)[2]	MCL or TT[1] (mg/L)[2]	Potential Health Effects from Ingestion of Water	Sources of Contaminant in Drinking Water
Ethylene dibromide	zero	0.00005	Problems with liver, stomach, reproductive system, or kidneys; increased risk of cancer	Discharge from petroleum refineries
Glyphosate	0.7	0.7	Kidney problems; reproductive difficulties	Runoff from herbicide use
Heptachlor	zero	0.0004	Liver damage; increased risk of cancer	Residue of banned termiticide
Heptachlor epoxide	zero	0.0002	Liver damage; increased risk of cancer	Breakdown of heptachlor
Hexachlorobenzene	zero	0.001	Liver or kidney problems; reproductive difficulties; increased risk of cancer	Discharge from metal refineries and agricultural chemical factories
Hexachlorocyclopentadiene	0.05	0.05	Kidney or stomach problems	Discharge from chemical factories
Lindane	0.0002	0.0002	Liver or kidney problems	Runoff/leaching from insecticide used on cattle, lumber, gardens
Methoxychlor	0.04	0.04	Reproductive difficulties	Runoff/leaching from insecticide used on fruits, vegetables, alfalfa, livestock
Oxamyl (Vydate)	0.2	0.2	Slight nervous system effects	Runoff/leaching from insecticide used on apples, potatoes, and tomatoes
Polychlorinated biphenyls (PCBs)	zero	0.0005	Skin changes; thymus gland problems; immune deficiencies; reproductive or nervous system difficulties; increased risk of cancer	Runoff from landfills; discharge of waste chemicals
Pentachlorophenol	zero	0.001	Liver or kidney problems; increased cancer risk	Discharge from wood preserving factories

Table 23.5. (continued) National Drinking Water Regulations for Organic Chemicals

Organic Chemicals	MCLG[1] (mg/L)[2]	MCL or TT[1] (mg/L)[2]	Potential Health Effects from Ingestion of Water	Sources of Contaminant in Drinking Water
Picloram	0.5	0.5	Liver problems	Herbicide runoff
Simazine	0.004	0.004	Problems with blood	Herbicide runoff
Styrene	0.1	0.1	Liver, kidney, or circulatory system problems	Discharge from rubber and plastic factories; leaching from landfills
Tetrachloroethylene	zero	0.005	Liver problems; increased risk of cancer	Discharge from factories and dry cleaners
Toluene	1	1	Nervous system, kidney, or liver problems	Discharge from petroleum factories
Toxaphene	zero	0.003	Kidney, liver, or thyroid problems; increased risk of cancer	Runoff/leaching from insecticide used on cotton and cattle
2,4,5-TP (Silvex)	0.05	0.05	Liver problems	Residue of banned herbicide
1,2,4-Trichlorobenzene	0.07	0.07	Changes in adrenal glands	Discharge from textile finishing factories
1,1,1-Trichloroethane	0.20	0.2	Liver, nervous system, or circulatory problems	Discharge from metal degreasing sites and other factories
1,1,2-Trichloroethane	0.003	0.005	Liver, kidney, or immune system problems	Discharge from industrial chemical factories
Trichloroethylene	zero	0.005	Liver problems; increased risk of cancer	Discharge from metal degreasing sites and other factories
Vinyl chloride	zero	0.002	Increased risk of cancer	Leaching from PVC pipes; discharge from plastic factories
Xylenes (total)	10	10	Nervous system damage	Discharge from petroleum factories; discharge from chemical factories

207

Table 23.6. National Drinking Water Regulations for Radionuclides

Radionuclides	MCLG[1] (mg/L)[2]	MCL or TT[1] (mg/L)[2]	Potential Health Effects from Ingestion of Water	Sources of Contaminant in Drinking Water
Alpha particles	none[7] zero	15 pico-curies per Liter (pCi/L)	Increased risk of cancer	Erosion of natural deposits of certain minerals that are radioactive and may emit a form of radiation known as alpha radiation
Beta particles and photon emitters	none[7] zero	4 milli-rems per year	Increased risk of cancer	Decay of natural and man-made deposits of certain minerals that are radioactive and may emit forms of radiation known as photons and beta radiation
Radium 226 and Radium 228 (combined)	none[7] zero	5 pCi/L	Increased risk of cancer	Erosion of natural deposits
Uranium	zero	30 µg/L as of 12/08/03	Increased risk of cancer, kidney toxicity	Erosion of natural deposits

Notes to Tables

1. Definitions:

    Maximum Contaminant Level (MCL): The highest level of a contaminant that is allowed in drinking water. MCLs are set as close to MCLGs as feasible using the best available treatment technology and taking cost into consideration. MCLs are enforceable standards.

    Maximum Contaminant Level Goal (MCLG): The level of a contaminant in drinking water below which there is no known or expected risk to health. MCLGs allow for a margin of safety and are non-enforceable public health goals.

    Maximum Residual Disinfectant Level (MRDL): The highest level of a disinfectant allowed in drinking water. There is convincing evidence that addition of a disinfectant is necessary for control of microbial contaminants.

    Maximum Residual Disinfectant Level Goal (MRDLG): The level of a drinking water disinfectant below which there is no known or expected risk to health. MRDLGs do not reflect the benefits of the use of disinfectants to control microbial contaminants.

Treatment Technique: A required process intended to reduce the level of a contaminant in drinking water.

2. Units are in milligrams per liter (mg/L) unless otherwise noted. Milligrams per liter are equivalent to parts per million.

3. EPA's surface water treatment rules require systems using surface water or ground water under the direct influence of surface water to (1) disinfect their water, and (2) filter their water or meet criteria for avoiding filtration so that the following contaminants are controlled at the following levels:

    Cryptosporidium (as of 1/1/02 for systems serving >10,000 and 1/14/05 for systems serving <10,000) 99% removal.

    Giardia lamblia: 99.9% removal/inactivation

    Viruses: 99.99% removal/inactivation

    Legionella: No limit, but EPA believes that if *Giardia* and viruses are removed/inactivated, *Legionella* will also be controlled.

    Turbidity: At no time can turbidity (cloudiness of water) go above 5 nephelolometric turbidity units (NTU); systems that filter must ensure that the turbidity go no higher than 1 NTU (0.5 NTU for conventional or direct filtration) in at least 95% of the daily samples in any month. As of January 1, 2002, turbidity may never exceed 1 NTU, and must not exceed 0.3 NTU in 95% of daily samples in any month.

    HPC: No more than 500 bacterial colonies per milliliter.

    Long Term 1 Enhanced Surface Water Treatment (Effective Date: January 14, 2005); Surface water systems or (GWUDI) systems serving fewer than 10,000 people must comply with the applicable Long Term 1 Enhanced Surface Water Treatment Rule provisions (e.g. turbidity standards, individual filter monitoring, *Cryptosporidium* removal requirements, updated watershed control requirements for unfiltered systems).

    Filter Backwash Recycling; The Filter Backwash Recycling Rule requires systems that recycle to return specific recycle flows through all processes of the system's existing conventional or direct filtration system or at an alternate location approved by the state.

4. More than 5.0% samples total coliform-positive in a month. (For water systems that collect fewer than 40 routine samples per month, no more than one sample can be total coliform-positive per month.) Every sample that has total coliform must be analyzed for either fecal coliforms or *E. coli* if two consecutive TC-positive samples, and one is also positive for *E. coli* fecal coliforms, system has an acute MCL violation.

5. Fecal coliform and *E. coli* are bacteria whose presence indicates that the water may be contaminated with human or animal wastes. Disease-causing microbes (pathogens) in these wastes can cause diarrhea, cramps, nausea, headaches, or other symptoms. These pathogens may pose a special health risk for infants, young children, and people with severely compromised immune systems.

6. Although there is no collective MCLG for this contaminant group, there are individual MCLGs for some of the individual contaminants:

> Trihalomethanes: bromodichloromethane (zero); bromoform (zero); dibromochloromethane (0.06 mg/L). Chloroform is regulated with this group but has no MCLG.

> Haloacetic acids: dichloroacetic acid (zero); trichloroacetic acid (0.3 mg/L). Monochloroacetic acid, bromoacetic acid, and dibromoacetic acid are regulated with this group but have no MCLGs.

7. MCLGs were not established before the 1986 Amendments to the Safe Drinking Water Act. Therefore, there is no MCLG for this contaminant.

8. Lead and copper are regulated by a Treatment Technique that requires systems to control the corrosiveness of their water. If more than 10% of tap water samples exceed the action level, water systems must take additional steps. For copper, the action level is 1.3 mg/L, and for lead is 0.015 mg/L.

9. Each water system must certify, in writing, to the state (using third-party or manufacturer's certification) that when acrylamide and epichlorohydrin are used in drinking water

systems, the combination (or product) of dose and monomer level does not exceed the levels specified, as follows:

Acrylamide = 0.05% dosed at 1 mg/L (or equivalent)

Epichlorohydrin = 0.01% dosed at 20 mg/L (or equivalent)

National Secondary Drinking Water Regulations

National Secondary Drinking Water Regulations (NSDWRs or secondary standards) are non-enforceable guidelines regulating contaminants that may cause cosmetic effects (such as skin or tooth discoloration) or aesthetic effects (such as taste, odor, or color) in drinking water. EPA recommends secondary standards to water systems but does not require systems to comply. However, states may choose to adopt them as enforceable standards.

Table 23.7. National Secondary Drinking Water Regulations

Contaminant	Secondary Standard
Aluminum	0.05 to 0.2 mg/L
Chloride	250 mg/L
Color	15 (color units)
Copper	1.0 mg/L
Corrosivity	noncorrosive
Fluoride	2.0 mg/L
Foaming Agents	0.5 mg/L
Iron	0.3 mg/L
Manganese	0.05 mg/L
Odor	3 threshold odor number
pH	6.5-8.5
Silver	0.10 mg/L
Sulfate	250 mg/L
Total Dissolved Solids	500 mg/L
Zinc	5 mg/L

Chapter 24

Contaminants in Drinking Water

Drinking water, including bottled water, may reasonably be expected to contain at least small amounts of some contaminants. The presence of contaminants does not necessarily indicate that water poses a health risk. EPA sets standards for approximately 90 contaminants in drinking water.

Following is detailed information on specific contaminants that may be found in drinking water.

Microbes

Coliform bacteria are common in the environment and are generally not harmful. However, the presence of these bacteria in drinking water is usually a result of a problem with the treatment system or the pipes which distribute water, and indicates that the water may be contaminated with germs that can cause disease.

Fecal Coliform and E. coli are bacteria whose presence indicates that the water may be contaminated with human or animal wastes. Microbes in these wastes can cause short-term effects, such as diarrhea, cramps, nausea, headaches, or other symptoms.

Turbidity has no health effects. However, turbidity can interfere with disinfection and provide a medium for microbial growth. Turbidity

"Drinking Water Contaminants," an undated fact sheet produced by the U.S. Environmental Protection Agency (EPA). Available online at http://www. epa.gov/safewater/hfacts.html. Cited February 2003.

213

may indicate the presence of disease causing organisms. These organisms include bacteria, viruses, and parasites that can cause symptoms such as nausea, cramps, diarrhea, and associated headaches.

Cryptosporidium is a parasite that enters lakes and rivers through sewage and animal waste. It causes cryptosporidiosis, a mild gastrointestinal disease. However, the disease can be severe or fatal for people with severely weakened immune systems. EPA and CDC have prepared advice for those with severely compromised immune systems who are concerned about *Cryptosporidium*.

Giardia lamblia is a parasite that enters lakes and rivers through sewage and animal waste. It causes gastrointestinal illness (e.g. diarrhea, vomiting, cramps).

Radionuclides

Alpha emitters. Certain minerals are radioactive and may emit a form of radiation known as alpha radiation. Some people who drink water containing alpha emitters in excess of EPA's standard over many years may have an increased risk of getting cancer.

Beta/photon emitters. Certain minerals are radioactive and may emit forms of radiation known as photons and beta radiation. Some people who drink water containing beta and photon emitters in excess of EPA's standard over many years may have an increased risk of getting cancer.

Combined Radium 226/228. Some people who drink water containing radium 226 or 228 in excess of EPA's standard over many years may have an increased risk of getting cancer.

Radon gas can dissolve and accumulate in underground water sources, such as wells, and in the air in your home. Breathing radon can cause lung cancer. Drinking water containing radon presents a risk of developing cancer. Radon in air is more dangerous than radon in water.

Inorganic Contaminants

Arsenic. Some people who drink water containing arsenic in excess of EPA's standard over many years could experience skin damage or problems with their circulatory system, and may have an increased risk of getting cancer.

Fluoride. Many communities add fluoride to their drinking water to promote dental health. Each community makes its own decision about whether or not to add fluoride. EPA has set an enforceable drinking water standard for fluoride of 4 mg/L (some people who drink water containing fluoride in excess of this level over many years could get bone disease, including pain and tenderness of the bones). EPA has also set a secondary fluoride standard of 2 mg/L to protect against dental fluorosis. Dental fluorosis, in its moderate or severe forms, may result in a brown staining and/or pitting of the permanent teeth. This problem occurs only in developing teeth, before they erupt from the gums. Children under nine should not drink water that has more than 2 mg/L of fluoride.

Lead typically leaches into water from plumbing in older buildings. Lead pipes and plumbing fittings have been banned since August 1998. Children and pregnant women are most susceptible to lead health risks. For advice on avoiding lead, see EPA's lead in your drinking water fact sheet.

Other inorganic contaminants include:

- Antimony
- Asbestos
- Barium
- Beryllium
- Cadmium
- Chromium
- Copper
- Cyanide
- Mercury
- Nitrate
- Nitrite
- Selenium
- Thallium

Technical fact sheets on inorganic contaminants are available on the EPA website at http://www.epa.gov/safewater/dwh/t-ioc.html.

Synthetic Organic Contaminants, Including Pesticides and Herbicides

Technical fact sheets on the following synthetic organic contaminants are available on the EPA website at http://www.epa.gov/safewater/dwh/t-soc.html.

- 2,4-D
- 2,4,5-TP (Silvex)
- Acrylamide
- Alachlor
- Atrazine
- Benzoapyrene
- Carbofuran
- Chlordane
- Dalapon
- Di 2-ethylhexyl adipate

- Di 2-ethylhexyl phthalate
- Dibromochloropropane
- Dinoseb
- Dioxin (2,3,7,8-TCDD)
- Diquat
- Endothall
- Endrin
- Epichlorohydrin
- Ethylene dibromide
- Glyphosate
- Heptachlor
- Heptachlor epoxide

- Hexachlorobenzene
- Hexachlorocyclopentadiene
- Lindane
- Methoxychlor
- Oxamyl [Vydate]
- PCBs [Polychlorinated biphenyls]
- Pentachlorophenol
- Picloram
- Simazine
- Toxaphene

Volatile Organic Contaminants

Technical fact sheets on volatile organic contaminants are available on the EPA website at http://www.epa.gov/safewater/dwh/t-voc.html.

- Benzene
- Carbon Tetrachloride
- Chlorobenzene
- o-Dichlorobenzene
- p-Dichlorobenzene
- 1,1-Dichloroethylene
- cis-1,2-Dichloroethylene
- trans-1,2-Dicholoroethylene
- Dichloromethane
- 1,2-Dichloroethane
- 1,2-Dichloropropane

- Ethylbenzene
- Styrene
- Tetrachloroethylene
- 1,2,4-Trichlorobenzene
- 1,1,1-Trichloroethane
- 1,1,2-Trichloroethane
- Trichloroethylene
- Toluene
- Vinyl Chloride
- Xylenes

Disinfectants

Many water suppliers add a disinfectant to drinking water to kill germs such as *Giardia* and *E. coli*. Especially after heavy rainstorms, your water system may add more disinfectant to guarantee that these germs are killed.

Chlorine. Some people who use drinking water containing chlorine well in excess of EPA's standard could experience irritating effects to their eyes and nose. Some people who drink water containing chlorine well in excess of EPA's standard could experience stomach discomfort.

Chloramine. Some people who use drinking water containing chloramines well in excess of EPA's standard could experience irritating effects to their eyes and nose. Some people who drink water containing chloramines well in excess of EPA's standard could experience stomach discomfort or anemia.

Chlorine Dioxide. Some infants and young children who drink water containing chlorine dioxide in excess of EPA's standard could experience nervous system effects. Similar effects may occur in fetuses of pregnant women who drink water containing chlorine dioxide in excess of EPA's standard. Some people may experience anemia.

Disinfection Byproducts

Disinfection byproducts form when disinfectants added to drinking water to kill germs react with naturally occurring organic matter in water.

Total Trihalomethanes. Some people who drink water containing trihalomethanes in excess of EPA's standard over many years may experience problems with their liver, kidneys, or central nervous systems, and may have an increased risk of getting cancer.

Haloacetic Acids. Some people who drink water containing haloacetic acids in excess of EPA's standard over many years may have an increased risk of getting cancer.

Bromate. Some people who drink water containing bromate in excess of EPA's standard over many years may have an increased risk of getting cancer.

Chlorite. Some infants and young children who drink water containing chlorite in excess of EPA's standard could experience nervous system effects. Similar effects may occur in fetuses of pregnant women who drink water containing chlorite in excess of EPA's standard. Some people may experience anemia.

MTBE is a fuel additive, commonly used in the United States to reduce carbon monoxide and ozone levels caused by auto emissions. Due to its widespread use, reports of MTBE detections in the nation's ground and surface water supplies are increasing. The Office of Water and other EPA offices are working with a panel of leading experts to focus on issues posed by the continued use of MTBE and other oxygenates in gasoline. EPA is currently studying the implications of setting a drinking water standard for MTBE.

Health advisories provide additional information on certain contaminants. Health advisories are guidance values based on health effects other than cancer. These values are set for different durations of exposure (e.g., one-day, ten-day, longer-term, and lifetime).

Chapter 25

Chlorination of Drinking Water: Its Benefits and Risks

For over 90 years, chlorination has played a critical role in protecting America's drinking water supply from diseases that can be passed through water.

Before the use of chlorine as a disinfectant in drinking water, cholera and typhoid outbreaks were common in major cities such as New York, Boston and New Orleans. In the early 1900s, Great Britain began disinfecting water with chlorine and saw a sharp reduction in typhoid deaths.

Shortly after this dramatic success, chlorination and filtration were introduced into the U.S., resulting in the virtual elimination of waterborne diseases such as cholera, typhoid, dysentery and hepatitis A. Today, over 98% of U.S. water treatment facilities disinfect with chlorine and chlorine-based chemicals.

We know that chlorine's chief benefit is the protection of public health through the control of waterborne diseases. But in addition to controlling the growth of germs and other microorganisms, chlorine also eliminates many chemicals, resulting in drinking water that tastes and smells better. And, chlorine has lasting effects.

A major benefit of chlorine-based compounds is that they protect against microbial contamination long after the water has left the treatment plant. Chlorine reduces the level of disease-causing micro-organisms in drinking water to almost immeasurable levels. However, during the water treatment process chlorine reacts with organic matter in the water and disinfection by-products (DBPs) form. While there has been concern that the presence of these compounds in drinking water may present potential health risks, the World Health Organization (WHO) notes that "the risks to health from DBPs are extremely small in comparison with the risks associated with inadequate disinfection, and it is important that disinfection should not be compromised in attempting to control such by-products."

Alternatives to chlorination have been suggested. But all alternative methods, with the possible exception of ultraviolet radiation, also form by-products. In addition, because alternative disinfectants cannot provide the residual protection of chlorine based disinfectants, they must be used in combination with chlorine or chloramines to provide a complete disinfection system.

The World Health Organization, in its *Guidelines for Drinking Water Quality*, supports the necessity for water disinfection; "Disinfection is unquestionably the most important step in the treatment of water for public supply."

Chlorination is, one of the most significant advances in public health protection and is vital in drinking water treatment. The need for water systems to provide proper water treatment and disinfection at all times cannot be overstated.

Questions and Answers

Should I worry about the safety of my drinking water?

Drinking water in the U.S. is among the safest and most regulated in the world. In most instances, outbreaks of waterborne disease occur in water systems with inadequate or no treatment. Still, certain segments of the population may be more vulnerable to waterborne illnesses. These segments include pregnant women, infants, the elderly and those whose immune systems are compromised by cancer, AIDS or the drugs used to treat these and other conditions.

Is it safe to use chlorine to disinfect drinking water?

Chlorination of drinking water is an important public health intervention in the fight against microbial disease. Safe and reliable use of chlorine in the disinfection process can be achieved in treatment plants or all sizes.

Why should we use chlorine as the disinfectant?

To date, chlorine has emerged as the disinfectant of choice primarily because of its effectiveness, efficiency, affordability, convenience and lasting effect as a disinfectant.

Why should we disinfect our drinking water system?

The primary goal of drinking water disinfection is to kill or render harmless microbial organisms that cause disease. Chlorine has a lasting effect as a disinfectant in the water distribution system and can protect against contamination that might occur after the water leaves the treatment plant.

Should I be concerned about disinfectant byproducts in my water?

Potential harmful levels of disinfection by-products are extremely rare in treated drinking water. Nonetheless, since disinfection byproducts were first discovered over 20 years ago, water utilities have been continuously working to lower the levels of DBPs while maintaining microbial protection.

Terms to Know

Ammonia: A chemical compound used in the treatment of water with chlorine to form chloramines.

Chloramination: The process in water treatment in which a chlorine/ammonia compound is used as the disinfecting agent.

Chloramines: The product of the reaction between chlorine and ammonia compounds.

Chlorination: The process in water treatment of adding chlorine for purposes of disinfection.

Chlorine: The element that produces hypo-chlorous acid on reaction with water.

Disinfection Byproducts (DBPS): The reaction produced between chlorine and organic components in water. The by-products are known as trihalomethanes (THMS) and haloacetic acids.

Hydrolysis: The reaction of chlorine with water.

Hypochlorous Acid: The reaction product of hydrolysis that actually disinfects.

Telephone Numbers to Know

The Chlorine Institute, Inc.
Tel: 202-775-2790

Chemical Manufacturers Association Responsible Care Initiative
Tel: 703-741-5000

Chlorine Chemistry Council
Toll Free: 800-254-6361

U.S. Department of Energy's Office of Health and Environmental Research
Tel: 505-586-5430

The American Water Works Association
Tel: 303-794-7711

EPA Safe Drinking Water Hotline
Toll Free: 800-426-4791

Chapter 26

Lead in Drinking Water

Lead is a common metal found in our environment. Before we knew its dangers, lead was used in many items such as paint, gasoline and fertilizers. Lead is rarely found in sources of drinking water. However, it can enter public and private drinking water systems through corrosion that occurs in lead service lines, plumbing and faucets.

You are most likely to have high levels of lead in your water if your water is soft or acidic and you have lead pipes, copper pipes with lead solder or faucets containing lead. Additionally, lead may leach into your drinking water if your water sits several hours in plumbing that contains lead materials.

What are the dangers of lead poisoning?

Lead can cause a variety of adverse health conditions when people are exposed to it at elevated levels. Short term exposure can cause interference with red blood cell chemistry and cause delays in normal physical and mental development in babies and young children. Long term exposure to lead can cause stroke, kidney disease and cancer. Children and pregnant women are at highest risk for the damaging effects of lead. It's important to know if there is lead in your drinking water.

"The Facts about Lead in Drinking Water," from South Carolina Department of Health and Environmental Control, 2001. For additional information, visit www.scdhec.net/water.

How do I have my water tested for lead?

Ask your public water provider for information on how to have your water tested for lead.

How can I remove lead from my drinking water?

If a water test indicates that the drinking water drawn from a tap in your home contains lead above 15 parts per billion or .015 milligrams per liter (mg/l), you should take the following actions to treat for the elevated level.

- Flush each tap before using water from it for drinking or cooking purposes. To flush your tap, let the water run about 30 seconds to allow the release of water that has been standing in the lines. This water can be used to water plants or wash dishes. Lead is not absorbed through the skin, so don't be concerned about bathing and showering with water that might contain lead. Try to use cold tap water for drinking and cooking. Do not cook with or drink water from the hot water tap. Hot water can dissolve lead more quickly than cold water. If you need hot water, draw it from the cold tap and heat it on the stove.

- Remove loose solder and debris from the plumbing in new homes or areas where plumbing recently has been replaced. This can be done by removing the faucet strainers from all taps and running the water for three to five minutes. Periodically remove the strainers and flush out any debris that has accumulated.

- Replace lead materials with lead-free ones. If your copper pipes have been joined with lead solder since its ban in 1988, notify the plumber who did the work and ask to have it replaced. Lead solder initially looks dull gray, but turns shiny when scratched with a key.

- Find out whether the service line that connects your home or apartment to the water main is made of lead. A licensed plumber can check to see if your home's plumbing contains lead solder, lead pipes, or pipe fittings that contain lead.

- Have an electrician check your wiring. If grounding wires from the electrical system are attached to your pipes, it can increase corrosion. Check with a licensed electrician or your local electric code to determine if wiring can be grounded elsewhere. Do not attempt to change the wiring yourself. Improper grounding can cause electrical shock and fire hazards.

If you find your water has high lead levels and you are concerned that your child might be affected, contact your private physician or your county health department for information on how to get a blood lead test.

Treatment of Lead in a Public Water System

Public water systems are working to control the corrosiveness of their water if the level of lead at home taps exceeds the .015 mg/l action level. The systems are implementing an optimum corrosion control treatment plan. Corrosion control allows for a decrease in the amount of lead that is leached from a piping system. This decrease is accomplished by adjusting pH, and alkalinity, or calcium in an effort to make the water less corrosive or by adding a phosphate or silica-based inhibitor to form a protective film on the interior of pipes and fixtures.

Potential Causes of Lead in Drinking Water

- Lead pipes
- Copper pipes with lead solder
- Water sitting in lead or lead soldered pipes for several hours
- Soft, acidic water in conjunction with lead pipes or lead solder
- Lead in source water (occurs in rare instances)

You are most likely to have high levels of lead in your water if your water is soft or acidic and you have lead pipes, copper pipes with lead solder or faucets containing lead.

Chapter 27

MTBE (Methyl-Tert-Butyl Ether) in Drinking Water

MTBE in Drinking Water

What Is MTBE?

MTBE (methyl-*tert*-butyl ether) is a member of a group of chemicals commonly known as fuel oxygenates. Oxygenates are added to fuel to increase its oxygen content. MTBE is used in gasoline throughout the United States to reduce carbon monoxide and ozone levels caused by auto emissions. MTBE replaces the use of lead as an octane enhancer since 1979.

How does MTBE contaminate water supplies?

Releases of MTBE to ground and surface water can occur through leaking underground storage tanks and pipelines, spills, emissions from marine engines into lakes and reservoirs, and to some extent from air deposition.

How do I know if I have MTBE in my water?

You can determine if your water contains MTBE the following ways. If your drinking water is supplied by a public water system, you can

"MTBE in Drinking Water," an undated fact sheet produced by the U.S. Environmental Protection Agency (EPA). Available online at http://www.epa.gov/safe water/mtbe.html. Cited February 2003; And "Frequently Asked Questions (FAQs) about MTBE and USTs," and undated fact sheet produced by the EPA. Available online at http://www.epa.gov/swerust1/mtbe/mtbefaqs.html. Cited February 2003.

contact the system directly and ask whether they monitor for MTBE and what levels, if any, have been detected. As of 2001, public water systems serving most of the population are required to monitor for MTBE. If you have a private well, your local health department may be able to tell you if MTBE has been found in water in your area. If you want to get your water tested, call the Safe Drinking Water Hotline (800-426-4791) or go to http://www.epa.gov/safewater/faq/sco.html to get the phone number for the office in your state that certifies drinking water laboratories.

How can I remove MTBE from my water?

Public water systems can use existing technologies such as air stripping, granular activated carbon (GAC), and advanced oxidation to remove MTBE contamination. Some home treatment units can also remove MTBE in tap water. The EPA does not certify the effectiveness of home treatment units since it only regulates public water supplies. NSF International has a respected certification program for home treatment systems. They do certify home treatment systems for MTBE and other regulated contaminants. Another source of information on home treatment devices is the Water Quality Association. The Underwriters Laboratories, Inc. website also provides further insight into home treatment devices.

What is the Office of Water doing to address MTBE concerns?

Due to its widespread use, reports of MTBE detections in the nation's ground and surface water supplies are increasing. The Office of Water is actively involved in identifying the issues and addressing the concerns over the potential presence of MTBE in our water supplies. The Office of Water is participating in MTBE projects in the following areas:

Blue Ribbon Panel: EPA has established a panel of leading experts in the fields of public health, the scientific community, automotive fuels, water utilities, and local and State environmental officials to focus on the issues posed by the continued use of MTBE and other oxygenates in gasoline. The panel will look at the role of oxygenates in meeting clean air standards; evaluate its efficiency and other alternatives; assess the behavior of oxygenates in the environment; review known health effects; look at the cost of production and use and the product's availability; study causes of ground and drinking water contamination from motor vehicle fuels; and examine cleanup technologies for water and soil. In September 1999, the panel released its final report on the findings and recommendations on how best to ensure public health and environmental protection while maintaining clean air and water benefits.

In response to the recommendations of the Blue Ribbon Panel, the Office of Water issued a memo to the States regarding concerns about MTBE and how to protect sources of drinking water. The memo encourages early MTBE monitoring under the Unregulated Contaminant Monitoring Rule and assessing the impact of MTBE sources into source water assessments, and highlights the development of a secondary drinking water standard.

MTBE and the Safe Drinking Water Act: As part of implementing the Safe Drinking Water Act Amendments of 1996, the Office of Water has placed MTBE on the drinking water Contaminant Candidate List (CCL) for further evaluation to determine whether or not regulation with a National Primary Drinking Water Regulation (NPDWR) is necessary. The CCL divided the contaminants among those which are priorities for additional research, those which need additional occurrence data, and those which are priorities for consideration for rulemaking. The Agency determined that MTBE needs more health effects research and occurrence data before a regulatory determination can be made. Information gathered from the Agency's research and data collection efforts will assist our regulatory determination.

In addition, MTBE has been included in the final Unregulated Contaminant Monitoring Regulation that will require all large public water systems and a statistical sampling of small and medium public water systems to monitor and report the presence of MTBE in their water supplies.

As an additional interim measure, EPA responded to requests for guidance by reviewing and updating an advisory for MTBE in December 1997. This *Drinking Water Advisory: Consumer Acceptability and Health Effects Analysis* provides guidance to communities that may become exposed to drinking water contaminated with MTBE. The advisory recommends control levels that prevent adverse taste and odor (i.e. 20 to 40 parts per billion). Managing water supplies to avoid the unpleasant taste and odor effects at levels in this range also provides protection against any potential adverse health effects with a very large margin of safety.

Research

To facilitate the advancement of crucial scientific knowledge needed for MTBE and other fuel oxygenates in the environment, the Office of Water has participated in an agency-wide task force on an "Oxygenates in Water: Critical Information and Research Needs" (NEEDS) document. The Needs document identifies key issues and information needed to support risk assessment and risk management of MTBE and other oxygenates in water, and lists more than 40 projects that are currently underway or anticipated. EPA is conducting a key pharmacokinetic study that will help clarify the potential health risks from MTBE in drinking water more quickly than the amount of time (likely more than four years) it would require to conduct and analyze a two-year drinking water study in rodents.

Occurrence

The Agency is very concerned and has been closely following the increasing detections of MTBE in the ground and surface water supplies throughout the nation. While most MTBE detections typically occur at levels below those recommended in EPA's Drinking Water Advisory, there have been instances of contamination at much higher levels of potential health concern. We are working together with the U.S. Geological Survey to assess the frequency and levels of MTBE occurrence in geographic regions using MTBE as part of the Reformulated Gasoline (RFG) program. This study, as well as an upcoming national occurrence survey sponsored by American Water Works Association Research Foundation and increased monitoring studies by many states, will help clarify the extent to which MTBE may threaten the nation's water supplies.

Frequently Asked Questions (FAQs) about MTBE and USTs

When was gasoline that contains MTBE first stored in USTs?

Gasoline containing MTBE has been stored in underground storage tanks (USTs) since the 1970s. MTBE was first used as an octane-enhancing replacement for lead, primarily in mid- and high-grade gasoline at concentrations as high as 7% (by volume). Now, however, MTBE is mainly used as a fuel oxygenate at higher concentrations (11% to 15% by volume) as part of the Federal RFG and Wintertime Oxyfuel programs. The Oxyfuel and RFG Programs were initiated by the U.S. EPA in 1992 and 1995, respectively, to meet requirements of the 1990 Clean Air Act Amendments.

What is the difference between Oxyfuel and RFG?

The Oxyfuel Program requires the use of gasoline with 2.7-percent oxygen (by weight) in areas with high levels of carbon monoxide during the fall and winter. When MTBE is used to meet this requirement, it is used at a concentration of 15 percent (by volume) in gasoline. Because ethanol has a higher oxygen content, it can meet this requirement with a concentration of 7.3 percent (by volume). The RFG Program requires 2.0-percent oxygen (by weight) throughout the year in the most polluted metropolitan areas. MTBE meets this level with an 11-percent (by volume) concentration, and ethanol can be used with a 5.4-percent (by volume) concentration.

Where are USTs which store gasoline containing MTBE located?

MTBE is a common and widely used additive in gasoline. MTBE has been used in conventional gasoline to boost the octane since the 1970s. Given MTBE's widespread use as a gasoline additive and the large volumes of gasoline that are stored, transported, and used in all areas of the country, MTBE could have been (or is now) in virtually any UST anywhere in the U.S., not just areas required to use RFG or Oxyfuel.

Studies by the U.S. Geological Survey have found that water supplies are more likely to be contaminated with MTBE in areas where RFG or Oxyfuel is required than in other areas. The Clean Air Act (CAA) mandates that reformulated gasoline (RFG) be sold in the 10 largest metropolitan areas with the most severe summertime ozone levels. The CAA also allows any other area classified as a marginal, moderate, or serious ozone nonattainment area to opt into the RFG program. In addition to the RFG program, certain areas in the nation that have not attained the National Ambient Air Quality Standards (NAAQS) for carbon monoxide are required under the CAA to implement the Wintertime Oxyfuel program. EPA's Office of Transportation and Air Quality (OTAQ) maintains a "List of Reformulated Gasoline Program Areas" which are required to use oxygenated fuels at least part of the year.

Other than regulated USTs, what are some other sources of MTBE releases?

As a large industrialized nation, the United States produces, distributes, and consumes extensive quantities of gasoline, and much of

231

that gasoline contains MTBE. After production, gasoline may travel through thousands of miles of pipelines, or be transported by truck, to any of roughly 10,000 terminals and bulk stations. From there it may be distributed to one of 180,000 retail outlets and fleet storage facilities, or to any of hundreds of thousands of above ground or underground tanks at farms, industrial facilities, businesses, and homes. Finally, gasoline is removed from bulk storage into individualized storage units associated with such products as cars, trucks, boats, planes, lawn mowers, brush cutters, and chain saws. Residual gasoline in transport conduits may contaminate different types of fuels (e.g., home heating oil) that is transported through the same conduits at different times. There are opportunities for leaks wherever gasoline (or a product containing gasoline) is stored and there are opportunities for spills whenever fuel is transported or transferred from one container to another. Gasoline is released to the environment every day.

Although releases (through leaks, spills, and overfills) from underground storage tank systems is a major source of MTBE contamination there are many other potential sources. Other potential sources of MTBE releases include: farm and residential tanks of 1,100 gallons or less, home heating oil tanks, tanks in basements, tanks of 110 gallons or less, emergency spill and overfill tanks, above ground tanks, automobile accidents, tank truck spills, consumer disposal of old gasoline, spills during refueling operations, motorized water craft, and storm water runoff.

Is funding available for LUST (Leaking Underground Storage Tank) prevention and remediation projects?

The Office of Water has produced a fact sheet about the Clean Water State Revolving Fund (CWSRF) program that addresses this question.

Chapter 28

Drinking Water: Microbial and Disinfection Byproducts

Disinfection of drinking water is one of the major public health advances in the 20th century. One hundred years ago, typhoid and cholera epidemics were common throughout American cities. Disinfection was a major factor in reducing these epidemics, and it is an essential part of drinking water treatment today. However, the disinfectants themselves can react with naturally occurring materials in the water to form unintended organic and inorganic byproducts which may pose health risks.

Over the past ten years, we have also learned that there are specific microbial pathogens, such as *Cryptosporidium*, that are highly resistant to traditional disinfection practices. In 1993, *Cryptosporidium* caused 400,000 people in Milwaukee to experience intestinal illness. More than 4,000 were hospitalized, and at least 50 deaths have been attributed to the disease. There have also been cryptosporidiosis outbreaks in Nevada, Oregon, and Georgia over the past several years.

A major challenge for water suppliers is how to balance the risks from microbial pathogens and disinfection byproducts. It is important to provide protection from these microbial pathogens while simultaneously ensuring decreasing health risks to the population from disinfection byproducts (DBPs). The 1996 Safe Drinking Water Act (SDWA) Amendments require EPA to develop rules to achieve these goals.

"Drinking Water Priority Rulemaking: Microbial and Disinfection Byproduct Rules," a fact sheet produced by the U.S. Environmental Protection Agency (EPA), 2001. Available online at http://www.epa.gov/safewater/mdbp/mdbpfactsheet.pdf.

Table 28.1. Schedule of M-DBP Rules

November 1998—Final Rule	Interim Enhanced Surface Water Treatment Rule & Stage 1 Disinfection Byproduct Rule
Early 2001—Final Rule	Filter Backwash Recycling Rule
Early 2001—Final Rule	Long Term 1 Enhanced Surface Water Treatment Rule
Summer 2001—Final Rule	Ground Water Rule
May 2002—Final Rule	Stage 2 Disinfection Byproduct Rule & Long Term 2 Enhanced Surface Water Treatment Rule

Public Health Concerns

Most Americans drink tap water that meets all existing health standards all the time. These new rules will further strengthen existing drinking water standards and thus increase protection for many water systems.

EPA's Science Advisory Board concluded in 1990 that exposure to microbial contaminants such as bacteria, viruses, and protozoa (e.g., *Giardia lamblia* and *Cryptosporidium*) was likely the greatest remaining health risk management challenge for drinking water suppliers. Acute health effects from exposure to microbial pathogens are documented and associated illness can range from mild to moderate cases lasting only a few days to more severe infections that can last several weeks and may result in death for those with weakened immune systems.

In addition, while disinfectants are effective in controlling many microorganisms, they react with natural organic and inorganic matter in source water and distribution systems to form potentially harmful DBPs. Many of these DBPs have been shown to cause cancer and reproductive and developmental effects in laboratory animals. More than 200 million people consume water that has been disinfected. Because of the large population exposed, health risks associated with DBPs, even if small, need to be taken seriously.

Existing Regulations

Microbial Contaminants: The Surface Water Treatment Rule, promulgated in 1989, applies to all public water systems using surface water sources or ground water sources under the direct influence of surface water. It establishes maximum contaminant level goals (MCLGs) for viruses, bacteria and *Giardia lamblia*. It also includes treatment technique requirements for filtered and unfiltered systems that are specifically designed to protect against the adverse health effects of exposure to these microbial pathogens. The Total Coliform Rule, revised in 1989, applies to all public water systems (PWSs) and establishes a maximum contaminant level (MCL) for total coliforms.

Disinfection Byproducts: In 1979, EPA set an interim MCL for total trihalomethanes of 0.10 mg/l as an annual average. This applies to any community water system serving at least 10,000 people that adds a disinfectant to the drinking water during any part of the treatment process.

Information Collection Rule

To support the M-DBP rulemaking process, the Information Collection Rule required large public water systems serving at least 100,000 people to monitor and collect data on microbial contaminants, disinfectants and disinfection byproducts for 18 months. The data provide EPA with information about disinfection byproducts, disease-causing microorganisms, including *Cryptosporidium*, and engineering data to control these contaminants. Drinking Water Microbial and Disinfection Byproduct Information collected for the ICR is available in EPA's Envirofacts Warehouse.

Interim Enhanced Surface Water Treatment Rule and Stage 1 Disinfectants and Disinfection Byproducts Rule

EPA finalized the Interim Enhanced Surface Water Treatment Rule and Stage 1 Disinfectants and Disinfection Byproducts Rule in November 1998, as required by the 1996 Amendments to the Safe Drinking Water Act, Section 1412(b)(2)(C). The final rules resulted from formal regulatory negotiations with a wide range of stakeholders that took place in 1992-93 and 1997. On Jan 16, 2001, EPA published final revisions to the IESWTR and Stage 1DBPR.

Interim Enhanced Surface Water Treatment Rule

The Interim Enhanced Surface Water Treatment Rule applies to systems using surface water, or ground water under the direct influence of surface water, that serve 10,000 or more persons. The rule also includes provisions for states to conduct sanitary surveys for surface water systems regardless of system size. The rule builds upon the treatment technique requirements of the Surface Water Treatment Rule with the following key additions and modifications:

- Maximum contaminant level goal (MCLG) of zero for *Cryptosporidium*

- 2-log *Cryptosporidium* removal requirements for systems that filter

- Strengthened combined filter effluent turbidity performance standards

- Individual filter turbidity monitoring provisions

- Disinfection profiling and benchmarking provisions

- Systems using ground water under the direct influence of surface water now subject to the new rules dealing with *Cryptosporidium*

- Inclusion of *Cryptosporidium* in the watershed control requirements for unfiltered public water systems

- Requirements for covers on new finished water reservoirs

- Sanitary surveys, conducted by states, for all surface water systems regardless of size

The Interim Enhanced Surface Water Treatment Rule, with tightened turbidity performance criteria and required individual filter monitoring, is designed to optimize treatment reliability and to enhance physical removal efficiencies to minimize the *Cryptosporidium* levels in finished water. In addition, the rule includes disinfection benchmark provisions to assure continued levels of microbial protection while facilities take the necessary steps to comply with new DBP standards.

Stage 1 Disinfectants and Disinfection Byproducts Rule

The final Stage 1 Disinfectants and Disinfection Byproducts Rule applies to community water systems and non-transient non-community systems, including those serving fewer than 10,000 people, that add a disinfectant to the drinking water during any part of the treatment process.

The final Stage 1 Disinfectants and Disinfection Byproducts Rule includes the following key provisions:

- Maximum residual disinfectant level goals (MRDLGs) for chlorine (4 mg/L), chloramines (4 mg/L), and chlorine dioxide (0.8 mg/L);

- Maximum contaminant level goals (MCLGs) for four trihalomethanes (chloroform [zero], bromodichloromethane [zero], dibromochloromethane (0.06 mg/L), and bromoform [zero]), two haloacetic acids (dichloroacetic acid [zero] and trichloroacetic acid [0.3 mg/L]), bromate (zero), and chlorite (0.8 mg/L); EPA subsequently removed the zero MCLG for chloroform from its National Primary Drinking Water Regulations, effective May 30, 2000, in accordance with an order of the U.S. Court of Appeals for the District of Columbia Circuit.

- MRDLs for three disinfectants (chlorine [4.0 mg/L], chloramines [4.0 mg/L], and chlorine dioxide [0.8 mg/L]);

- MCLs for total trihalomethanes—a sum of the four listed previously (0.080 mg/L), haloacetic acids (HAA5) (0.060 mg/L)—a sum of the two listed above plus monochloroacetic acid and mono- and dibromoacetic acids), and two inorganic disinfection byproducts (chlorite [1.0 mg/L]) and bromate [0.010 mg/L]); and

- A treatment technique for removal of DBP precursor material.

The terms MRDLG and MRDL, which are not included in the SDWA, were created during the negotiations to distinguish disinfectants (because of their beneficial use) from contaminants. The final rule includes monitoring, reporting, and public notification requirements for these compounds. This final rule also describes the best available technology (BAT) upon which the MRDLs and MCLs are based.

Filter Backwash Recycling Rule

The Filter Backwash Recycling Rule (FBRR) requires public water systems (PWSs) to review their backwash water recycling practices to ensure that they do not compromise microbial control. Under the FBRR, recycled filter backwash water, sludge thickener supernatant, and liquids from dewatering processes must be returned to a location such that all processes of a system's conventional or direct filtration including coagulation, flocculation, sedimentation (conventional filtration only) and filtration, are employed. Systems may apply to the State for approval to recycle at an alternate location. The Filter Backwash Rule applies to all public water systems, regardless of size.

Long Term 1 Enhanced Surface Water Treatment Rule

While the Stage 1 Disinfectants and Disinfection Byproducts Rule rule applies to systems of all sizes, the Interim Enhanced Surface Water Treatment Rule only applies to systems serving 10,000 or more people. The Long Term 1 Enhanced Surface Water Treatment Rule, promulgated in January 2002, will strengthen microbial controls for small systems i.e., those systems serving fewer than 10,000 people. The rule will also prevent significant increase in microbial risk where small systems take steps to implement the Stage 1 Disinfectants and Disinfection Byproducts Rule.

EPA believes that the rule will generally track the approaches in the Interim Enhanced Surface Water Treatment Rule for improved turbidity control, including individual filter monitoring and reporting. The rule will also address disinfection profiling and benchmarking. The Agency is considering what modifications of some large system requirements may be appropriate for small systems.

Future M-DBP Rules

Ground Water Rule

EPA has proposed a Ground Water Rule that specifies the appropriate use of disinfection while addressing other components of ground water systems to ensure public health protection. There are more than 158,000 public ground water systems. Almost 89 million people are served by community ground water systems, and 20 million people are served by non-community ground water systems. Ninety-nine percent (157,000) of ground water systems serve fewer than 10,000 people. However, systems serving more than 10,000 people serve 55% (more than 60 million) of all people who get their drinking water from public ground water systems. The Ground Water Rule will be promulgated summer 2001.

Long Term 2 Enhanced Surface Water Treatment Rule and Stage 2 Disinfectants and Disinfection Byproducts Rule

The SDWA, as amended in 1996, requires EPA to finalize a Stage 2 Disinfectants and Disinfection Byproducts Rule by May 2002. Although the 1996 Amendments do not require EPA to finalize a Long

Term 2 Enhanced Surface Water Treatment Rule along with the Stage 2 Disinfectants and Disinfection Byproducts Rule, EPA believes it is important to finalize these rules together to ensure a proper balance between microbial and DBP risks.

EPA begun discussions with stakeholders in December 1998 on the direction for these rules. EPA anticipates proposing these rules in 2001. The intent of the rules is to provide additional public health protection, if needed, from DBPs and microbial pathogens.

Chapter 29

Drinking Water from Household Wells

If your family gets drinking water from your own well, do you know if your water is safe to drink? What health risks could you and your family face? Where can you go for help or advice? This chapter helps answer these questions. It gives you general information about drinking water from home wells (also considered private drinking water sources). It describes types of activities in your area that can create threats to your water supply. It also describes problems to look for and offers maintenance suggestions.

All of us need clean water to drink. We can go for weeks without food, but only days without water. Contaminated water can be a threat to anyone's health, but especially to young children. About 15 percent of Americans have their own sources of drinking water, such as wells, cisterns, and springs. Unlike public drinking water systems serving many people, they do not have experts regularly checking the water's source and its quality before it is sent through pipes to the community.

To help protect families with their own wells, almost all states license or register water-well installers. Most also have construction standards for home wells. In addition, some city and county health departments have local rules and permitting. All this helps make sure the well is built properly. But what about checking to see that it is working correctly and the water is always healthy to drink? That is the job of the well owner, and it takes some work and some knowledge.

"Drinking Water from Household Wells," a brochure produced by the U.S. Environmental Protection Agency (EPA), EPA 816-K-02-003, 2002. Available online at http://www.epa.gov/safewater/consumer/household_wells.pdf.

What Is Ground Water and How Can It Be Polluted?

Ground water is a resource found under the earth's surface. Most ground water comes from rain and melting snow soaking into the ground. Water fills the spaces between rocks and soils, making an aquifer. About half of our nation's drinking water comes from ground water. Most is supplied through public drinking water systems. But many families rely on private, household wells and use ground water as their source of fresh water.

Ground water—its depth from the surface, quality for drinking water, and chance of being polluted—varies from place to place. Generally, the deeper the well, the better the ground water. The amount of new water flowing into the area also affects ground water quality.

Ground water may contain some natural impurities or contaminants, even with no human activity or pollution. Natural contaminants can come from many conditions in the watershed or in the ground. Water moving through underground rocks and soils may pick up magnesium, calcium and chlorides. Some ground water naturally contains dissolved elements such as arsenic, boron, selenium, or radon, a gas formed by the natural breakdown of radioactive uranium in soil. Whether these natural contaminants are health problems depends on the amount of the substance present.

In addition to natural contaminants, ground water is often polluted by human activities such as:

- Improper use of fertilizers, animal manures, herbicides, insecticides, and pesticides
- Improperly built or poorly located and/or maintained septic systems for household wastewater
- Leaking or abandoned underground storage tanks and piping
- Storm-water drains that discharge chemicals to ground water
- Improper disposal or storage of wastes
- Chemical spills at local industrial sites

Suburban growth is bringing businesses, factories and industry (and potential sources of pollution) into once rural areas where families often rely on household wells. Growth is also pushing new home developments onto the edge of rural and agricultural areas. Often municipal water and sewer lines do not extend to these areas. Many new houses rely on wells and septic tanks. But the people buying them may not have any experience using these systems.

Most U.S. ground water is safe for human use. However, ground water contamination has been found in all 50 states, so well owners have reason to be vigilant in protecting their water supplies. Well owners need to be aware of potential health problems. They need to test their water regularly and maintain their wells to safeguard their families' drinking water.

Quick Reference List of Noticeable Problems

Visible

- Scale or scum from calcium or magnesium salts in water
- Unclear/turbid water from dirt, clay salts, silt or rust in water
- Green stains on sinks or faucets caused by high acidity
- Brown-red stains on sinks, dishwasher, or clothes in wash points to dissolved iron in water
- Cloudy water that clears upon standing may have air bubbles from poorly working pump or problem with filters.

Tastes

- Salty or brackish taste from high sodium content in water
- Alkali/soapy taste from dissolved alkaline minerals in water
- Metallic taste from acidity or high iron content in water
- Chemical taste from industrial chemicals or pesticides

Smell

- A rotten egg odor can be from dissolved hydrogen sulfide gas or certain bacteria in your water. If the smell only comes with hot water it is likely from a part in your hot water heater.
- A detergent odor and water that foams when drawn could be seepage from septic tanks into your ground water well.
- A gasoline or oil smell indicates fuel oil or gasoline likely seeping from a tank into the water supply
- Methane gas or musty/earthy smell from decaying organic matter in water
- Chlorine smell from excessive chlorination.

Note: Many serious problems (bacteria, heavy metals, nitrates, radon, and many chemicals) can only be found by laboratory testing of water.

Where Do Ground Water Pollutants Come From?

Understanding and spotting possible pollution sources is important. It's the first step to safeguard drinking water for you and your family. Some threats come from nature. Naturally occurring contaminants such as minerals can present a health risk. Other potential sources come from past or present human activity—things that we do, make, and use—such as mining, farming and using chemicals. Some of these activities may result in the pollution of the water we drink.

Several sources of pollution are easy to spot by sight, taste, or smell. However many serious problems can only be found by testing your water. Knowing the possible threats in your area will help you decide on the kind of tests you need.

What Are Some Naturally Occurring Sources of Pollution?

Microorganisms: Bacteria, viruses, parasites and other microorganisms are sometimes found in water. Shallow wells—those with water close to ground level—are at most risk. Runoff, or water flowing over the land surface, may pick up these pollutants from wildlife and soils. This is often the case after flooding. Some of these organisms can cause a variety of illnesses. Symptoms include nausea and diarrhea. These can occur shortly after drinking contaminated water. The effects could be short-term yet severe (similar to food poisoning) or might recur frequently or develop slowly over a long time.

Radionuclides: Radionuclides are radioactive elements such as uranium and radium. They may be present in underlying rock and ground water. Radon—a gas that is a natural product of the breakdown of uranium in the soil—can also pose a threat. Radon is most dangerous when inhaled and contributes to lung cancer. Although soil is the primary source, using household water containing Radon contributes to elevated indoor Radon levels. Radon is less dangerous when consumed in water, but remains a risk to health.

Nitrates and Nitrites: Although high nitrate levels are usually due to human activities, they may be found naturally in ground water. They come from the breakdown of nitrogen compounds in the soil. Flowing ground water picks them up from the soil. Drinking large amounts of nitrates and nitrites is particularly threatening to infants (for example, when mixed in formula).

244

Heavy Metals: Underground rocks and soils may contain arsenic, cadmium, chromium, lead, and selenium. However, these contaminants are not often found in household wells at dangerous levels from natural sources.

Fluoride: Fluoride is helpful in dental health, so many water systems add small amounts to drinking water. However, excessive consumption of naturally occurring fluoride can damage bone tissue. High levels of fluoride occur naturally in some areas. It may discolor teeth, but this is not a health risk.

What Human Activities Can Pollute Ground Water?

Bacteria and Nitrates: These pollutants are found in human and animal wastes. Septic tanks can cause bacterial and nitrate pollution. So can large numbers of farm animals. Both septic systems and animal manures must be carefully managed to prevent pollution. Sanitary landfills and garbage dumps are also sources. Children and some adults are at extra risk when exposed to water-born bacteria. These include the elderly and people whose immune systems are weak due to AIDS or treatments for cancer. Fertilizers can add to nitrate problems. Nitrates cause a health threat in very young infants called "blue baby" syndrome. This condition disrupts oxygen flow in the blood.

Concentrated Animal Feeding Operations (CAFOs): The number of CAFOs, often called "factory farms," is growing. On these farms thousands of animals are raised in a small space. The large amounts of animal wastes/manures from these farms can threaten water supplies. Strict and careful manure management is needed to prevent pathogen and nutrient problems. Salts from high levels of manures can also pollute groundwater.

Heavy Metals: Activities such as mining and construction can release large amounts of heavy metals into nearby ground water sources. Some older fruit orchards may contain high levels of arsenic, once used as a pesticide. At high levels, these metals pose a health risk.

Fertilizers and Pesticides: Farmers use fertilizers and pesticides to promote growth and reduce insect damage. These products are also used on golf courses and suburban lawns and gardens. The chemicals in these products may end up in ground water. Such pollution depends on the types and amounts of chemicals used and how they are applied.

245

Local environmental conditions (soil types, seasonal snow and rainfall) also affect this pollution. Many fertilizers contain forms of nitrogen that can break down into harmful nitrates. This could add to other sources of nitrates mentioned previously. Some underground agricultural drainage systems collect fertilizers and pesticides. This polluted water can pose problems to ground water and local streams and rivers. In addition, chemicals used to treat buildings and homes for termites or other pests may also pose a threat. Again, the possibility of problems depends on the amount and kind of chemicals. The types of soil and the amount of water moving through the soil also play a role.

Industrial Products and Wastes: Many harmful chemicals are used widely in local business and industry. These can become drinking water pollutants if not well managed. The most common sources of such problems are:

- Local Businesses: These include nearby factories, industrial plants, and even small businesses such as gas stations and dry cleaners. All handle a variety of hazardous chemicals that need careful management. Spills and improper disposal of these chemicals or of industrial wastes can threaten ground water supplies.

- Leaking Underground Tanks and Piping: Petroleum products, chemicals, and wastes stored in underground storage tanks and pipes may end up in the ground water. Tanks and piping leak if they are constructed or installed improperly. Steel tanks and piping corrode with age. Tanks are often found on farms. The possibility of leaking tanks is great on old, abandoned farm sites. Farm tanks are exempt from the EPA rules for petroleum and chemical tanks.

- Landfills and Waste Dumps: Modern landfills are designed to contain any leaking liquids. But floods can carry them over the barriers. Older dumpsites may have a wide variety of pollutants that can seep into ground water.

- Household Wastes: Improper disposal of many common products can pollute ground water. These include cleaning solvents, used motor oil, paints, and paint thinners. Even soaps and detergents can harm drinking water. These are often a problem from faulty septic tanks and septic leaching fields.

- Lead and Copper: Household plumbing materials are the most common source of lead and copper in home drinking water. Corrosive water may cause metals in pipes or soldered joints to leach into your tap water. Your water's acidity or alkalinity (often measured as pH) greatly affects corrosion. Temperature and mineral content also affect how corrosive it is. They are often used in pipes, solder, or plumbing fixtures. Lead can cause serious damage to the brain, kidneys, nervous system, and red blood cells. The age of plumbing materials—in particular, copper pipes soldered with lead—is also important. Even in relatively low amounts these metals can be harmful. EPA rules under the Safe Drinking Water Act limit lead in drinking water to 15 parts per billion. Since 1988 the Act only allows "lead free" pipe, solder, and flux in drinking water systems. The law covers both new installations and repairs of plumbing. For more information on avoiding lead in drinking water, visit the EPA Website at www.epa.gov/safewater/Pubs/lead1.html.

- Water Treatment Chemicals: Improper handling or storage of water-well treatment chemicals (disinfectants, corrosion inhibitors, etc.) close to your well can cause problems.

Should I Be Concerned?

You should be aware because the Safe Drinking Water Act does not protect private wells. EPA's rules only apply to "public drinking water systems"—government or privately run companies supplying water to 25 people or 15 service connections. While most states regulate private household wells, most have limited rules. Individual well owners have primary responsibility for the safety of the water drawn from their wells. They do not benefit from the government's health protections for water systems serving many families.

These must comply with federal and state regulations for frequent analysis, testing, and reporting of results. Instead, household well owners should rely on help from local health departments. They may help you with yearly testing for bacteria and nitrates. They may also oversee the placement and construction of new wells to meet state and local regulations. Most have rules about locating drinking water wells near septic tanks, drain fields, and livestock. But remember, the final responsibility for constructing your well correctly, protecting it from pollution, and maintaining it falls on you, the well owner.

How Much Risk Can I Expect?

The risk of having problems depends on how good your well is—how well it was built and located, and how well you maintain it. It

247

also depends on your local environment. That includes the quality of the aquifer from which you draw your water and the human activities going on in your area that can affect your well water.

Some questions to consider in protecting your drinking water and maintaining your well are:

- What distance should my well be from sources of human wastes such as septic systems?

- How far should it be from animal feedlots or manure spreading?

- What are the types of soil and underlying rocks? Does water flow easily or collect on the surface?

- How deep must a well be dug to avoid seasonal changes in ground water supply?

- What activities in my area (farming, mining, industry) might affect my well?

- What is the age of my well, its pump, and other parts?

- Is my water distribution system protected from cross connections and backflow problems?

What Should I Do?

Following are the six basic steps you should take to maintain the safety of your drinking water. After the list you'll find "how to" suggestions for each point to help you protect your well and your drinking water.

1. Identify potential problem sources.

2. Talk with local experts.

3. Have your water tested periodically.

4. Have the test results interpreted and explained clearly.

5. Set a regular maintenance schedule for your well, do the scheduled maintenance and keep accurate, up-to-date records.

6. Remedy any problems.

Protecting Your Ground Water Supply

When building, modifying, or closing a well:

- Hire a certified well driller for any new well construction or modification.

- Slope well area so surface runoff drains away.

- When closing a well:

  Do not cut off the well casing below the land surface.

  Hire a certified well contractor to fill or seal the well.

To prevent problems:

- Install a locking well cap or sanitary seal to prevent unauthorized use of, or entry into, the well.

- Do not mix or use pesticides, fertilizers, herbicides, degreasers, fuels, and other pollutants near the well.

- Never dispose of wastes in dry wells or in abandoned wells.

- Pump and inspect septic systems as often as recommended by your local health department.

- Never dispose of hazardous materials in a septic system.

- Take care in working or mowing around your well.

To maintain your well:

- Each month check visible parts of your system for problems such as:

  Cracking or corrosion,

  Broken or missing well cap,

  Settling and cracking of surface seals.

- Have the well tested once a year for coliform bacteria, nitrates, and other contaminants.

- Keep accurate records in a safe place, including:

  Construction contract or report

  Maintenance records, such as disinfection or sediment removal

  Any use of chemicals in the well

  Water testing results

After a flood—concerns and advisories:

- Stay away from the well pump while flooded to avoid electric shock.

- Do not drink or wash from the flooded well to avoid becoming sick.

- Get assistance from a well or pump contractor to clean and turn on the pump.

- After the pump is turned back on, pump the well until the water runs clear to rid the well of flood water.

- If the water does not run clear, get advice from the county or state health department or extension service.

- For additional information go to http://www.epa.gov/safewater/consumer/whatdo.htm

How Can I Spot Potential Problems?

The potential for pollution entering your well is affected by its placement and construction—how close is your well to potential sources of pollution? Local agricultural and industrial activities, your area's geology and climate also matter. Because ground water contamination is usually localized, the best way to identify potential contaminants is to consult a local expert. For example, talk with a geologist at a local college or someone from a nearby public water system. They'll know about conditions in your area.

Have Your Well Water Tested

Test your water every year for total coliform bacteria, nitrates, total dissolved solids, and pH levels. If you suspect other contaminants, test for these also. Chemical tests can be expensive. Limit them to possible problems specific to your situation.

Again, local experts can tell you about possible impurities in your area. Often county health departments do tests for bacteria and nitrates. For other substances, health departments, environmental offices, or county governments should have a list of state certified laboratories. Your State Laboratory Certification Officer can also provide one. Call EPA's Safe Drinking Water Hotline, 800-426-4791, for the name and phone number of your state's certification officer.

Before taking a sample, contact the lab that will perform your tests. Ask for instructions and sampling bottles. Follow the instructions carefully so you will get correct results. The first step is getting a good water sample. It is also important to follow advice about storing the samples. Ask how soon they must be taken to the lab for testing. These instructions can be very different for each substance being tested.

Remember to test your water after replacing or repairing any part of the well system (piping, pump, or the well itself.) Also test if you notice a change in your water's look, taste, or smell.

Understanding Your Test Results

Have your well water tested for any possible contaminants in your area. Use a state-approved testing lab. Do not be surprised if a lot of substances are found and reported to you.

The amount of risk from a drinking water contaminant depends on the specific substance and the amount in the water. The health of the person also matters. Some contaminant cause immediate and severe effects. It may take only one bacterium or virus to make a weak person sick. Another person may not be affected. For very young children, taking in high levels of nitrate over a relatively short period of time can be very dangerous. Many other contaminants pose a long-term or chronic threat to your health—a little bit consumed regularly over a long time could cause health problems such as trouble having children and other effects.

EPA drinking water rules for public water systems aim to protect people from both short and long term health hazards. The amounts of contaminants allowed are based on protecting people over a lifetime of drinking water. Public water systems are required to test their water regularly before delivery. They also treat it so that it meets drinking water standards, notify customers if water does not meet standards and provide annual water quality reports.

Compare your well's test results to federal and state drinking water standards. (You can find these standards at www.epa.gov/safewater/mcl.html or call the Safe Drinking Water Hotline 800-426-4791. In some cases, the laboratory will give a very helpful explanation. But you may have to rely on other experts to aid you in understanding the results.

Well Construction and Maintenance

Proper well construction and continued maintenance are keys to the safety of your water supply. Your state water-well contractor licensing agency, local health department, or local water system professional can provide information on well construction.

Water-well drillers and pump-well installers are listed in your local phone directory. The contractor should be bonded and insured. Make certain your ground water contractor is registered or licensed in your state, if required. If your state does not have a licensing/registration program contact the National Ground Water Association. They have a voluntary certification program for contractors. (In fact, some states use the Association's exams as their test for licensing.) For a list of

Table 29.1. Reasons to Test Your Water

Conditions or Nearby Activities:	Test for:
Recurring gastrointestinal illness	Coliform bacteria
Household plumbing contains lead	pH, lead, copper
Radon in indoor air or region is radon rich	Radon
Corrosion of pipes, plumbing	Corrosion, pH, lead
Nearby areas of intensive agriculture	Nitrate, pesticides, coliform bacteria
Coal or other mining operations nearby	Metals, pH, corrosion
Gas drilling operations nearby	Chloride, sodium, barium, strontium
Dump, junkyard, landfill, factory, gas station, or dry-cleaning operation nearby	Volatile organic compounds, total dissolved solids, pH, sulfate, chloride, metals
Odor of gasoline or fuel oil, and near gas station or buried fuel tanks	Volatile organic compounds
Objectionable taste or smell	Hydrogen sulfide, corrosion, metals
Stained plumbing fixtures, laundry	Iron, copper, manganese
Salty taste and seawater, or a heavily salted roadway nearby	Chloride, total dissolved solids, sodium
Scaly residues, soaps don't lather	Hardness
Rapid wear of water treatment equipment	pH, corrosion
Water softener needed to treat hardness	Manganese, iron
Water appears cloudy, frothy, or colored	Color, detergents

certified contractors in your state contact the Association at 614-898-7791 or 800-551-7379. There is no cost for mailing or faxing the list to you.

Many homeowners tend to forget the value of good maintenance until problems reach crisis levels. That can be expensive. It's better to maintain your well, find problems early, and correct them to protect your well's performance. Keep up-to-date records of well installation and repairs plus pumping and water tests. Such records can help spot changes and possible problems with your water system. If you have problems, ask a local expert to check your well construction and maintenance records. He or she can see if your system is okay or needs work.

Protect your own well area. Be careful about storage and disposal of household and lawn care chemicals and wastes. Good farmers and gardeners minimize the use of fertilizers and pesticides. Take steps to reduce erosion and prevent surface water runoff. Regularly check underground storage tanks that hold home heating oil, diesel, or gasoline. Make sure your well is protected from the wastes of livestock, pets, and wildlife.

Talk with Local Experts

Good sources of information and advice can be found close to home. The following list tells about some local experts:

- The local health department's registered sanitarian is a health specialist. He or she likely knows the most about any problems with private wells.

- Local water-well contractors can tell you about well drilling and construction. They are also familiar with local geology and water conditions. Look in the yellow pages of your phone book or contact the agency in your state that licenses water well contractors. Call the National Ground Water Association (NGWA) at 614-898-7791 or 800-551-7379 to find NGWA-certified water-well contractors in your area.

- Officials at the nearest public water system may explain any threats to local drinking water and may be developing plans to address potential threats. They may advise you on taking samples and understanding tests done on your water. Ask the local health department or look in your phone book for the name and address of the closest system.

- Local county extension agents will know about local farming and forestry activities that can affect your water. They may also have information about water testing.

- The Natural Resources Conservation Service (NRCS) replaced the old U.S. Soil Conservation Service. It is part of the U.S. Department of Agriculture. The NRCS and the U.S. Geological Survey have information about local soils and ground water. They can tell you where a local water supply is located and how it is recharged or replenished. They would know of any pollution threats and if radon is a problem in the area. Look for both in the blue pages of your local phone book.

- Local or county planning commissions can be good sources. They know about past and present land uses in your area that affect water.

- Your public library may also have records and maps that can provide useful information. Nearby colleges and universities have research arms that can provide facts and expertise. They may also have a testing lab.

Fix Problems Immediately

If you find that your well water is polluted, fix the problem as soon as possible. You may need to disinfect your water, have a new well drilled, replumb or repair your system. Consider hooking into a nearby community water system (if one is available). If you have a new well drilled or connect to a community water system, the old well must be closed properly. Consult local experts for help. You might consider installing a water treatment device to remove impurities.

Find Out More

To find out more about your watershed and its ground water visit "Surf Your Watershed" at www.epa.gov/surf. Also look at the "Index of Watershed Indicators" at www.epa.gov/iwi. These websites can also tell you possible sources of problems. Companies with permits to release their wastewaters in your area are listed. You can see if they meet pollution control laws. You can also learn how your watershed compares to others in the country.

The U.S. Department of Agriculture and EPA support a program to help farmers, ranchers and rural homeowners.

Definitions

Aquifer—An underground formation or group of formations in rocks and soils containing enough ground water to supply wells and springs.

Backflow—A reverse flow in water pipes. A difference in water pressures pulls water from sources other than the well into a home's water system, for example waste water or flood water. Also called back siphonage.

Bacteria—Microscopic living organisms; some are helpful and some are harmful. Good bacteria aid in pollution control by consuming and breaking down organic matter and other pollutants in septic systems, sewage, oil spills, and soils. However, bad bacteria in soil, water, or air can cause human, animal, and plant health problems.

Confining layer—Layer of rock that keeps the ground water in the aquifer below it under pressure. This pressure creates springs and helps supply water to wells.

Contaminant—Anything found in water (including microorganisms, minerals, chemicals, radionuclides, etc.) which may be harmful to human health.

Cross-connection—Any actual or potential connection between a drinking (potable) water supply and a source of contamination.

Heavy metals—Metallic elements with high atomic weights, such as, mercury chromium cadmium, arsenic, and lead. Even at low levels these metals can damage living things. They do not break down or decompose and tend to build up in plants, animals, and people causing health concerns.

Leaching field—The entire area where many materials (including contaminants) dissolve in rain, snowmelt, or irrigation water and are filtered through the soil.

Microorganisms—Also called microbes. Very tiny life forms such as bacteria, algae, diatoms, parasites, plankton, and fungi. Some can cause disease.

Nitrates—Plant nutrient and fertilizer that enters water supply sources from fertilizers, animal feed lots, manures, sewage, septic systems, industrial wastewaters, sanitary landfills, and garbage dumps.

Protozoa—One-celled animals, usually microscopic, that are larger and more complex than bacteria. May cause disease.

Radon—A colorless, odorless naturally occurring radioactive gas formed by the breakdown or decay of radium or uranium in soil or rocks like granite. Radon is fairly soluble in water, so well water may contain radon.

Radionuclides—Distinct radioactive particles coming from both natural sources and human activities. Can be very long lasting as soil or water pollutants.

Recharge area—The land area through or over which rainwater and other surface water soaks through the earth to replenish an aquifer, lake, stream, river, or marsh. Also called a watershed.

Saturated zone—The underground area below the water table where all open spaces are filled with water. A well placed in this zone will be able to pump ground water.

Unsaturated zone—The area above the ground water level or water table where soil pores are not fully saturated, although some water may be present.

Viruses—Submicroscopic disease-causing organisms that grow only inside living cells.

Watershed—The land area that catches rain or snow and drains it into a local water body (such as a river, stream, lake, marsh, or aquifer) and affects its flow, and the local water level. Also called a recharge area.

Water table—The upper level of the saturated zone. This level varies greatly in different parts of the country and also varies seasonally depending on the amount of rain and snowmelt.

Well cap—A tight-fitting, vermin-proof seal designed to prevent contaminants from flowing down inside of the well casing.

Well casing—The tubular lining of a well. Also a steel or plastic pipe installed during construction to prevent collapse of the well hole.

Wellhead—The top-of a structure built over a well. Term also used for the source of a well or stream.

Chapter 30

Swimming Water Hazards

Beach Pollution

The water at the beach looks clean, but is it? It may be worth your while to find out before you or your children go swimming. The water at most beaches is safe for swimming, most of the time. However, you cannot be sure the beach water is safe unless it is tested because your beach water may contain disease-causing microorganisms that you cannot see.

Monitoring of beach water quality by local health and environmental officials is necessary to warn citizens when there is a problem. With the passage of the Beaches Environmental Assessment and Coastal Health (BEACH) Act on October 10, 2000, the Clean Water Act was amended to include significant new beach protection provisions. This new law authorizes a national grant program to assist state, tribal, and local governments in developing and implementing monitoring and public notification programs for their coastal recreation waters. It also requires states to adopt improved water quality standards for pathogens and pathogen indicators and requires EPA to conduct studies and develop improved microbiological water quality criteria guidance. In addition, the law requires EPA to develop performance criteria for monitoring, notification, and public information databases and requires other federal agencies to establish certain programs.

"Before You Go to the Beach..." a brochure produced by the U.S. Environmental Protection Agency (EPA), EPA 823-F-02-004, 2002. Available online at http://www.epa.gov/waterscience/beaches/30cwabeach.pdf.

How does beach pollution affect you and your family?

Water can be polluted by different things. Trash, such as picnic plates, plastic bags and bottles, and cigarette butts is easy to see. It is often the things we can't see, such as bacteria and other microorganisms that we need to be more concerned about. If you or your family are exposed to these disease-causing organisms, they may make you sick.

Swimming or playing in unsafe water may result in minor illnesses such as sore throats or diarrhea. It also might result in more serious illnesses that may last longer than your vacation at the beach. Children, the elderly, and people with weakened immune systems have a greater chance of getting sick when they come in contact with contaminated water.

Where does this pollution come from?

The most frequent sources of disease-causing microorganisms are sewage overflows, polluted storm water runoff, sewage treatment plant malfunctions, boating wastes, and malfunctioning septic systems. Pollution in beach water is often much higher during and immediately after rainstorms because water draining into the beach may be carrying sewage from over-flowing sewage treatment systems. Rainwater also flows to our beaches after running off lawns, farms, streets, construction sites, and other urban areas, picking up animal waste, fertilizer, pesticides, trash, and many other pollutants. Many of these pollutants can end up in the water at our beaches.

BEACH Program

The BEACH Program will help reduce health risks to you and your family by minimizing your exposure to disease-causing microorganisms in the water where you swim or play. The BEACH Program is ensuring public access to information about the quality of their beach water. In addition, EPA is working with state, tribal, and local health and environmental officials to encourage use of faster tests to detect pollution as well as develop methods that will help predict when pollution may occur. With advance warning provided by the local authorities, you will be able to decide when and where to swim.

How do I get information about my beach?

State, tribal, and local health and environmental protection officials are responsible for monitoring the quality of water at our nation's beaches. When they find a beach is contaminated they may post warnings or close the beach. Your local public health or environmental office can tell you if and when the water at your beach is monitored, who does it, and where the results are posted. Check with EPA's Beach Watch website at www.epa.gov/OST/beaches or contact your city, county, or other local health officials listed in your local telephone book.

Questions to ask your local beach health monitoring official.

- Which beaches do you monitor and how often?
- What do you test for?
- Where can I see the test results and who can explain them to me?
- What are the primary sources of pollution that affect this beach?

What to do if your beach is not monitored regularly.

- Avoid swimming after a heavy rain.
- Look for storm drains along the beach. Don't swim near them.
- If the waters of your beach have been designated as a no-discharge zone for vessel sewage, check to see if boat pump-out facilities are available and working.

Table 30.1. Disease-Causing Microorganisms in Sewage

Microorganisms	Some Illnesses and Symptoms
Bacteria	Gastroenteritis (includes diarrhea and abdominal pain), salmonellosis (food poisoning), cholera.
Viruses	Fever, common colds, gastroenteritis, diarrhea, respiratory infections, hepatitis.
Protozoa	Gastroenteritis, cryptosporidiosis and giardiasis (including diarrhea and abdominal cramps), dysentery.
Worms	Digestive disturbances, vomiting, restlessness, coughing, chest pain, fever, diarrhea.

- Look for trash and such other signs of pollution as oil slicks in the water. These kinds of pollutants may indicate the presence of disease-causing microorganisms that may also have been washed into the water.

- If you think your beach water is contaminated, contact your local health or environmental protection officials. It is important for them to know about suspected beach water contamination so they can protect citizens from exposure.

- Work with your local authorities to create a monitoring program.

Part Four

Chemical Hazards

Chapter 31

Dioxins

About Dioxin

Dioxin is the common name used to refer to the chemical 2,3,7,8-tetrachlorodibenzo-p-dioxin or TCDD. In addition to dioxin itself there are other compounds, such as the polychlorinated dibenzodioxins (PCDDs), polychlorinated dibenzofurans (PCDFs) and some polychlorinated biphenyls (PCBs), that have similar structures and activity as dioxin. These are often commonly referred to as dioxin-like compounds or dioxins.

How are dioxins formed?

Dioxins are chemical contaminants that have no commercial usefulness by themselves. They are formed during combustion processes, such as waste incineration, forest fires and backyard trash burning, and during manufacturing processes such as herbicide manufacture and paper manufacture, e.g. dioxin was a contaminant of the herbicide Agent Orange used as a defoliant by U.S. forces in Vietnam.

"Dioxin Research at the National Institute of Environmental Health Sciences (NIEHS)," a fact sheet produced by the National Institute of Environmental Health Sciences (NIEHS), reviewed for currency April 24, 2001. Available online at http://www.niehs.nih.gov/oc/factsheets/dioxin.htm.

Why are dioxins of concern?

People are constantly exposed to dioxins through ingestion of dioxins that are present at low levels as environmental contaminants in food. Although they are at low levels in food, some dioxins are very slowly removed from the body and therefore they accumulate in our fat tissue. In laboratory animals, dioxins are highly toxic, cause cancer, and alter reproductive, developmental and immune function.

What are the health effects of dioxin on humans?

Studies have shown that dioxin exposure at high levels in exposed chemical workers leads to an increase in cancer. Other studies in highly exposed people show that dioxin exposure can lead to reproductive and developmental problems, increased heart disease and increased diabetes. Dioxins ability to cause birth defects (teratogenicity) has not been established in humans but studies in mice have shown that dioxin and similar chemicals can produce congenital defects.

In general the effects of dioxin on humans were only observed in populations that were highly exposed. The effect of the long-term low level exposure that is normally experienced by the general population is not known. The long-term effects of dioxin exposure on human immunity, reproduction and development, and other organs and systems remain focal points for ongoing research, as are the molecular and cellular mechanisms by which dioxin causes these health effects.

What are the biological mechanisms of dioxin's toxicity?

The way in which dioxin affects cells is similar in some way to the way in which hormones such as estrogen work. Dioxin enters a cell and binds to a protein present in cells known as the Ah receptor. The receptor when bound to dioxin can then bind to DNA and alter the expression of some genes. This can lead to alterations in the level of specific proteins and enzymes in the cell. While it is not known exactly how changes in the levels of these different proteins cause the toxicity of dioxin, it is believed by most scientists that the initial binding of dioxin the Ah receptor is the first step.

Ongoing Dioxin Research by the National Institute of Environmental Health Sciences

The health effects of dioxin on humans are the subject of ongoing studies at a number of research centers including the National Institute of Environmental Health Sciences in Research Triangle Park, North Carolina. In addition, NIEHS-supported researchers have studied the health effects of dioxin for more than 20 years and their efforts are reported in a large number of articles published in the scientific literature.

Dioxin and Cancer

The ability of dioxin to cause cancer (carcinogenicity) in laboratory animals is well established. The way in which dioxin cause cancer in animals and humans however is not fully understood, nor is it known if other dioxin-like compounds cause cancer. Humans are exposed to mixtures of dioxins and regulatory agencies such as the EPA regulate dioxin-like compounds together. Ongoing research at NIEHS is being conducted to examine the carcinogenicity of different dioxins, mixtures of these compounds, and the biological mechanisms responsible.

Dioxin and Agent Orange

Researchers are examining the effect of long term exposure to dioxin as a result of exposure to a Agent Orange, a defoliant used by U.S. forces in Vietnam. These studies have shown an elevation in diabetes in serviceman exposed to dioxin contaminated Agent Orange.

Dioxin and Endometriosis

Studies have shown that dioxin exposure can increases the occurrence of endometriosis in monkeys exposed to low levels of dioxins. NIEHS grantees are extending these studies to examine the consequence of long-term exposure to dioxins on the incidence of endometriosis in women exposed to dioxin during a chemical accident in Seveso, Italy.

Dioxin and Immune Function

One of the primary toxic effects of dioxin in laboratory animals is immune suppression, which results in decreased resistance to infectious agents and some cancers. The mechanisms and relationship between altered host resistance and immune dysfunction is complex, poorly defined, but extremely important to understanding health effects. NIEHS researchers are examining the mechanisms of immune suppression. Other studies are examining alterations in immune cell function in several human populations exposed to dioxin at both high levels and at low levels similar to that seen in the general U.S. population.

Human Response to Dioxin

The increased knowledge of the changes occurring in cells after exposure to dioxin allow us to examine if those effects are occurring in humans. Ongoing studies using state of the art molecular techniques are examining the effect of dioxins on the levels of specific genes in humans exposed long term to both high and low levels of dioxins. These studies will determine if there are individuals that are more responsive to dioxin and if these differences indicate that they are at higher risk of developing health problems.

Chapter 32

Lead and Your Health

Did you know the following facts about lead?

FACT: Lead exposure can harm young children and babies even before they are born.

FACT: Even children who seem healthy can have high levels of lead in their bodies.

FACT: You can get lead in your body by breathing or swallowing lead dust, or by eating soil or paint chips containing lead.

FACT: You have many options for reducing lead hazards. In most cases, lead-based paint that is in good condition is not a hazard.

FACT: Removing lead-based paint improperly can increase the danger to your family.

If you think your home might have lead hazards, read on to learn about lead and some simple steps to protect your family.

Health Effects of Lead

In the United States, about 900,000 children ages 1 to 5 have a blood-lead level above the level of concern. Even children who appear healthy can have dangerous levels of lead in their bodies.

"Lead in Paint, Dust, and Soil: Basic Information," an undated fact sheet produced by the U.S. Environmental Protection Agency (EPA). Available online at http://www.epa.gov/lead/leadinfo.htm. Cited February 2003.

People can get lead in their body if they:

- Put their hands or other objects covered with lead dust in their mouths.

- Eat paint chips or soil that contains lead.

- Breathe in lead dust (especially during renovations that disturb painted surfaces).

Lead is even more dangerous to children than adults because:

- Babies and young children often put their hands and other objects in their mouths. These objects can have lead dust on them.

- Children's growing bodies absorb more lead.

- Children's brains and nervous systems are more sensitive to the damaging effects of lead.

If not detected early, children with high levels of lead in their bodies can suffer from:

- Damage to the brain and nervous system
- Behavior and learning problems (such as hyperactivity)
- Slowed growth
- Hearing problems
- Headaches

Lead is also harmful to adults. Adults can suffer from:

- Difficulties during pregnancy
- Other reproductive problems (in both men and women)
- High blood pressure
- Digestive problems
- Nerve disorders
- Memory and concentration problems
- Muscle and joint pain

Where Lead Is Found

- *Paint:* In general, the older your home, the more likely it has lead-based paint. Many homes built before 1978 have lead-based paint. The federal government banned lead-based paint from housing in 1978. Some states stopped its use even earlier. Lead can be found:

- In homes in the city, country, or suburbs.
- In apartments, single-family homes, and both private and public housing.
- Inside and outside of the house.
- *In soil around a home.* (Soil can pick up lead from exterior paint, or other sources such as past use of leaded gas in cars.)
- *Household dust.* (Dust can pick up lead from deteriorating lead-based paint or from soil tracked into a home.)
- *Drinking water.* Your home might have plumbing with lead or lead solder. Call your local health department or water supplier to find out about testing your water. You cannot see, smell, or taste lead, and boiling your water will not get rid of lead. If you think your plumbing might have lead in it:
  - Use only cold water for drinking and cooking.
  - Run water for 15 to 30 seconds before drinking it, especially if you have not used your water for a few hours.
- *The job.* If you work with lead, you could bring it home on your hands or clothes. Shower and change clothes before coming home. Launder your work clothes separately from the rest of your family's clothes.
- *Old painted toys and furniture.*
- *Food and liquids* stored in lead crystal or lead-glazed pottery or porcelain.
- *Lead smelters* or other industries that release lead into the air.
- *Hobbies* that use lead, such as making pottery or stained glass, or refinishing furniture.
- *Folk remedies* that contain lead, such as greta and azarcon used to treat an upset stomach.

Where Lead Is Likely to Be a Hazard

Lead from paint chips, which you can see, and lead dust, which you can't always see, can be serious hazards. Peeling, chipping, chalking, or cracking lead-based paint is a hazard and needs immediate attention. Lead-based paint may also be a hazard when found on surfaces that children can chew or that get a lot of wear-and-tear. These areas include:

- Windows and window sills.
- Doors and door frames.
- Stairs, railings, and banisters.
- Porches and fences.

Note: Lead-based paint that is in good condition is usually not a hazard.

Lead dust can form when lead-based paint is dry scraped, dry sanded, or heated. Dust also forms when painted surfaces bump or rub together. Lead chips and dust can get on surfaces and objects that people touch. Settled lead dust can re-enter the air when people vacuum, sweep, or walk through it.

Lead in soil can be a hazard when children play in bare soil or when people bring soil into the house on their shoes. Contact the National Lead Information Center (NLIC) to find out about testing soil for lead.

Checking Your Family and Home for Lead

Get your children and home tested if you think your home has high levels of lead. Just knowing that a home has lead-based paint may not tell you if there is a hazard. To reduce your child's exposure to lead, get your child checked, have your home tested (especially if your home has paint in poor condition and was built before 1978), and fix any hazards you may have.

Your Family

Children's blood lead levels tend to increase rapidly from 6 to 12 months of age, and tend to peak at 18 to 24 months of age. Consult your doctor for advice on testing your children. A simple blood test can detect high levels of lead. Blood tests are important for:

- Children at ages 1 and 2.
- Children and other family members who have been exposed to high levels of lead.

270

- Children who should be tested under your state or local health screening plan.

Your doctor can explain what the test results mean and if more testing will be needed.

Your Home

You can get your home checked in one of two ways, or both:

- A paint inspection tells you the lead content of every different type of painted surface in your home. It won't tell you whether the paint is a hazard or how you should deal with it.

- A risk assessment tells you if there are any sources of serious lead exposure (such as peeling paint and lead dust). It also tells you what actions to take to address these hazards.

Have qualified professionals do the work. There are standards in place for certifying lead-based paint professionals to ensure the work is done safely, reliably, and effectively. Contact the National Lead Information Center (NLIC) for a list of contacts in your area.

Trained professionals use a range of methods when checking your home, including:

- Visual inspection of paint condition and location.
- A portable x-ray fluorescence (XRF) machine.
- Lab tests of paint samples.
- Surface dust tests.

Note: Home test kits for lead are available, but studies suggest that they are not always accurate. Consumers should not rely on these tests before doing renovations or to assure safety.

What You Can do to Protect Your Family

If you suspect that your house has lead hazards, you can take some immediate steps to reduce your family's risk.

- If you rent, notify your landlord of peeling or chipping paint.
- Clean up paint chips immediately.
- Clean floors, window frames, window sills, and other surfaces weekly. Use a mop, sponge, or paper towel with warm water and

a general all-purpose cleaner or a cleaner made specifically for lead. Remember: **Never mix ammonia and bleach products together since they can form a dangerous gas.**

- Thoroughly rinse sponges and mop heads after cleaning dirty or dusty areas.

- Wash children's hands often, especially before they eat and before nap time and bed time.

- Keep play areas clean. Wash bottles, pacifiers, toys, and stuffed animals regularly.

- Keep children from chewing window sills or other painted surfaces.

- Clean or remove shoes before entering your home to avoid tracking in lead from soil.

- Make sure children eat nutritious, low-fat meals high in iron and calcium, such as spinach and dairy products. Children with good diets absorb less lead.

In addition to day-to-day cleaning and good nutrition:

- You can temporarily reduce lead hazards by taking actions such as repairing damaged painted surfaces and planting grass to cover soil with high lead levels. These actions (called interim controls) are not permanent solutions and will need ongoing attention.

- To permanently remove lead hazards, you must hire a certified lead abatement contractor. Abatement (or permanent hazard elimination) methods include removing, sealing, or enclosing lead-based paint with special materials. Just painting over the hazard with regular paint is not enough.

- Always hire a person with special training for correcting lead problems—someone who knows how to do this work safely and has the proper equipment to clean up thoroughly. Certified contractors will employ qualified workers and follow strict safety rules set by their state or the federal government.

- Contact the National Lead Information Center (NLIC) for help with locating certified contractors in your area and to see if financial assistance is available.

Are You Planning to Buy or Rent a Home Built before 1978?

Many houses and apartments built before 1978 have paint that contains lead (called lead-based paint). Lead from paint, chips, and dust can pose serious health hazards if not taken care of properly.

Federal law requires that individuals receive certain information before renting or buying a pre-1978 housing:

Residential Lead-Based Paint Disclosure Program

Landlords have to disclose known information on lead-based paint and lead-based paint hazards before leases take effect. Leases must include a disclosure form about lead-based paint.

Sellers have to disclose known information on lead-based paint and lead-based paint hazards before selling a house. Sales contracts must include a disclosure form about lead-based paint. Buyers have up to 10 days to check for lead hazards.

Remodeling or Renovating a Home with Lead-Based Paint

If not conducted properly, certain types of renovations can release lead from paint and dust into the air. Many houses and apartments built before 1978 have paint that contains lead (called lead-based paint). Lead from paint, chips, and dust can pose serious health hazards if not taken care of properly.

Federal law requires that contractors provide lead information to residents before renovating a pre-1978 housing:

- Pre-Renovation Education Program (PRE)

- Renovators have to give you a pamphlet titled "Protect Your Family from Lead in Your Home," before starting work.

Take precautions before your contractor or you begin remodeling or renovations that disturb painted surfaces (such as scraping off paint or tearing out walls):

- Have the area tested for lead-based paint.

- Do not use a belt-sander, propane torch, heat gun, dry scraper, or dry sandpaper to remove lead-based paint. These actions create large amounts of lead dust and fumes.

- Lead dust can remain in your home long after the work is done.

- Temporarily move your family (especially children and pregnant women) out of the apartment or house until the work is done and the area is properly cleaned. If you can't move your family, at least completely seal off the work area.

- Follow other safety measures to reduce lead hazards. You can find out about other safety measures in the EPA brochure titled "Reducing Lead Hazards When Remodeling Your Home." This brochure explains what to do before, during, and after renovations.

- If you have already completed renovations or remodeling that could have released lead-based paint or dust, get your young children tested and follow the steps outlined to protect your family.

Chapter 33

Health Hazards of Malathion

Uses

Malathion is an organophosphate (OP) insecticide used on a variety of agricultural food and feed crops. There are nonagricultural uses on commodities such as Christmas trees and agricultural premises.

Malathion has registered residential uses on lawns, gardens, and ornamental trees, shrubs, and plants.

Malathion is also used for public health mosquito control, and in government programs such as the USDA Boll Weevil Eradication Program.

Malathion is applied by many methods, such as aircraft (fixed wing), duster, fogger, helicopter, irrigation, shaker can, shovel, sprayer, and spreader.

Approximately 16.7 million pounds of active ingredient are used annually, most of which is applied to cotton in the Boll Weevil Eradication Program (11.2 million pounds).

Health Effects

As with all OPs, malathion is a cholinesterase inhibitor. Cholinesterase inhibition in humans can overstimulate the nervous system

---

"Malathion Summary," a fact sheet produced by the U.S. Environmental Protection Agency (EPA), 2000. Available online at http://www.epa.gov/pesticides/op/malathion/summary.htm.

causing nausea, dizziness, confusion, and, at very high exposures (e.g. accidents, major spills), respiratory paralysis and death.

Risks

Dietary Risk

The dietary risk from food treated with malathion is low and not of concern.

Drinking Water Risks

Acute and chronic exposure from surface and ground drinking water sources are low and not of concern.

Surface drinking water concentrations are based on modeling estimates, and ground drinking water concentrations are based on limited monitoring data.

Residential Risks

Adult applicator exposure and toddler post-application exposure to turf treatments are of risk concern. All other home and garden uses are not of risk concern.

Bystander risks from public health mosquito control and the USDA Boll Weevil Eradication Program are low and not of concern.

Aggregate Dietary Risk

Aggregate acute and chronic risk (food and water) are not of concern. There are a few residential uses of malathion for which the Agency has risk concerns (i.e., application and post-application exposure to turf treatments). These residential uses pose problems when combined with food and drinking water exposure.

Aggregate risk from dietary (food and water) and residential bystander pathways (from public health mosquito abatement control and the Boll Weevil Eradication Program) are low and not of concern.

Worker Risks

Risks to mixers/loaders/applicators are not of concern with some additional personal protective equipment (PPE) or engineering controls.

The current restricted entry interval (REI) of 12 hours is not sufficiently protective for most reentry scenarios. For some post-application activities, the REI is as high as 6 days.

Ecological Risks

Risks to birds and mammals are low from acute dietary exposure.

Chronic exposure to birds and mammals is low, but there could be concern if maximum rates and shortest application intervals are used. There is concern for acute and chronic risk to fish and aquatic invertebrates.

Drift from ultra low volume (ULV) applications and the fate of the degradate malaoxon in the environment are of concern.

How the Risk Picture May Change

At this time, the Agency does not anticipate that the risk assessments will change significantly.

Chapter 34

Health Hazards of Mercury

How Mercury Harms Humans

Elemental (metallic) mercury and its compounds are toxic and exposure to excessive levels can permanently damage or fatally injure the brain and kidneys. Elemental mercury can also be absorbed through the skin and cause allergic reactions. Ingestion of inorganic mercury compounds can cause severe renal and gastrointestinal toxicity. Organic compounds of mercury such as methyl mercury are considered the most toxic forms of the element. Exposures to very small amounts of these compounds can result in devastating neurological damage and death.

For fetuses, infants and children, the primary health effects of mercury are on neurological development. Even low levels of mercury exposure such as result from mother's consumption methyl-mercury in dietary sources can adversely affect the brain and nervous system. Impacts on memory, attention, language and other skills have been found in children exposed to moderate levels in the womb.

How People Get Exposed to Mercury

Metallic mercury slowly evaporates when exposed to the air. The air in a room can reach contamination levels just from the mercury

"Mercury Health Hazards," a fact sheet produced by the Division of Safety, Office of Research Services (ORS), National Institutes of Health (NIH). Reviewed and updated by the NIH in April, 2001. Available online at http://www.nih.gov/od/ors/ds/nomercury/health.htm.

in a broken thermometer. Air borne mercury is highly toxic when inhaled.

Mercury may be released into the air when coal, oil, or wood are burned as fuel or when mercury-containing wastes are incinerated. The resulting mercury concentrations in outdoor air are usually low and of little direct concern. However, mercury in the air can fall to the ground with rain and snow, landing on soil or in bodies of water, causing contamination. Lakes and rivers are also contaminated when there is a direct discharge of mercury-laden industrial or municipal waste into the water.

When mercury enters bodies of water, biological processes transform it to methyl-mercury, a highly toxic and bioaccumulative form. Fish can absorb methyl-mercury from their food and directly from water as it passes over their gills. The cycle of mercury in nature is complex. Methyl-mercury accumulates at the higher levels of the food chain and becomes concentrated in fish and animals that eat fish.

1. Methyl-mercury in the water and sediment is taken up by tiny animals and plants known as plankton.

2. Minnows and juvenile fish eat large quantities of plankton over time.

3. Larger predatory fish consume many smaller fish, accumulating methyl-mercury in their tissues. The older and larger the fish, the greater the potential for high mercury levels in their bodies.

4. Fish are caught and eaten by humans and animals, causing methyl-mercury to accumulate in human tissues.

Most people are exposed to mercury by eating fish containing mercury. Since mercury is tightly bound to proteins in all fish tissue, including muscle, there is no method of cooking or cleaning them that will reduce the amount of mercury in a meal.

From the mid-1950s to the 1970s, several mass poisonings took place in Japan and in Canada involving methyl-mercury from consumption of fish from contaminated waters. Although instances of poisoning from fish consumption in the U.S. have not been reported, the possibility of such poisoning has been a subject of concern. In the U.S., the number of states that have issued health advisories limiting consumption of fish has risen steadily from 27 states in 1993 to 41 states in 1999.

Currently, concern is focused on the health impacts of chronic exposures to low levels of mercury from dietary sources. Preliminary estimates of mercury levels in hair and blood samples from the 1999 National Health and Nutrition Examination Survey suggest that approximately 10% of women have mercury levels within one tenth of potentially hazardous levels indicating a narrow margin of safety for some women. The National Research Council (NRC) issued a report estimating that as many as 60,000 newborns a year in the U.S. are now at risk for adverse neurodevelopmental effects from dietary mercury. These studies strongly support efforts to reduce methylmercury exposure.

Occupational Health Hazards in Biomedical Facilities

The most common potential mode of occupational exposure to mercury in biomedical facilities is probably via inhalation of vapors. If not cleaned up properly, spills of even small amounts of elemental mercury, such as may result from breakage of thermometers, can contaminate indoor air above recommended limits and lead to serious health consequences.

Some organic mercury compounds such as methyl-mercury, find limited use in biomedical research procedures such as gel electrophoresis and as a reference in nuclear magnetic spectroscopy. At least two fatal exposures have occurred in laboratories. The most recently reported incident involved a chemistry professor with an interest in the toxicology of heavy metals. During an experiment performed in a fume hood, she accidentally spilled several drops of methyl-mercury onto a gloved hand. The spill was considered inconsequential and cleaned up without special measures. Approximately two months later, the professor began to develop symptoms of neurotoxicity. She died despite receiving aggressive chelation therapy and medical support.

Chapter 35

Pesticides

What Is a Pesticide?

A pesticide is any substance or mixture of substances intended for preventing, destroying, repelling, or mitigating any pest. Pests can be insects, mice and other animals, unwanted plants (weeds), fungi, or microorganisms like bacteria and viruses. Though often misunderstood to refer only to insecticides, the term pesticide also applies to herbicides, fungicides, and various other substances used to control pests. Under United States law, a pesticide is also any substance or mixture of substances intended for use as a plant regulator, defoliant, or desiccant.

Many household products are pesticides. Did you know that all of these common products are considered pesticides?

- Cockroach sprays and baits.
- Insect repellents for personal use.
- Rat and other rodent poisons.

Text in this chapter is from "What Is a Pesticide," an undated fact sheet produced by the Environmental Protection Agency (EPA), available online at http:// www.epa.gov/pesticides/whatis.htm, cited February 2003; "What Are Antimicrobial Pesticides?" an undated fact sheet produced by the EPA, available online at http://www.epa.gov/oppad001/ad_info.htm, cited February 2003; "What Are Biopesticides?" an undated fact sheet produced by EPA, available online at http://www.epa.gov/pesticides/biopesticides/what_are_biopesticides.htm, cited February 2003; and "Larvicides For Mosquito Control," a fact sheet produced by EPA, 2002, available online at http://www.epa.gov/pesticides/citizens/ larvicides4mosquitos.htm

- Flea and tick sprays, powders, and pet collars.
- Kitchen, laundry, and bath disinfectants and sanitizers.
- Products that kill mold and mildew.
- Some lawn and garden products, such as weed killers.
- Some swimming pool chemicals.

By their very nature, most pesticides create some risk of harm to humans, animals, or the environment because they are designed to kill or otherwise adversely affect living organisms. At the same time, pesticides are useful to society because of their ability to kill potential disease-causing organisms and control insects, weeds, and other pests. In the United States, the Office of Pesticide Programs of the Environmental Protection Agency is chiefly responsible for regulating pesticides. Biologically-based pesticides, such as pheromones and microbial pesticides, are becoming increasingly popular and often are safer than traditional chemical pesticides.

Here are some common kinds of pesticides and their function:

- *Algicides:* Control algae in lakes, canals, swimming pools, water tanks, and other sites.

- *Antifouling agents:* Kill or repel organisms that attach to underwater surfaces, such as boat bottoms.

- *Antimicrobials:* Kill microorganisms (such as bacteria and viruses).

- *Attractants:* Attract pests (for example, to lure an insect or rodent to a trap). (However, food is not considered a pesticide when used as an attractant.)

- *Biocides:* Kill microorganisms.

- *Disinfectants and sanitizers:* Kill or inactivate disease-producing microorganisms on inanimate objects.

- *Fungicides:* Kill fungi (including blights, mildews, molds, and rusts).

- *Fumigants:* Produce gas or vapor intended to destroy pests in buildings or soil.

- *Herbicides:* Kill weeds and other plants that grow where they are not wanted.

- *Insecticides:* Kill insects and other arthropods.

- *Miticides (also called acaricides):* Kill mites that feed on plants and animals.

- *Microbial pesticides:* Microorganisms that kill, inhibit, or out compete pests, including insects or other microorganisms.

- *Molluscicides:* Kill snails and slugs.

- *Nematicides:* Kill nematodes (microscopic, worm-like organisms that feed on plant roots).

- *Ovicides:* Kill eggs of insects and mites.

- *Pheromones:* Biochemicals used to disrupt the mating behavior of insects.

- *Repellents:* Repel pests, including insects (such as mosquitoes) and birds.

- *Rodenticides:* Control mice and other rodents.

The term pesticide also includes these substances:

- *Defoliants:* Cause leaves or other foliage to drop from a plant, usually to facilitate harvest.

- *Desiccants:* Promote drying of living tissues, such as unwanted plant tops.

- *Insect growth regulators:* Disrupt the molting, maturity from pupal stage to adult, or other life processes of insects.

- *Plant growth regulators:* Substances (excluding fertilizers or other plant nutrients) that alter the expected growth, flowering, or reproduction rate of plants.

What about pest control devices?

EPA also has a role in regulating devices used to control pests. More specifically, a device is any instrument or contrivance (other than a firearm) intended for trapping, destroying, repelling, or mitigating any pest. A black light trap is an example of a device. Unlike pesticides, EPA does not require devices to be registered with the Agency. Devices are subject to certain labeling, packaging, record keeping, and import/export requirements, however.

What is not a pesticide?

The U.S. definition of pesticides is quite broad, but it does have some exclusions:

- Drugs used to control diseases of humans or animals (such as livestock and pets) are not considered pesticides; such drugs are regulated by the Food and Drug Administration.

- Fertilizers, nutrients, and other substances used to promote plant survival and health are not considered plant growth regulators and thus are not pesticides.

- Biological control agents, except for certain microorganisms, are exempted from regulation by EPA. (Biological control agents include beneficial predators such as birds or ladybugs that eat insect pests.)

- Products which contain certain low-risk ingredients, such as garlic and mint oil, have been exempted from Federal registration requirements, although State regulatory requirements may still apply. For a list of ingredients which may be exempt, and a discussion of allowable label claims for such products, see EPA's Pesticide Registration Notice 2000-6, "Minimum Risk Pesticides Exempted under FIFRA Section 25(b)."

What Are Antimicrobial Pesticides?

Antimicrobial pesticides, such as disinfectants and sanitizers, are pesticides that are intended to "(i) disinfect, sanitize, reduce, or mitigate growth or development of microbiological organisms; or (ii) protect inanimate objects (for example floors and walls), industrial processes or systems, surfaces, water, or other chemical substances from contamination, fouling, or deterioration caused by bacteria, viruses, fungi, protozoa, algae, or slime." This category does not include certain pesticides intended for food use; but does encompass pesticides with a wide array of other uses. For example, antimicrobial pesticides act as preserving agents in paints, metalworking fluids, wood supports, and many other products to prevent their deterioration.

Antimicrobials are especially important because many are public health pesticides. They help to control microorganisms (viruses, bacteria, and other microorganisms) that can cause human disease. Antimicrobial public health pesticides are used as disinfectants in medical settings, where they are present in products used in cleaning cabinets, floors, walls, toilets, and other surfaces. Proper use of these disinfectants is an important part of infection control activities employed by hospitals and other medical establishments.

What Are Biopesticides?

Biopesticides are certain types of pesticides derived from such natural materials as animals, plants, bacteria, and certain minerals. For example, canola oil and baking soda have pesticidal applications and are considered biopesticides. At the end of 2001, there were approximately 195 registered biopesticide active ingredients and 780 products. Biopesticides fall into three major classes:

(1) Microbial pesticides consist of a microorganism (e.g., a bacterium, fungus, virus or protozoan) as the active ingredient. Microbial pesticides can control many different kinds of pests, although each separate active ingredient is relatively specific for its target pest[s]. For example, there are fungi that control certain weeds, and other fungi that kill specific insects.

The most widely used microbial pesticides are subspecies and strains of *Bacillus thuringiensis*, or *Bt*. Each strain of this bacterium produces a different mix of proteins, and specifically kills one or a few related species of insect larvae. While some *Bt*s control moth larvae found on plants, other *Bt*s are specific for larvae of flies and mosquitoes. The target insect species are determined by whether the particular *Bt* produces a protein that can bind to a larval gut receptor, thereby causing the insect larvae to starve.

(2) Plant-Incorporated-Protectants (PIPs) are pesticidal substances that plants produce from genetic material that has been added to the plant. For example, scientists can take the gene for the *Bt* pesticidal protein, and introduce the gene into the plant's own genetic material. Then the plant, instead of the *Bt* bacterium, manufactures the substance that destroys the pest. The protein and its genetic material, but not the plant itself, are regulated by EPA.

(3) Biochemical pesticides are naturally occurring substances that control pests by non-toxic mechanisms. Conventional pesticides, by contrast, are generally synthetic materials that directly kill or inactivate the pest. Biochemical pesticides include

substances, such as insect sex pheromones, that interfere with mating, as well as various scented plant extracts that attract insect pests to traps. Because it is sometimes difficult to determine whether a substance meets the criteria for classification as a biochemical pesticide, EPA has established a special committee to make such decisions.

What are the advantages of using biopesticides?

Biopesticides are usually inherently less toxic than conventional pesticides. Biopesticides generally affect only the target pest and closely related organisms, in contrast to broad spectrum, conventional pesticides that may affect organisms as different as birds, insects, and mammals. Biopesticides often are effective in very small quantities and often decompose quickly, thereby resulting in lower exposures and largely avoiding the pollution problems caused by conventional pesticides.

When used as a component of Integrated Pest Management (IPM) programs, biopesticides can greatly decrease the use of conventional pesticides, while crop yields remain high. To use biopesticides effectively, however, users need to know a great deal about managing pests.

How does EPA encourage the development and use of biopesticides?

In 1994, the Biopesticides and Pollution Prevention Division was established in the Office of Pesticide Programs to facilitate the registration of biopesticides. This Division promotes the use of safer pesticides, including biopesticides, as components of IPM programs. The Division also coordinates the Pesticide Environmental Stewardship Program (PESP). Since biopesticides tend to pose fewer risks than conventional pesticides, EPA generally requires much less data to register a biopesticide than to register a conventional pesticide. In fact, new biopesticides are often registered in less than a year, compared with an average of more than 3 years for conventional pesticides.

While biopesticides require less data and are registered in less time than conventional pesticides, EPA always conducts rigorous reviews to ensure that pesticides will not have adverse effects on human health or the environment. For EPA to be sure that a pesticide is safe, the Agency requires that registrants submit a variety of data about the composition, toxicity, degradation, and other characteristics of the pesticide.

Larvicides for Mosquito Control

The Environmental Protection Agency (EPA) evaluates and registers (licenses) pesticides to ensure that they can be used safely. These pesticides include products used in the mosquito control programs that states and communities have established. To evaluate any pesticide, EPA assesses a wide variety of tests to determine whether a pesticide has the potential to cause adverse effects on humans, wildlife, fish and plants, including endangered species and non-target organisms.

Officials responsible for mosquito control programs make decisions to use pesticides based on an evaluation of the risks to the general public from diseases transmitted by mosquitoes or on an evaluation of the nuisance level that communities can tolerate from a mosquito infestation. Based on surveillance and monitoring, mosquito control officials select specific pesticides and other control measures that best suit local conditions in order to achieve effective control of mosquitoes with the least impact on human health and the environment. It is especially important to conduct effective mosquito prevention programs by eliminating breeding habitats or applying pesticides to control the early life stages of the mosquito. Prevention programs, such as elimination of any standing water that could serve as a breeding site, help reduce the adult mosquito population and the need to apply other pesticides for adult mosquito control. Since no pesticide can be considered 100 percent safe, pesticide applicators and the general public should always exercise care and follow specified safety precautions during use to reduce risks.

What is the mosquito life cycle?

The mosquito goes through four distinct stages during its life cycle:

* egg—hatches when exposed to water;
* larva (plural = larvae)—lives in the water; molts several times; most species surface to breathe air;
* pupa (plural = pupae)—does not feed; stage just prior to emerging as adult;
* adult—flies short time after emerging and after its body parts have hardened.

289

What are larvicides?

Larvicides kill mosquito larvae. Larvicides include biological insecticides, such as the microbial larvicides *Bacillus sphaericus* and *Bacillus thuringiensis israelensis*. Larvicides include other pesticides, such as temephos, methoprene, oils, and monomolecular films. Larvicide treatment of breeding habitats help reduce the adult mosquito population in nearby areas.

How are larvicides used in mosquito control?

State and local agencies in charge of mosquito control typically employ a variety of techniques in an Integrated Pest Management (IPM) program. An IPM approach includes surveillance, source reduction, larviciding and adulticiding to control mosquito populations. Since mosquitoes must have water to breed, source reduction can be as simple as turning over trapped water in a container to undertaking large-scale engineering and management of marsh water levels. Larviciding involves applying pesticides to breeding habitats to kill mosquito larvae. Larviciding can reduce overall pesticide usage in a control program. Killing mosquito larvae before they emerge as adults can reduce or eliminate the need for ground or aerial application of pesticides to kill adult mosquitoes.

What are microbial larvicides?

Microbial larvicides are bacteria that are registered as pesticides for control of mosquito larvae in outdoor areas such as irrigation ditches, flood water, standing ponds, woodland pools, pastures, tidal water, fresh or saltwater marshes, and storm water retention areas. Duration of effectiveness depends primarily on the mosquito species, the environmental conditions, the formulation of the product, and water quality. Microbial larvicides may be used along with other mosquito control measures in an IPM program. The microbial larvicides used for mosquito control are *Bacillus thuringiensis israelensis* (*Bti*) and *Bacillus sphaericus* (*B. sphaericus*).

Bacillus thuringiensis israelensis is a naturally occurring soil bacterium registered for control of mosquito larvae. *Bti* was first registered by EPA as an insecticide in 1983. Mosquito larvae eat the *Bti* product that is made up of the dormant spore form of the bacterium and an associated pure toxin. The toxin disrupts the gut in the mosquito by binding to receptor cells present in insects, but not in mammals. There are 26 *Bti* products registered for use in the United States.

Aquabac, Teknar, Vectobac, and LarvX are examples of common trade names for the mosquito control products.

Bacillus sphaericus is a naturally occurring bacterium that is found throughout the world. *B. sphaericus* was initially registered by EPA in 1991 for use against various kinds of mosquito larvae. Mosquito larvae ingest the bacteria, and as with *Bti*, the toxin disrupts the gut in the mosquito by binding to receptor cells present in insects but not in mammals. VectoLex CG and WDG are registered *B. sphaericus* products and are effective for approximately one to four weeks after application.

Do microbial larvicides pose risks to human health?

The microbial pesticides have undergone extensive testing prior to registration. They are essentially nontoxic to humans, so there are no concerns for human health effects with *Bti* or *B. sphaericus* when they are used according to label directions.

Do microbial larvicides pose risks to wildlife or the environment?

Extensive testing shows that microbial larvicides do not pose risks to wildlife, nontarget species, or the environment, when used according to label directions.

What is methoprene?

Methoprene is a compound first registered by EPA in 1975 that mimics the action of an insect growth-regulating hormone and prevents the normal maturation of insect larvae. It is applied to water to kill mosquito larvae, and it may be used along with other mosquito control measures in an IPM program. Altosid is the name of the methoprene product used in mosquito control and is applied as briquets (similar in form to charcoal briquets), pellets, sand granules, and liquids. The liquid and pelletized formulations can be applied by helicopter and fixed-wing aircraft.

Does methoprene pose risks to human health?

Methoprene, used for mosquito control according to its label directions, does not pose unreasonable risks to human health. In addition to posing low toxicity to mammals, there is little opportunity for human exposure, since the material is applied directly to ditches, ponds, marshes, or flooded areas that are not drinking water sources.

Does methoprene pose risks to wildlife or the environment?

Methoprene used in mosquito control programs does not pose unreasonable risks to wildlife or the environment. Toxicity of methoprene to birds and fish is low, and it is nontoxic to bees. Methoprene breaks down quickly in water and soil and will not leach into ground water. Methoprene mosquito control products present minimal acute and chronic risk to freshwater fish, freshwater invertebrates, and estuarine species.

What is temephos?

Temephos is an organophosphate (OP) pesticide registered by EPA in 1965 to control mosquito larvae, and it is the only organophosphate with larvicidal use. It is an important resistance management tool for mosquito control programs; its use helps prevent mosquitoes from developing resistance to the bacterial larvicides. Temephos is used in areas of standing water, shallow ponds, swamps, marshes, and intertidal zones. It may be used along with other mosquito control measures in an IPM program. Abate is the trade name of the temephos product used for mosquito control. Temephos is applied most commonly by helicopter but can be applied by backpack sprayers, fixed-wing aircraft, and right-of-way sprayers in either liquid or granular form.

Does temephos pose risks to human health?

Temephos, applied according to the label for mosquito control, does not pose unreasonable risks to human health. It is applied to water, and the amount of temephos is very small in relation to the area covered, less than 1 ounce of active ingredient per acre for the liquid and 8 ounces per acre for the granular formulations. Temephos breaks down within a few days in water, and post-application exposure is minimal. However, at high dosages, temephos, like other OPs, can overstimulate the nervous system causing nausea, dizziness, and confusion.

Does temephos pose risks to wildlife or the environment?

Because temephos is applied directly to water, it is not expected to have a direct impact on terrestrial animals or birds. Current mosquito larviciding techniques pose some risk to nontarget aquatic species and the aquatic ecosystem. Although temephos presents relatively low risk to birds and terrestrial species, available information suggests that it is more toxic to aquatic invertebrates than alternative larvicides.

For this reason, EPA is limiting temephos use to areas where less-hazardous alternatives would not be effective, specifying intervals between applications, and limiting the use of high application rates.

What is the current regulatory status of temephos?

As part of its responsibility to reassess all older pesticides registered before 1984, EPA completed its revised risk assessments for temephos in July 2001, and has issued risk management decisions in the final re-registration eligibility decision (RED). The RED document is available on the EPA Web site at: www.epa.gov/oppsrrd1/REDs/temephos_red.htm.

What are monomolecular films?

Monomolecular films are low-toxicity pesticides that spread a thin film on the surface of the water that makes it difficult for mosquito larvae, pupae, and emerging adults to attach to the water's surface, causing them to drown. Films may remain active typically for 10-14 days on standing water, and have been used in the United States in floodwaters, brackish waters, and ponds. They may be used along with other mosquito control measures in an IPM program. They are also known under the trade names Arosurf MSF and Agnique MMF.

Do monomolecular films pose risks to human health?

Monomolecular films, used according to label directions for larva and pupa control, do not pose a risk to human health. In addition to low toxicity, there is little opportunity for human exposure, since the material is applied directly to ditches, ponds, marshes, or flooded areas that are not drinking water sources.

Do films pose risks to wildlife or the environment?

Monomolecular films, used according to label directions for larva and pupa control, pose minimal risks to the environment. They do not last very long in the environment, and are usually applied only to standing water, such as roadside ditches, woodland pools, or containers which contain few nontarget organisms.

What are oils?

Oils, like films, are pesticides used to form a coating on top of water to drown larvae, pupae, and emerging adult mosquitoes. They are specially derived from petroleum distillates and have been used for many years in the United States to kill aphids on crops and orchard trees, and to control mosquitoes. They may be used along with other mosquito control measures in an IPM program. Trade names for oils used in mosquito control are Bonide, BVA2, and Golden Bear-1111, (GB-1111).

Do oils pose risks to human health?

Oils, used according to label directions for larva and pupa control, do not pose a risk to human health. In addition to low toxicity, there is little opportunity for human exposure, since the material is applied directly to ditches, ponds, marshes, or flooded areas that are not drinking water sources.

Do oils pose risks to wildlife or the environment?

Oils, if misapplied, may be toxic to fish and other aquatic organisms. For that reason, EPA has established specific precautions on the label to reduce such risks.

Chapter 36

Protecting People Who Work with Pesticides

Basic Principles of the Worker Protection Standard

The 1992 Worker Protection Standard protects over three and a half million people who work with pesticides at over 560,000 workplaces. The Worker Protection Standard represents a major strengthening of national efforts to safeguard the health of agricultural workers and pesticide handlers. Effective implementation of the WPS will substantially lower the risk of pesticide poisonings among agricultural workers and pesticide handlers.

Summary of WPS Requirements

Protection during applications: Applicators are prohibited from applying a pesticide in a way that will expose workers or other persons. Workers are excluded from areas while pesticides are being applied.

Restricted-entry intervals: Restricted-entry intervals must be specified on all agricultural plant pesticide product labels. Workers are excluded from entering a pesticide treated area during the restricted entry interval, with only narrow exceptions.

"Basic Principles of the Worker Protection Standard," and "Worker Safety and Training: Who and What Are Covered?" undated fact sheets produced by the U.S. Environmental Protection Agency (EPA), available online at http://www.epa.gpv/oppfead1/safety/workers, cited February 2003.

295

Personal protective equipment: Personal protective equipment must be provided and maintained for handlers and early-entry workers.

Notification of workers: Workers must be notified about treated areas so they may avoid inadvertent exposures.

Decontamination supplies: Handlers and workers must have an ample supply of water, soap, and towels for routine washing and emergency decontamination.

Emergency assistance: Transportation must be made available to a medical care facility if a worker or handler may have been poisoned or injured. Information must be provided about the pesticide to which the person may have been exposed.

Pesticide safety training and safety posters: Training is required for all workers and handlers, and a pesticide safety poster must be displayed.

Access to labeling and site specific information: Handlers and workers must be informed of pesticide label requirements. Central posting of recent pesticide applications is required.

Who and What Are Covered?

The Worker Protection Standard protects employees on farms, forests, nurseries, and greenhouses from occupational exposure to agricultural pesticides. The regulation covers two types of employees:

Pesticide handlers—those who mix, load, or apply agricultural pesticides; clean or repair pesticide application equipment; or assist with the application of pesticides in any way.

Agricultural workers—those who perform tasks related to the cultivation and harvesting of plants on farms or in greenhouses, nurseries, or forests. Workers include anyone employed for any type of compensation (including self-employed) doing tasks, such as carrying nursery stock, repotting plants, or watering, related to the production of agricultural plants on an agricultural establishment.

Workers do not include such employees as office employees, truck drivers, mechanics, and any other workers not engaged in worker/

handler activities. Some requirements do, however, apply to all persons; and some requirements apply to anyone who handles pesticide application equipment or cleans or launders pesticide-contaminated personal protective equipment.

The WPS does not apply when pesticides are applied on an agricultural establishment in the following circumstances:

- For mosquito abatement, Mediterranean fruit fly eradication, or similar wide-area public pest control programs sponsored by governmental entities. The WPS does apply to cooperative programs in which the growers themselves make or arrange for pesticide applications.

- On livestock or other animals, or in or about animal premises.

- On plants grown for other than commercial or research purposes, which may include plants in habitations, home fruit and vegetable gardens, and home greenhouses.

- On plants that are in ornamental gardens, parks, and public or private lawns and grounds that are intended only for aesthetic purposes or climatic modification.

- By injection directly into agricultural plants. Direct injection does not include "hack and squirt," "frill and spray," chemigation, soil-incorporation, or soil-injection.

- In a manner not directly related to the production of agricultural plants, such as structural pest control, control of vegetation along rights-of-way and in other noncrop areas, and pasture and rangeland use.

- For control of vertebrate pests.

- As attractants or repellents in traps.

- On the harvested portions of agricultural plants or on harvested timber.

- For research uses of unregistered pesticides.

Chapter 37

Pesticides and Mosquito Control

Mosquito-borne diseases affect millions of people worldwide each year. In the United States, some species of mosquitoes can transmit diseases such as encephalitis, dengue fever, and malaria to humans, and a variety of diseases to wildlife and domestic animals. To combat mosquitoes and the public health hazards they present, many states and localities have established mosquito control programs. These programs, which are based on surveillance, can include nonchemical forms of prevention and control as well as ground and aerial application of chemical and biological pesticides.

The mission of the Environmental Protection Agency (EPA) is to protect human health and the environment. EPA reviews and approves pesticides and their labeling to ensure that the pesticides used to protect public health are applied by methods that minimize the risk of human exposure and adverse health and environmental effects. In relation to mosquito control, the Agency also serves as a source of information about pesticide and nonpesticide controls to address the concerns of the general public, news media, and the state and local agencies dealing with outbreaks of infectious diseases or heavy infestations of mosquitoes. The following questions and answers provide some basic information on mosquito control, safety precautions, and information on insecticides used for mosquito control programs.

"Pesticides and Mosquito Control," a fact sheet produced by the U.S. Environmental Protection Agency (EPA), 2002. Available online at http://www.epa. gov/pesticides/citizens/pesticides4mosquitos.htm.

How does EPA ensure the safest possible use of pesticides?

EPA must evaluate and register pesticides before they may be sold, distributed, or used in the United States. The Agency is also in the process of reassessing, and reregistering when appropriate, all older pesticides (those registered prior to 1984) to ensure that they meet current scientific standards. To evaluate a pesticide for either registration or re-registration, EPA assesses a wide variety of potential human health and environmental effects associated with use of the product. The producer of the pesticide must provide data from tests done according to EPA guidelines. These tests determine whether a pesticide has the potential to cause adverse effects on humans, wildlife, fish, and plants, including endangered species and non-target organisms. Other tests help to assess the risks of contaminating surface water or ground water from leaching, runoff, or spray drift. If a pesticide meets EPA requirements, the pesticide is approved for use in accordance with label directions. However, no pesticide is 100 percent safe and care must be exercised in the use of any pesticide.

How are mosquitoes controlled with pesticides and other methods?

The first step in mosquito control is surveillance. Mosquito specialists conduct surveillance for diseases harbored by domestic and non-native birds, including sentinel chickens (used as virus transmission indicators), and mosquitoes. Surveillance for larval habitats is conducted by using maps and aerial photographs, and by evaluating larval populations. Other techniques include various light traps, biting counts, and analysis of reports from the public. Mosquito control programs also put high priority on trying to prevent a large population of adult mosquitoes from developing so that additional controls may not be necessary. Since mosquitoes must have water to breed, methods of prevention may include controlling water levels in lakes, marshes, ditches, or other mosquito breeding sites, eliminating small breeding sites if possible, and stocking bodies of water with fish species that feed on larvae. Both chemical and biological measures may be employed to kill immature mosquitoes during larval stages. Larvicides target larvae in the breeding habitat before they can mature into adult mosquitoes and disperse. Larvicides include the bacterial insecticides *Bacillus thuringiensis israelensis* and *Bacillus sphaericus*, the insect growth inhibitor methoprene, and the organophosphate insecticide temephos. Mineral oils and other materials form a thin film on the surface of the water which cause larvae and pupae to drown. Liquid larvicide products are applied directly to water using backpack sprayers and truck or aircraft-mounted sprayers. Tablet, pellet, granular, and briquet formulations of larvicides are also applied by mosquito controllers to breeding areas.

Adult mosquito control may be undertaken to combat an outbreak of mosquito-borne disease or a very heavy nuisance infestation of mosquitoes in a community. Pesticides registered for this use are adulticides and are applied either by aircraft or on the ground employing truck-mounted sprayers. State and local agencies commonly use the organophosphate insecticides malathion and naled and the synthetic pyrethroid insecticides permethrin, resmethrin, and sumithrin for adult mosquito control.

Mosquito adulticides are applied as ultra-low volume (ULV) sprays. ULV sprayers dispense very fine aerosol droplets that stay aloft and kill flying mosquitoes on contact. ULV applications involve small quantities of pesticide active ingredient in relation to the size of the area treated, typically less than 3 ounces per acre, which minimizes exposure and risks to people and the environment.

What can I do to reduce the number of mosquitoes in and around my home?

The most important step is to eliminate potential breeding habitats for mosquitoes. Get rid of any standing water around the home, including water in potted plant dishes, garbage cans, old tires, gutters, ditches, wheelbarrows, bird baths, hollow trees, and wading pools. Any standing water should be drained, including abandoned or unused swimming pools. Mosquitoes can breed in any puddle that lasts more than 4 days. Make sure windows and screen doors are bug tight. Replace outdoor lights with yellow bug lights. Wear head nets, long-sleeved shirts, and long pants if venturing into areas with high mosquito populations, such as salt marshes or wooded areas. Use mosquito repellents when necessary, always following label instructions.

Should I take steps to reduce exposure to pesticides during mosquito control spraying?

Generally, there is no need to relocate during mosquito control spraying. The pesticides have been evaluated for this use and found to pose minimal risks to human health and the environment when used according to label directions. For example, EPA has estimated the exposure and risks to both adults and children posed by ULV aerial and ground applications of the insecticides malathion and naled. For all the exposure scenarios considered, exposures ranged from 100 to 10,000 times below an amount of pesticide that might pose a health concern. These estimates assumed several spraying events over a period of weeks, and also assumed that a toddler would ingest some soil and grass in addition to dermal exposure. Other mosquito control pesticides pose similarly low risks. Although mosquito control pesticides pose low risks, some people may prefer to avoid or further minimize exposure. Some common sense steps to help reduce possible exposure to pesticides include:

- Pay attention to the local media for announcements about spraying and remain indoors during applications in the immediate area.

- People who suffer from chemical sensitivities or feel spraying may aggravate a preexisting health condition, may consult their physician or local health department and take special measures to avoid exposure.

- Close windows and turn off window-unit air conditioners when spraying is taking place in the immediate area.

- Do not let children play near or behind truck-mounted applicators when they are in use.

Chapter 38

DEET
(N,N-Deithyl-Meta-Toluamide)

What Is DEET?

DEET (short for N,N-diethyl-meta-toluamide) is a commonly used insect repellent for several types of biting and sucking insects, including mosquitoes, files and ticks.

DEET is one of the few pesticides that can be applied to human skin or clothes.

DEET does not actually kill insects, but repels them from treated areas.

How Does DEET Work?

Even though it has been in use for over 40 years, scientists are not completely sure how DEET repels biting insects.

DEET most likely affects the insect's ability to locate animals to feed on. Scientists believe that DEET disturbs the function of special receptors in mosquito antennae that sense chemicals that are produced by humans and other animals.[1]

Reprinted with permission from "DEET: General Fact Sheet," produced by the National Pesticide Information Center (NPIC), March 2000. © National Pesticide Information Center. For the most recent version of this fact sheet, or additional information about pesticides, visit http://npic.orst.edu, or call 800-858-7378. NPIC is a cooperative effort of Oregon State University and the U.S. Environmental Protection Agency.

What Products Contain DEET?

- Aerosol products that are intended for use on human skin and clothing.

- Liquid products for human skin and clothing.

- Skin lotions.

- Impregnated materials such as towelettes, wristbands, and tablecloths.

How Toxic Is DEET?

Animals

DEET is slightly toxic to rats when ingested or applied to skin. DEET is very low in toxicity when rats breathe in the vapors.[2]

DEET does not cause permanent eye damage in rabbits, although it causes some irritation. DEET does not cause skin irritation or skin sensitization.[2]

In long term toxicity studies, dogs and rats fed low levels of DEET daily in the diet do not suffer any long term health effects.[2]

Animals of both sexes fed high levels of DEET exhibit weight loss and excessive salivation.[2]

Humans

Because DEET is used directly on human skin, scientists have thoroughly studied it toxicity.[2] Over its long use history, relatively few confirmed incidents have been reported when DEET is used properly.[2]

Exposure

Effects of DEET on human health and the environment depend on how much DEET is present and the length and frequency of exposure. Effects also depend on the health of a person and/or certain environmental factors.

Laboratory Testing

Before pesticides are registered by the U.S. Environmental Protection Agency (EPA), they must undergo laboratory testing for short-term and long-term health effects. Laboratory animals are purposely fed high enough doses to cause toxic effects. These tests help scientists judge how these chemicals might affect humans, domestic animals, and wildlife in cases of overexposure. When pesticide products are used according to the label directions, toxic effects are not likely to occur because the amount of pesticide that people and pets may be exposed to is low compared to the does fed to laboratory animals.

LD50/LC50

A common measure of toxicity is the lethal dose (LD50) or lethal concentration (LC50) which causes death (resulting from a single or limited exposure) in 50 percent of the treated animals. LD50 is generally expressed as the dose in milligrams (mg) of chemical per kilogram (kg) of body weight. LC50 is often expressed as mg of chemical per volume (e.g., liter (l) of medium—i.e., air or water) the organism is exposed to. Chemicals are considered highly toxic when the LD50/LC50 is small and practically non-toxic when the value is large. However, the LD50/LC50 does not reflect any effects from long-term exposure (i.e., cancer, birth defects or reproductive toxicity), which may occur at doses below those used in short-term studies.

Does DEET Cause Developmental or Birth Defects?

Animals

DEET does not cause birth defects in rats.[3]

Rats and rabbits suffer no adverse birth complications except when fed high doses of DEET. Pups experience reduced body weights at high doses.[3] Unborn and baby rats suffer increased mortality rates when exposed to high doses of DEET.[4]

DEET causes birth defects in chicks when injected directly into chicken eggs.[4]

Humans

Scientists have gathered no evidence that indicates DEET causes harmful reproductive effects to users.

Does DEET Cause Cancer?

Animals

Rats and mice did not develop cancer when fed high daily doses of DEET over their lifetime.[2]

Humans

No direct relationship between DEET use and carcinogenicity in humans has been established.[2]

U.S. EPA has classified DEET as a group D carcinogen (not classifiable as to human carcinogenicity). The U.S. EPA need further animal testing data to completely evaluate DEET.[2]

The U.S. EPA has strict guidelines that require testing of pesticides for their potential to cause cancer. These studies involve feeding laboratory animals large daily doses of the pesticide over most of the lifetime of the animal. Based on these tests, and any other available information, EPA gives the pesticide a rating for its potential to cause cancer in humans. For example, if a pesticide does not cause cancer in animal tests, then the EPA considers it unlikely the pesticide will cause cancer in humans. Testing for cancer has not been done on human subjects.

Does DEET Break Down and Leave the Body?

Animals

For a wide variety of test animals, DEET in the body is broken down and eliminated. Mice eliminate the majority of DEET absorbed through their skin in 1 to 3 days. Trace amounts of DEET were discovered in the mouse tissue 1 to 3 months after application.[4]

DEET is a broken down in the body prior to elimination. Elimination occurs mostly in the urine.[4]

Humans

DEET can penetrate through human skin. Once in the body, it is eliminated in the urine. Peak concentrations in the urine occur several hours after application. Based on this information and animal studies, DEET is not expected to accumulate in the body.[3]

What Happens to DEET in the Environment?

Because of its limited use pattern, EPA has required very little testing to be done on environmental fate of DEET.[2]

DEET does not readily degrade by hydrolysis at environmental pHs.[2]

DEET that is released into the soil breaks down fairly slowly.[4]

Residues of DEET in the atmosphere degrade fairly quickly.[3]

DEET has a moderate potential to move through soil and into groundwater.[4]

Table 38.1. Toxicity Category (*Single Word*)

	High Toxicity (*Danger*)	Moderate Toxicity (*Warning*)	Low Toxicity (*Caution*)	Very Low Toxicity (*Caution*)
Oral LD50	Less Than 50 mg/kg	50-500 mg/kg	500-5000 mg/kg	Greater Than 5000 mg/kg
Inhalation LC50	Less Than 0.2 mg/l	0.2-2 mg/l	2-20 mg/l	Greater Than 20 mg/l
Dermal LD50	Less Than 200 mg/kg	200-2000 mg/kg	2000-5000 mg/kg	Greater Than 5000 mg/kg
Eye Effects	Corrosive	Irritation Persisting for 7 Days	Irritation Reversible within 7 Days	No Irritation
Skin Effects	Corrosive	Severe Irritation at 72 Hours	Moderate Irritation At 72 Hours	Mild or Slight Irritation At 72 Hours

Table 38.2. Half-Life Values

Half Life is the time required for half of the compound to degrade.

1 half-life	=	50% degraded
2 half-lives	=	75% degraded
3 half-lives	=	88% degraded
4 half-lives	=	94% degraded
5 half-lives	=	97% degraded

Remember that the amount of chemical remaining after a half-life will always depend on the amount of the chemical originally applied.

What Effect Does DEET Have on Wildlife?

- DEET is slightly toxic to fish, birds, and aquatic invertebrates.[2]
- DEET is practically non-toxic to mammals.[2]
- Based on information from a study of carp fish, scientists believe DEET will not bio-accumulate in a food chain.[3]

References

1. McIver, S.B., A model for the mechanism of action of the repellant DEET N,N-diethyl-meta-toluamide on *Aedes aegypti* (dipteria: Culicidae). *Journal of Medical Entomology* 1981, Vol. 18, pp. 357-361.

2. *DEET: Reregistration Eligibility Decision*, U.S. Environmental Protection Agency (EPA), Office of Pesticide Programs, U.S. Government Printing Office: Washington D.C., 1998.

3. DEET. In *Hazardous Substances Data Bank (HSDB)* [CD-ROM]; Department of Health and Human Services; Bethesda, MD, July 1999.

4. *Handbook of Pesticide Toxicology;* Hayes, W. J., Jr.; Laws, E.R.J., Eds.; Academic Press, Inc.: San Diego, CA, 1991, Vol. 2., pp. 816-822.

Chapter 39

Chemical Hazards in the Workplace

Hazardous substances are used in many workplaces today. Working people are discovering that they need to know more about the health effects of chemicals which they use or may be exposed to on the job. Textbooks, fact sheets, and material safety data sheets (MSDSs) provide important information, but they are often written in technical language.

What Makes a Chemical Toxic?

The toxicity of a substance is its ability to cause harmful effects. These effects can strike a single cell, a group of cells, an organ system, or the entire body. A toxic effect may be visible damage, or a decrease in performance or function measurable only by a test. All chemicals can cause harm. When only a very large amount of the chemical can cause damage, the chemical is considered to be relatively non-toxic. When a small amount can be harmful, the chemical is considered toxic.

The toxicity of a substance depends on three factors: its chemical structure, the extent to which the substance is absorbed by the body, and the body's ability to detoxify the substance (change it into less toxic substances) and eliminate it from the body.

Reprinted with permission from *Understanding Toxic Substances: An Introduction to Chemical Hazards in the Workplace,* 1996 (revised 1999), Hazard Evaluation System and Information Service (HESIS), California Department of Health Services Occupational Health Branch. For additional information, about the health effects of occupational hazards, including online publications, visit the HESIS website at http://www.dhs.cahwnet.gov/ohb/HESIS/.

Are Toxic and Hazardous the Same?

No. The toxicity of a substance is the potential of that substance to cause harm, and is only one factor in determining whether a hazard exists. The hazard of a chemical is the practical likelihood that the chemical will cause harm. A chemical is determined to be a hazard depending on the following factors:

- _toxicity:_ how much of the substance is required to cause harm,
- _route of exposure:_ how the substance enters your body,
- _dose:_ how much enters your body,
- _duration:_ the length of time you are exposed,
- _reaction and interaction:_ other substances you are exposed to, and
- _sensitivity:_ how your body reacts to the substance compared to others.

Some chemicals are hazardous because of the risk of fire or explosion. These are important dangers, but are considered to be safety rather than toxic hazards. The factors of a toxic hazard are more fully explained later in this chapter.

Why Are Some Chemicals More Harmful Than Others?

The most important factor in toxicity is the chemical structure of a substance—what it is made of, what atoms and molecules it contains and how they are arranged. Substances with similar structures often cause similar health problems. However, slight differences in chemical structure can lead to large differences in the type of health effect produced. For example, silica in one form (amorphous) has little effect on health, and is allowed to be present in the workplace at relatively high levels. After it is heated, however, it turns into another form of silica (crystalline) that causes serious lung damage, and is allowed to be present only at very low levels (200 times lower than amorphous silica).

Routes of Exposure

How can chemicals enter the body?

Exposure normally occurs through inhalation, skin or eye contact, and ingestion.

Inhalation. The most common type of exposure occurs when you breathe a substance into the lungs. The lungs consist of branching airways (called bronchi) with clusters of tiny air sacs (called alveoli) at the ends of the airways. The alveoli absorb oxygen and other chemicals into the bloodstream.

Some chemicals are irritants and cause nose or throat irritation. They may also cause discomfort, coughing, or chest pain when they are inhaled and come into contact with the bronchi (chemical bronchitis). Other chemicals may be inhaled without causing such warning symptoms, but they still can be dangerous.

Sometimes a chemical is present in the air as small particles (dust or mist). Some of these particles, depending on their size, may be deposited in the bronchi and/or alveoli. Many of them may be coughed out, but others may stay in the lungs and may cause lung damage. Some particles may dissolve and be absorbed into the blood stream, and have effects elsewhere in the body.

Skin Contact. The skin is a protective barrier that helps keep foreign chemicals out of the body. However, some chemicals can easily pass through the skin and enter the bloodstream. If the skin is cut or cracked, chemicals can penetrate through the skin more easily. Also, some caustic substances, like strong acids and alkalis, can chemically burn the skin. Others can irritate the skin. Many chemicals, particularly organic solvents, dissolve the oils in the skin, leaving it dry, cracked, and susceptible to infection and absorption of chemicals.

Eye Contact. Some chemicals may burn or irritate the eye. Occasionally they may be absorbed through the eye and enter the bloodstream. The eyes are easily harmed by chemicals, so any eye contact with chemicals should be taken as a serious incident.

Ingestion. The least common source of exposure in the workplace is swallowing chemicals. Chemicals can be ingested if they are left on hands, clothing or beard, or accidentally contaminate food, drinks or cigarettes. Chemicals present in the workplace as dust, for example, metal dusts such as lead or cadmium, are easily ingested.

Dose: How Much Is Too Much?

In general, the greater the amount of a substance that enters your body, the greater is the effect on your body. This connection between amount and effect is called the dose-response relationship. For example, organic solvents such as toluene, acetone, and trichloroethylene all affect the brain in the same way, but to different degrees at different doses. The effects of these solvents are similar to those which result from drinking alcoholic beverages. At a low dose, you may feel nothing or a mild, sometimes pleasant ("high") sensation. A larger dose may cause dizziness or headache. With an even larger dose you may become drunk, pass out, or even stop breathing.

When you inhale a toxic chemical, the dose you receive depends on four factors: (1) the level (concentration) of chemical in the air; (2) how hard (fast and deep) you are breathing, which depends on your degree of physical exertion; (3) how much of the chemical that is inhaled stays in your lungs and is absorbed into your bloodstream; and (4) how long the exposure lasts.

It is safest to keep exposure to any toxic substance as low as possible. Since some chemicals are much more toxic than others, it is necessary to keep exposure to some substances lower than others. The threshold level is the lowest concentration that might produce a harmful effect. It is different for every chemical. The threshold for one chemical may differ from person to person. If the concentration of a chemical in the air is kept well below the threshold level, harmful effects probably will not occur. Levels above the threshold are too much. However, this means only that there is a possibility that health effects might occur, not that such effects definitely will occur.

Duration: How Long Is Too Long?

The longer you are exposed to a chemical, the more likely you are to be affected by it. The dose is still important—at very low levels you may not experience any effects no matter how long you are exposed. At higher concentrations you may not be affected following a short-term exposure, but repeated exposure over time may cause harm. Chemical exposure which continues over a long period of time is often particularly hazardous because some chemicals can accumulate in the body or because the damage does not have a chance to be repaired. The combination of dose and duration is called the rate of exposure.

The body has several systems, most importantly the liver, kidneys and lungs, that change chemicals to a less toxic form (detoxify) and eliminate them. If your rate of exposure to a chemical exceeds the rate at which you can eliminate it, some of the chemical will accumulate in your body. For example, if you work with a chemical for eight hours each day, you have the rest of the day (16 hours) to eliminate it from your body before you are exposed again the next day. If your body can't eliminate all the chemical in 16 hours and you continue to be exposed, the amount in the body will accumulate each day you are exposed. Illness that affects the organs for detoxification and elimination, such as hepatitis (inflammation of the liver), can also decrease their ability to eliminate chemicals from the body.

Accumulation does not continue indefinitely. There is a point where the amount in the body reaches a maximum and remains the same as long as your exposure remains the same. This point will be different for each chemical. Some chemicals, such as ammonia and formaldehyde, leave the body quickly and do not accumulate at all. Other chemicals are stored in the body for long periods. For instance, lead is stored in the bone, and calcium is stored in the liver and kidneys. There are a few substances, such as asbestos fibers, that, once deposited, remain in the body forever.

Latency: How Long Does it Take for a Toxic Effect to Occur?

The effects of toxic substances may appear immediately or soon after exposure, or they may take many years to appear. Acute exposure is a single exposure or a few exposures. Acute effects are those which occur following acute exposures. Acute effects can occur immediately, or be delayed and occur days or weeks after exposure. Chronic exposure is repeated exposure that occurs over months and years. Chronic effects are those which occur following chronic exposures, and so are always delayed.

A toxic chemical may cause acute effects, chronic effects or both. For example, if you inhale solvents on the job, you may experience acute effects such as headaches and dizziness which go away at the end of the day. Over months, you may begin to develop chronic effects such as liver and kidney damage.

The delay between the beginning of exposure and the appearance of disease caused by that exposure is called the latency period. Some chronic effects caused by chemicals, such as cancer, have very long latency periods. Cancer has been known to develop as long as 40 years after a worker's first exposure to a cancer-causing chemical.

The length of the latency period for chronic effects makes it difficult to establish the cause-and-effect relationship between the exposure and the illness. Since chronic diseases develop gradually, you may have the disease for some time before it is detected. It is, therefore, important for you and your physician to know what chronic effects might be caused by the substances you use on the job.

There are a few substances, such as asbestos fibers, that, once deposited, remain in the body forever.

Reaction and Interaction

What if you're exposed to more than one chemical?

Depending upon the job you have, you may be exposed to more than one chemical. If you are, you need to be aware of possible reactions and interactions between them. A reaction occurs when chemicals combine with each other to produce a new substance. The new substance may have properties different from those of the original substances, and it could be more hazardous. For example, when household bleach and lye (such as a drain cleaner) are mixed together, highly dangerous chlorine gas and hydrochloric acid are formed. The Material Safety Data Sheet (MSDS) for a chemical will often list its potential hazardous reactions and the substances which should not be mixed with it. Your employer is required by law to have an MSDS for each hazardous substance in the workplace, and make them available to you on request.

Table 39.1. The Differences between Acute and Chronic Effects

Acute	Chronic
Occurs immediately or soon after exposure (short latency).	Occurs over time or long after exposure (long latency)
Often involves a high exposure (large dose) over a short period.	Often involves low exposures (small doses) over a long period.
Often reversible after exposure stops.	Many effects are not reversible.
Can be minor or severe. For example, a small amount of ammonia can cause throat or eye irritation; larger amounts can be serious or even fatal.	Chronic effects are still unknown for many chemicals. For example, most chemicals have not been tested for cancer or reproductive effects.
Relationship between chemical exposure and symptoms is generally, although not always, obvious.	It may be difficult to establish the relationship between chemical exposure and illness because of the long time delay or latency period.
Knowledge often based on human exposure.	Knowledge often based on animal studies

314

An interaction occurs when exposure to more than one substance results in a health effect different from the effects of either one alone. One kind of interaction is called synergism, a process in which two or more chemicals produce an effect that is greater than the sum of their individual effects. For instance, carbon tetrachloride and ethanol (drinking alcohol) are both toxic to the liver. If you are overexposed to carbon tetrachloride and drink alcohol excessively, the damage to your liver may be much greater than the effects of the two chemicals added together.

Another example of synergism is the increased risk of developing lung cancer caused by exposures to both cigarette smoking and asbestos. By either smoking one pack of cigarettes per day or being heavily exposed to asbestos, you may increase your risk of lung cancer to six times higher than someone who does neither. But if you smoke a pack a day and are heavily exposed to asbestos, your risk may be 90 times higher than someone who does neither.

Another interaction is potentiation, which occurs when an effect of one substance is increased by exposure to a second substance which would not cause that effect by itself. For example, although acetone does not damage the liver by itself, it can increase carbon tetrachloride's ability to damage the liver.

Unfortunately, few chemicals have been tested to determine if interactions with other chemicals occur.

Sensitivity

Are some people more affected than others?

Yes. People vary widely in their sensitivity to the effects of a chemical. Many things determine how an individual will react to a chemical. These include age, sex, inherited traits, diet, pregnancy, state of health and use of medication, drugs or alcohol. Depending on these characteristics, some people will experience the toxic effects of a chemical at a lower (or higher) dose than other people.

People may also become allergic to a chemical. These people have a different type of response than those who are not allergic. This response frequently occurs at a very low dose. Not all chemicals can cause allergic reactions. Substances that are known to cause allergies are called allergens, or sensitizers.

For example, formaldehyde gas is very irritating. Everyone will experience irritation of the eyes, nose, and throat, with tears in the eyes and a sore throat, at some level of exposure. All people will experience irritation if exposed to high enough levels. A person may be more

315

sensitive to formaldehyde and have irritation at low levels of exposure. Formaldehyde also occasionally causes allergic reactions, such as allergic dermatitis, or hives. A few people may be allergic to formaldehyde and develop hives at very low levels, although most people will not get hives no matter how much they are exposed to formaldehyde.

How Can Toxic Substances Harm the Body?

When a toxic substance causes damage at the point where it first contacts the body, that damage is called a local effect. The most common points at which substances first contact the body are the skin, eyes, nose, throat and lungs. Toxic substances can also enter the body and travel in the bloodstream to internal organs. Effects that are produced this way are called systemic. The internal organs most commonly affected are the liver, kidneys, heart, nervous system (including the brain) and reproductive system.

A toxic chemical may cause local effects, systemic effects, or both. For example, if ammonia gas is inhaled, it quickly irritates the lining of the respiratory tract (nose, throat and lungs). Almost no ammonia passes from the lungs into the blood. Since damage is caused only at the point of initial contact, ammonia is said to exert a local effect. An epoxy resin is an example of a substance with local effects on the skin. On the other hand, if liquid phenol contacts the skin, it irritates the skin at the point of contact (a local effect) and can also be absorbed through the skin, and may damage the liver and kidneys (systemic effects).

Sometimes, as with phenols, the local effects caused by a chemical provide a warning that exposure is occurring. You are then warned that the chemical may be entering your body and producing systemic affects which you can't yet see or feel. Some chemicals, however, do not provide any warning at all, and so they are particularly hazardous. For example, glycol ethers (Cellosolve solvents) can pass through the skin and cause serious internal damage without producing any observable effect on the skin.

Do all toxic chemicals cause cancer?

No. Cancer—the uncontrolled growth and spread of abnormal cells in the body—is caused by some chemicals but not others. It is not true that everything causes cancer when taken in large enough doses. In fact, most substances do not cause cancer, no matter how high the dose. Only a relatively small number of the many thousands of chemicals in use today cause cancer.

Chemicals that can cause cancer are called carcinogens and the ability to cause cancer is called carcinogenicity. Evidence for carcinogenicity comes from either human or animal studies. There is enough evidence for about 30 chemicals to be called carcinogenic in humans. About 200 other chemicals are known to cause cancer in laboratory animals and are, therefore, likely to be human carcinogens.

Determining the causes of cancer in humans is difficult. There is usually a long latency period (10 to 40 years) between the start of exposure to a carcinogen and the appearance of cancer. Thus, a substance must be used for many years before enough people will be exposed to it long enough for researchers to see a pattern of increased cancer cases. It is often difficult to determine if an increase in cancer in humans is due to exposure to a particular substance, since exposure may have occurred many years before, and people are exposed to many different substances.

Since the study of cancer in humans is difficult and requires that people be exposed to carcinogenic chemicals and possibly get cancer, chemicals are tested for carcinogenicity using laboratory animals. If animals were exposed to the low levels typical of most human exposure, many hundreds of animals would be required for only a few to get cancer. To avoid this expense, animal cancer tests use large doses of chemicals in order to be able to detect an increase in cancer in a reasonable number of animals, such as 25-50. However, animal tests are still expensive, take about three years to perform, and are often inconclusive. When an animal cancer test is positive, the risk to a small number of rats at high doses must be used to try to predict the risk to humans at much lower doses. Chemicals that cause cancer in animals are considered likely to cause cancer in humans, even if the degree of risk is uncertain.

The issue of whether there is a safe dose for a carcinogen is controversial. Some scientists believe that any exposure, no matter how small, carries some risk. However, at very low exposures, the risk, if any, may be so small that it can be considered the same as no risk at all. Most carcinogens appear to require either exposure over a number of years or very high doses before the risk of developing cancer from exposure to them becomes of serious concern.

Do all toxic chemicals cause mutations?

Toxic chemicals can also cause genetic damage. The genetic material of a cell consists of genes, which exist in chromosomes. Genes and chromosomes contain the information that tells the cell how to function and how to reproduce (form new cells).

Some chemicals may change or damage the genes or chromosomes. This kind of change, or damage in a cell is called a mutation. Anything that causes a mutation is called a mutagen. Mutations may affect the way the cell functions or reproduces. The mutations can also be passed on to new cells that are formed from the damaged cell. This can lead to groups of cells that do not function or reproduce the same way the original cell did before the mutation occurred.

Some kinds of mutation result in cancer. Most chemicals that cause cancer also cause mutations. However, not all chemicals that cause mutations cause cancer. Tests for the ability of a chemical to cause a mutation take little time and are relatively easy to perform. If testing shows a chemical to be a mutagen, additional testing must be done to determine whether or not the chemical also causes cancer.

Can future generations be affected?

Exposure to chemical substances may affect your children or your ability to have children. Toxic reproductive effects include the inability to conceive children (infertility or sterility), lowered sex drive, menstrual disturbances, spontaneous abortions (miscarriages), stillbirths, and defects in children that are apparent at birth or later in the child's development.

Teratogens are chemicals which cause malformations or birth defects by directly damaging tissues in the fetus developing in the mother's womb. Other chemicals that harm the fetus are called fetotoxins. If a chemical causes health problems in the pregnant woman herself, the fetus may also be affected. Certain chemicals can damage the male reproductive system, resulting in sterility, infertility, or abnormal sperm.

There is not enough information on the reproductive toxicity of most chemicals. Most chemicals have not been tested for reproductive effects in animals. It is difficult to predict risk in humans using animal data. There may be safe levels of exposure to chemicals that affect the reproductive system. However, trying to determine a safe level is very difficult, if not impossible. It is even more difficult to study reproductive effects in humans than it is to study cancer. At this time, only a few industrial chemicals are known to cause birth defects or other reproductive effects in humans.

What Are the Different Forms of Toxic Materials?

Toxic materials can take the form of solids, liquids, gases, vapors, dusts, fumes, fibers and mists. How a substance gets into the body and what damage it causes depends on the form or the physical properties of the substance.

A toxic material may take different forms under varying conditions and each form may present a different type of hazard. For example, lead solder in solid form is not hazardous because it is not likely to enter the body. Soldering, however, turns the lead into a liquid, which may spill or come into contact with skin. When the spilled liquid becomes solid again, it may be in the form of small particles (dust) that may be inhaled or ingested and absorbed. If lead is heated to a very high temperature such as when it is welded, a fume may be created; a fume consists of very small particles which are extremely hazardous as they are easily inhaled and absorbed. It is thus important to know what form or forms a given substance takes in the workplace.

Solid. A solid is a material that retains its form, like stone. Most solids are generally not hazardous since they are not likely to be absorbed into the body, unless present as small particles such as dust.

Liquid. A liquid is a material that flows freely, like water. Many hazardous substances are in liquid form at normal temperatures. Some liquids can damage the skin. Some pass through the skin and enter the body and may or may not cause skin damage. Liquids may also evaporate (give off vapors), forming gases which can be inhaled.

Gas. A gas consists of individual chemical molecules dispersed in air, like oxygen, at normal temperature and pressure. Some gases are flammable, explosive, and/or toxic. The presence of a gas may be difficult to detect if it has no color or odor, and does not cause immediate irritation. Such gases, like carbon monoxide, may still be very hazardous.

Vapor. A vapor is the gas form of a substance that is primarily a liquid at normal pressure and temperature. Most organic solvents evaporate and produce vapors. Vapors can be inhaled into the lungs, and in some cases may irritate the eyes, skin or respiratory tract. Some are flammable, explosive and/or toxic. The term vapor pressure or evaporation rate is used to indicate the tendency for different liquids to evaporate.

Dust. A dust consists of small solid particles in the air. Dusts may be created when solids are pulverized or ground, or when powder (settled dust) becomes airborne. Dusts may be hazardous because they can be inhaled into the respiratory tract. Larger particles of dust are usually trapped in the nose and windpipe (trachea) where they can be expelled, but smaller particles (respirable dust) can reach and may damage the lungs. Some, like lead dust, may then enter the bloodstream through the lungs. Some organic dusts, such as grain dust, may explode when they reach high concentrations in the air.

Fume. A fume consists of very small, fine solid particles in the air which form when solid chemicals (often metals) are heated to very high temperatures, evaporate to vapor, and finally become solid again. The welding or brazing of metal, for example, produces metal fumes. Fumes are hazardous because they are easily inhaled. Many metal fumes can cause an illness called metal fume fever, consisting of fever, chills and aches like the flu. Inhalation of other metal fumes, such as lead, can cause poisoning without causing metal fume fever.

Fiber. A fiber is a solid particle whose length is at least three times its width. The degree of hazard depends upon the size of the fiber. Smaller fibers such as asbestos, can lodge in the lungs and cause serious harm. Larger fibers are trapped in the respiratory tract; and are expelled without reaching the lung.

Mist. A mist consists of liquid particles of various sizes which are produced by agitation or spraying of liquids. Mists can be hazardous when they are inhaled or sprayed on the skin. The spraying of pesticides and the machining of metals using metal working fluids are two situations where mists are commonly produced.

What Are Exposure Limits?

Exposure limits are established by health and safety authorities to control exposure to hazardous substances. Exposure limits usually represent the maximum amount (concentration) of a chemical which can be present in the air without presenting a health hazard. However, exposure limits may not always be completely protective, for the following reasons:

1. Although exposure limits are usually based on the best available information, this information, particularly for chronic (long-term) health effects, may be incomplete. Often we learn about chronic health effects only after workers have been exposed to a chemical for many years, and then as new information is learned, the exposure limits are changed.

2. Exposure limits are set to protect most workers. However, there may be a few workers who will be affected by a chemical at levels below these limits. Employees performing extremely heavy physical exertion breathe in more air and more of a chemical, and so may absorb an excessive amount.

3. Exposure limits do not take into account chemical interactions. When two or more chemicals in the workplace have the same health effects, industrial hygienists use a mathematical formula to adjust the exposure limits for those substances in that workplace. This formula applies to chemicals that have additive effects, but not to those with synergistic or potentiating effects.

4. Exposure limits usually apply to the concentration of a chemical in the air, and are established to limit exposure by inhalation. Limiting the concentration in air may not prevent excessive exposure through skin contact or ingestion. Chemicals that may produce health effects as a result of absorption through the skin have an "S" designation next to their numerical value in the PEL (Permissible Exposure Limit) table. Workers exposed to these chemicals must be provided with protective clothing to wear when overexposure through the skin is possible. Some chemicals, like lead and cadmium in dust form, may be ingested through contamination of hands, hair, clothes, food and cigarettes.

How Can Exposure Be Measured and Monitored?

When toxic chemicals are present in the workplace, your exposure can be estimated by measuring the concentration of a given chemical in the air and the duration of exposure. This measurement is called air or environmental monitoring or sampling and is usually done by industrial hygienists, using various types of instruments. The air is collected from your breathing zone (the air around your nose and mouth) so that the concentrations measured will accurately reflect the concentration you are inhaling. The exposure levels calculated from this monitoring can then be compared to the Permissible Exposure Level for that chemical.

Environmental monitoring is the most accurate way to determine your exposure to most chemicals. However, for chemicals that are absorbed by routes other than inhalation, such as through the skin and by ingestion, air monitoring may underestimate the amount of chemical you absorb. For these and some other chemicals, the levels of the chemical (or its breakdown products) in the body can sometimes be measured in the blood, urine or exhaled air. Such testing is called biological monitoring, and the results may give an estimate of the actual dose absorbed into the body. For one substance—lead—biological monitoring is required by law when air monitoring results are above a certain level. The American Conference of Governmental Industrial Hygienists (ACGIH) has recommended the exposure limits for biological monitoring for a small number of chemicals. These are called Biological Exposure Indices (BEIs) and are published together with TLVs (Threshold Limit Values).

Practical Clues to Exposure

Odor

If you smell a chemical, you are inhaling it. However, some chemicals can be smelled at levels well below those that are harmful, so that detecting an odor does not mean that you are inhaling harmful amounts. On the other hand, if you cannot smell a chemical, it may still be present. Some chemicals cannot be smelled even at levels that are harmful.

The odor threshold is the lowest level of a chemical that can be smelled by most people. If a chemical's odor threshold is lower than the amount that is hazardous, the chemical is said to have good warning properties. One example is ammonia. Most people can smell it at 5 ppm, below the PEL of 25 ppm. It is important to remember that for most chemicals, the odor thresholds vary widely from person to person. In addition, some chemicals, like hydrogen sulfide, cause you to rapidly lose your ability to smell them (called olfactory fatigue). With these cautions in mind, knowing a chemical's odor threshold may serve as rough guide to your exposure level.

Don't depend on odor to warn you. Remember that your sense of smell may be better or worse than average, that some very hazardous chemicals have no odor (carbon monoxide), some chemicals of low toxicity have very strong odors (mercaptans added to natural gas), and others produce olfactory fatigue.

Taste

If you inhale or ingest a chemical, it may leave a taste in your mouth. Some chemicals have a particular taste, which may be mentioned in an MSDS.

Particles in Nose or Mucous

If you cough up mucous (sputum or phlegm) with particles in it, or blow your nose and see particles on your handkerchief, then you have inhaled some chemical in particle form. Unfortunately, most particles which are inhaled into the lungs are too small to see.

Settled Dust or Mist

If chemical dust or mist is in the air, it will eventually settle on work surfaces or on your skin, hair and clothing. It is likely that you inhaled some of this chemical while it was in the air.

Immediate Symptoms

If you or your co-workers experience symptoms known to be caused by a chemical during or shortly after its use, you may have been over-exposed. Symptoms might include tears in your eyes; a burning sensation of skin, nose, or throat; a cough; dizziness or a headache.

Can You Be Tested for Health Effects of Exposure?

Sometimes. Medical surveillance is a program of medical examinations and tests designed to detect early warning signs of harmful exposure. A medical surveillance program may discover small changes in health before severe damage occurs. Testing for health effects is called medical monitoring. The type of testing needed in a surveillance program depends upon the particular chemical involved. Unfortunately, medical monitoring tests that accurately measure early health effects are available only for a small number of chemicals. A complete occupational surveillance program should consist of industrial hygiene monitoring, medical monitoring, and biological monitoring when appropriate. Tests for health effects when you are already sick are not part of medical surveillance, and must be selected by your physician on a case by case basis.

How Can Exposures Be Reduced?

The surest way to prevent toxic chemicals from causing harm is to minimize or prevent exposure.

Knowledge

Everyone who works with toxic substances should know the names, toxicity and other hazards of the substances they use. Employers are required by law to provide this information, along with training in how to use toxic substances safely. A worker may obtain information about a chemical's composition, physical characteristics, and toxicity from the Material Safety Data Sheet (MSDS).

Engineering Controls

Limiting exposure at the source is the preferred way to protect workers. The types of engineering controls, in order of effectiveness, are:

- *Substitution* is using a less hazardous substance. But before choosing a substitute, carefully consider its physical and health hazards. For example, mineral spirits (Stoddard Solvent) is less of a health hazard than perchlorethylene for dry cleaning, but is more of a fire hazard and an air pollutant.

- *Process or equipment enclosure* is the isolation of the source of exposure, often through automation. This completely eliminates the routine exposure of workers. For example, handling of radioactive materials is often done by mechanical arms or robots.

- *Local exhaust ventilation* is a hood or intake at or over the source of exposure to capture or draw contaminated air from its source before it spreads into the room and into your breathing zone.

- *General or dilution ventilation* is continual replacement and circulation of fresh air sufficient to keep concentrations of toxic substances diluted below hazardous levels. However, concentrations will be highest near the source, and overexposure may occur in this area. If the dilution air is not well mixed with the room air, pockets of high concentrations may exist.

Personal Protective Equipment

The following devices should be used only when engineering controls are not possible or are not sufficient to reduce exposure.

- *Respiratory protective equipment* consists of devices that cover the mouth and nose to prevent substances in the air from being inhaled. A respirator is effective only when used as part of a comprehensive program established by the employer, which includes measurement of concentrations of all hazardous substances, selection of the proper respirator, training the worker in its proper use, fitting of the respirator to the worker, maintenance, and replacement of parts when necessary.

- *Protective clothing* includes gloves, aprons, goggles, boots, face shields, and any other materials worn as protection. It should be made of material designed to resist penetration by the particular chemical being used. Such material may be called impervious to that chemical. The manufacturer of the protective clothing usually can provide some information regarding the substances that are effectively blocked.

- *Barrier creams* are used to coat the skin and prevent chemicals from reaching it. They may be helpful when the type of work prevents the use of gloves. However, barrier creams are not recommended as substitutes for gloves. General skin creams and lotions (such as moisturizing lotion) are not barrier creams.

Engineering Controls

Limiting exposure at the source is the preferred way to protect workers.

Checklist for Researching Toxic Substances Used on the Job

In order to determine the health risks of substances you use or may be exposed to on the job, and to find out how to work with them safely, you need to obtain information from many sources including material safety data sheets (MSDSs), medical and monitoring records; and reference materials. The law requires your employer to make much of this information available to you. The following checklist will help you gather facts which you can use along with the information in this pamphlet to get the answers you need.

- What is the substance? What's in it? How toxic is it? Are health effects acute, chronic, or both?

- Is there evidence based on research with animals or humans that the substance is a carcinogen? A mutagen? A teratogen or reproductive toxin?

- How does this substance enter the body (routes of entry): inhalation, skin absorption, ingestion?

- What is the legal exposure limit (PEL) or recommended TLV?

- To how much of the substance are you being exposed? What is the concentration of the substance in the workplace air? How long are you exposed?

- Are you exposed to other chemicals at the same time? Can they have a combined (additive or synergistic) effect?

- Do you have any medical conditions or take any drugs that might interact with chemicals?

- What controls are recommended to prevent overexposure?

- Is any type of medical testing recommended?

Chapter 40

Multiple Chemical Sensitivity Syndrome (MCS)

Multiple Chemical Sensitivities

Multiple chemical sensitivities (MCS) is a highly controversial entity. Some people believe that exposure to a chemical or chemicals triggers a symptom complex that has been called MCS. Those symptoms occur in many organ systems. No physical signs can be found consistently in MCS patients. There are a number of synonyms for MCS, including: 20th century disease, environmental illness, total allergy syndrome, idiopathic environmental illness, and chemical AIDS. MCS appears to affect young women at a proportionally greater rate than men or older women. Among the proposed theories are dysfunction of the immune system, and neurological abnormalities specifically chemical sensitization of the limbic system and various psychological theories. To date, no studies have validated any theory. Due to the lack of definite information on this subject evaluation must be performed by a physician knowledgeable of the symptoms of this condition.

Text in this chapter is from "Safety and Health Topics: Multiple Chemical Sensitivities," a fact sheet produced by the U.S. Department of Labor, 2002, available online at http://www.osha-slc.gov/SLCT/multiplechemicals ensitivities/index.html; and "Allergies—Multiple Chemical Sensitivity," an undated fact sheet produced by the National Institute of Environmental Health Sciences (NIEHS), available online at http://www.niehs.nih.gov/external/faq/allergy.htm, cited February 2003.

Control

Because the cause of MCS is not currently known, control methods could only be based on unproven theories. MCS is clearly not occupationally related.

Compliance

Limited information is available on effective control measures, exposure assessments, and regulations dealing with MCS; however, OSHA does regulate exposures to specific chemical hazards.

Allergies—Multiple Chemical Sensitivity

Question: Two years ago there was a chemical spill at my workplace, and many of my co-workers and I became ill immediately after the exposure. Since then, I haven't been the same. It feels like I can't think as clearly now, and I seem to be allergic to almost everything, including perfumes, cosmetics, detergents and household cleaning products. I heard about multiple chemical sensitivity (MCS) on a radio talk show, and I think I am chemically sensitive. When I asked my doctor about MCS, he didn't have much to say about it. What can you tell me about multiple chemical sensitivity?

Answer: Multiple chemical sensitivity (MCS) is something of a medical mystery. The medical community is divided over whether or not MCS actually exists.

Some physicians acknowledge MCS as a medical disorder that is triggered by exposures to chemicals in the environment, often beginning with a short term, severe chemical exposure (like a chemical spill) or with a longer term, small exposures (like a poorly ventilated office building). After the initial exposure, low levels of everyday chemicals such as those found in cosmetics, soaps, and newspaper inks can trigger physical reactions in MCS patients. These patients report a range of symptoms that often include headaches, rashes, asthma, depression, muscle and joint aches, fatigue, memory loss, and confusion.

Others in the medical community, however, do not accept MCS as a genuine medical disorder. The Centers for Disease Control, for example, do not recognize MCS as a clinical diagnosis. There is no official medical definition of MCS, partially because symptoms and chemical exposures are often unique and are widely varied between individuals. Some physicians are skeptical of concluding that low concentrations of the same chemicals that are tolerated by everyone else can cause dramatic symptoms in MCS patients. The American Medical Association denies that MCS is a clinical condition because conclusive scientific evidence is lacking.

For more information on multiple chemical sensitivities please see:

- A large number of papers on multiple chemical sensitivity that are located at http://www-rohan.sdsu.edu/staff/lhamilto/mcs/index2.html

- See what the Interagency Workgroup on Multiple Chemical Sensitivity had to say at http://web.health.gov/environment/mcs/toc.htm

- A report from the American Academy of Dermatology http://www.newswise.com/articles/2000/3/ALLERGY.AAD.html

Part Five

Radiation and Electromagnetic Field Hazards

Chapter 41

Understanding the Health Effects of Radiation Exposure

How Does Radiation Cause Health Effects?

Radioactive materials that decay spontaneously produce ionizing radiation, which has sufficient energy to strip away electrons from atoms (creating two charged ions) or to break some chemical bonds. Any living tissue in the human body can be damaged by ionizing radiation. The body attempts to repair the damage, but sometimes the damage is too severe or widespread, or mistakes are made in the natural repair process. The most common forms of ionizing radiation are alpha and beta particles, or gamma and x-rays.

What Kinds of Health Effects Occur from Exposure to Radionuclides?

In general, the amount and duration of radiation exposure affects the severity or type of health effect. There are two broad categories of health effects: stochastic and non-stochastic.

Stochastic Health Effects

Stochastic effects are associated with long-term, low-level (chronic) exposure to radiation. (Stochastic refers to the likelihood that something

"Understanding Radiation: Health Effects," an undated fact sheet produced by the U.S. Environmental Protection Agency (EPA), available online at http://www.epa.gov/radiation/understand/health_effects.htm. Cited February 2003.

will happen.) Increased levels of exposure make these health effects more likely to occur, but do not influence the type or severity of the effect.

Cancer is considered by most people the primary health effect from radiation exposure. Simply put, cancer is the uncontrolled growth of cells. Ordinarily, natural processes control the rate at which cells grow and replace themselves. They also control the body's processes for repairing or replacing damaged tissue. Damage occurring at the cellular or molecular level, can disrupt the control processes, permitting the uncontrolled growth of cells—cancer. This is why ionizing radiation's ability to break chemical bonds in atoms and molecules makes it such a potent carcinogen.

Other stochastic effects also occur. Radiation can cause changes in DNA, the blueprints that ensure cell repair and replacement produces a perfect copy of the original cell. Changes in DNA are called mutations.

Sometimes the body fails to repair these mutations or even creates mutations during repair. The mutations can be teratogenic or genetic. Teratogenic mutations affect only the individual who was exposed. Genetic mutations are passed on to offspring.

Non-Stochastic Health Effects

Non-stochastic effects appear in cases of exposure to high levels of radiation, and become more severe as the exposure increases. Short-term, high-level exposure is referred to as acute exposure.

Many non-cancerous health effects of radiation are non-stochastic. Unlike cancer, health effects from acute exposure to radiation usually appear quickly. Acute health effects include burns and radiation sickness. Radiation sickness is also called radiation poisoning. It can cause premature aging or even death. If the dose is fatal, death usually occurs within two months. The symptoms of radiation sickness include: nausea, weakness, hair loss, skin burns or diminished organ function.

Medical patients receiving radiation treatments often experience acute effects, because they are receiving relatively high bursts of radiation during treatment.

Is Any Amount of Radiation Safe?

There is no firm basis for setting a safe level of exposure above background for stochastic effects. Many sources emit radiation that is well below natural background levels. This makes it extremely difficult to isolate its stochastic effects.

Some scientists assert that low levels of radiation are beneficial to health (this idea is known as hormesis).

How Do We Know Radiation Causes Cancer?

Basically, we have learned through observation. When people first began working with radioactive materials, scientists didn't understand radioactive decay, and reports of illness were scattered.

As the use of radioactive materials and reports of illness became more frequent, scientists began to notice patterns in the illnesses. People working with radioactive materials and x-rays developed particular types of uncommon medical conditions. For example, scientists recognized as early at 1910 that radiation caused skin cancer. Scientists began to keep track of the health effects, and soon set up careful scientific studies of groups of people who had been exposed.

Among the best known long-term studies are those of Japanese atomic bomb blast survivors, other populations exposed to nuclear

Table 41.1. Threshold Exposures for the Various Non-Stochastic Health Effects

Exposure (rem)	Health Effect	Time to Onset
	radiation burns; more severe as exposure increases.	
5-10	changes in blood chemistry	
50	nausea	hours
	damage to bone marrow	
	fatigue	
	hair loss	2-3 weeks
	death from fatal doses	within 2 months
1,000	destruction of intestinal lining	
	internal bleeding	
	death	1-2 weeks
2,000	damage to central nervous system	
	loss of consciousness	minutes
	death	hours to days

testing fallout (for example, natives of the Marshall Islands), and uranium miners.

Aren't Children More Sensitive to Radiation Than Adults?

Yes, because children are growing more rapidly, there are more cells dividing and a greater opportunity for radiation to disrupt the process. EPA's radiation protection standards take into account the differences in the sensitivity due to age and gender.

Fetuses are also highly sensitive to radiation. However, the period during which they may be exposed is short.

Effects of Radiation Type and Exposure Pathway

Both the type of radiation to which the person is exposed and the pathway by which they are exposed influence health effects. Different types of radiation vary in their ability to damage different kinds of tissue.

Radiation and radiation emitters (radionuclides) can expose the whole body (direct exposure) or expose tissues inside the body when inhaled or ingested. All kinds of ionizing radiation can cause cancer and other health effects. The main difference in the ability of alpha and beta particles and gamma and x-rays to cause health effects is the amount of energy they have. Their energy determines how far they can penetrate into tissue. It also determines how much energy they are able to transmit directly or indirectly to tissues and the resulting damage.

Non-Radiation Health Effects of Radionuclides

Radioactive elements and compounds behave chemically exactly like their non-radioactive forms. For example, radioactive lead has the same chemical properties as non-radioactive lead. The public health protection question that EPA's scientists must answer is, "How do we best manage all the hazards a pollutant presents?"

Do Chemical Properties of Radionuclides Contribute to Radiation Health Effects?

The chemical properties of a radionuclide can determine where health effects occur. To function properly many organs require certain elements. They cannot distinguish between radioactive and non-radioactive forms of the element and accumulate one as quickly as the other.

Radioactive iodine concentrates in the thyroid. The thyroid needs iodine to function normally, and cannot tell the difference between stable and radioactive isotopes. As a result, radioactive iodine contributes to thyroid cancer more than other types of cancer.

Calcium, strontium-90, and radium-226 have similar chemical properties. The result is that strontium and radium in the body tend to collect in calcium rich areas, such as bones and teeth. They contribute to bone cancer.

Estimating Health Effects

What Is the Cancer Risk from Radiation? How Does It Compare to the Risk of Cancer from Other Sources?

Each radionuclide represents a somewhat different health risk. However, health physicists currently estimate that overall, if each person in a group of 10,000 people exposed to 1 rem of ionizing radiation, in small doses over a life time, we would expect 5 or 6 more people to die of cancer than would otherwise.

In this group of 10,000 people, we can expect about 2,000 to die of cancer from all non-radiation causes. The accumulated exposure to 1 rem of radiation would increase that number to about 2005 or 2006.

To give you an idea of the usual rate of exposure, most people receive about 3 tenths of a rem (300 mrem) every year from natural background sources of radiation (mostly radon).

What Are the Risks of Other Long-Term Health Effects?

Other than cancer, the most prominent long-term health effects are teratogenic and genetic mutations.

Teratogenic mutations result from the exposure of fetuses (unborn children) to radiation. They can include smaller head or brain size, poorly formed eyes, abnormally slow growth, and mental retardation. Studies indicate that fetuses are most sensitive between about eight to fifteen weeks after conception. They remain somewhat less sensitive between six and twenty-five weeks old.

The relationship between dose and mental retardation is not known exactly. However, scientists estimate that if 1,000 fetuses that were between eight and fifteen weeks old were exposed to one rem, four fetuses would become mentally retarded. If the fetuses were between sixteen and twenty-five weeks old, it is estimated that one of them would be mentally retarded.

Genetic effects are those that can be passed from parent to child. Health physicists estimate that about fifty severe hereditary effects will occur in a group of one million live-born children whose parents were both exposed to one rem. About one hundred twenty severe hereditary effects would occur in all descendants.

In comparison, all other causes of genetic effects result in as many as 100,000 severe hereditary effects in one million live-born children. These genetic effects include those that occur spontaneously (just happen) as well as those that have non-radioactive causes.

Protecting against Exposure

What Limits Does EPA Set on Exposure to Radiation?

Health physicists generally agree on limiting a person's exposure beyond background radiation to about 100 mrem per year from all sources. Exceptions are occupational, medical or accidental exposures. (Medical x-rays generally deliver less than 10 mrem). EPA and other regulatory agencies generally limit exposures from specific source to the public to levels well under 100 mrem. This is far below the exposure levels that cause acute health effects.

How Does EPA Protect against Radionuclides That Are Also Toxic?

In most cases, the radiation hazard is much greater than the chemical (toxic) hazard. Radiation protection limits are lower than the chemical hazard protection limits would be. By issuing radiation protection regulations, EPA can protect people from both the radiation and the chemical hazard. However, deciding which hazard is greater is not always straightforward. Several factors can tip the balance:

- toxicity of the radionuclide
- strength of the ionizing radiation
- how quickly the radionuclide emits radiation (half-life)
- relative abundance of the radioactive and non-radioactive forms

For example:

- Uranium-238 radioactive and very toxic. Its half-life of 4.5 billion years means that only a few atoms emit radiation at a time. A sample containing enough atoms to pose a radiation hazard contains enough atoms to pose a chemical hazard. As a result, EPA regulates uranium-238 as both a chemical and a radiation hazard.

- Radioactive isotopes of lead are both radioactive and toxic. In spite of the severe effects of lead on the brain and the nervous system, the radiation hazard is greater. However, the radioactive forms of lead are so uncommon that paint or other lead containing products do not contain enough radioactive lead to present a radiation hazard. As a result, EPA regulates lead as a chemical hazard.

Chapter 42

Radon

Radon is estimated to cause between 15,000 and 22,000 lung can-cer deaths per year according to the National Academy of Sciences 1998 data. The numbers of deaths from other causes are taken from 2001 National Safety Council reports.

Radon is a cancer-causing, radioactive gas. You can't see radon. And you can't smell it or taste it. But it may be a problem in your home. Radon is estimated to cause many thousands of deaths each year. That's because when you breathe air containing radon, you can get lung cancer. In fact, the Surgeon General has warned that radon is the second leading cause of lung cancer in the United States today. Only smoking causes more lung cancer deaths. If you smoke and your home has high radon levels, your risk of lung cancer is especially high.

Radon Can Be Found All over the U.S.

Radon comes from the natural (radioactive) breakdown of uranium in soil, rock and water and gets into the air you breathe. Radon can be found all over the U.S. It can get into any type of building—homes, offices, and schools—and result in a high indoor radon level. But you

"A Citizen's Guide to Radon: The Guide to Protect Yourself and Your Family from Radon (4th Edition)," a brochure produced by the U.S. Environmental Pro-tection Agency (EPA), U.S. Department of Health and Human Services (DHHS), and the U.S. Public Health Service Office of Air and Radiation, Indoor Envi-ronments Division (6609J), EPA Document 402-K02-006. Revised May 2002. Available online at http://www.epa.gov/iaq/radon/pubs/citguide.html.

and your family are most likely to get your greatest exposure at home. That's where you spend most of your time.

Testing for Radon in Your Home

Testing is the only way to know if you and your family are at risk from radon. EPA and the Surgeon General recommend testing all homes below the third floor for radon. EPA also recommends testing in schools.

Testing is inexpensive and easy—it should only take a few minutes of your time. Millions of Americans have already tested their homes for radon.

Fixing the Problem of Radon in Your Home

There are simple ways to fix a radon problem that aren't too costly. Even very high levels can be reduced to acceptable levels.

New homes can be built with radon-resistant features. Radon-resistant construction techniques can be effective in preventing radon entry. When installed properly and completely, these simple and inexpensive techniques can help reduce indoor radon levels in homes. In addition, installing them at the time of construction makes it easier and less expensive to reduce radon levels further if these passive techniques don't reduce radon levels to below 4 pCi/L. Every new home should be tested after occupancy, even if it was built radon-resistant.

How Does Radon Get into Your Home?

Radon is a radioactive gas. It comes from the natural decay of uranium that is found in nearly all soils. It typically moves up through the ground to the air above and into your home through cracks and other holes in the foundation. Your home traps radon inside, where it can build up. Any home may have a radon problem. This means new and old homes, well-sealed and drafty homes, and homes with or without basements.

Radon from soil gas is the main cause of radon problems. Sometimes radon enters the home through well water. In a small number of homes, the building materials can give off radon, too. However, building materials rarely cause radon problems by themselves.

Radon gets in through:

- Cracks in solid floors

- Construction joints
- Cracks in walls
- Gaps in suspended floors
- Gaps around service pipes
- Cavities inside walls
- The water supply

Nearly 1 out of every 15 homes in the U.S. is estimated to have elevated radon levels. Elevated levels of radon gas have been found in homes in your state. Contact your state radon office for general information about radon in your area. While radon problems may be more common in some areas, any home may have a problem. The only way to know about your home is to test.

Radon can be a problem in schools and workplaces, too. Ask your state radon office about radon problems in schools, daycare and childcare facilities, and workplaces in your area.

How to Test Your Home

You can't see radon, but it's not hard to find out if you have a radon problem in your home. All you need to do is test for radon. Testing is easy and should only take a few minutes of your time. The amount of radon in the air is measured in "picoCuries per liter of air," or "pCi/L." Sometimes test results are expressed in Working Levels (WL) rather than picoCuries per liter (pCi/L). There are many kinds of low-cost do-it-yourself radon test kits you can get through the mail and in hardware stores and other retail outlets. If you prefer, or if you are buying or selling a home, you can hire a qualified tester to do the testing for you. You should contact your state radon office about obtaining a list of qualified testers. You can also contact a private radon proficiency program for lists of privately certified radon professionals serving your area.

There are two general ways to test for radon:

Short-term testing: The quickest way to test is with short-term tests. Short-term tests remain in your home for two days to 90 days, depending on the device. Charcoal canisters, alpha track, electret ion chamber, continuous monitors, and charcoal liquid scintillation detectors are most commonly used for short-term testing. Because radon levels tend to vary from day to day and season to season, a short-term test is less likely than a long-term test to tell you your year-round average radon level. If you need results quickly, however, a short-term test followed by a second short-term test may be used to decide whether to fix your home.

Long-term testing: Long-term tests remain in your home for more than 90 days. Alpha track and electret detectors are commonly used for this type of testing. A long-term test will give you a reading that is more likely to tell you your home's year-round average radon level than a short-term test.

How to Use a Test Kit

Follow the instructions that come with your test kit. If you are doing a short-term test, close your windows and outside doors and keep them closed as much as possible during the test. Heating and air-conditioning system fans that re-circulate air may be operated. Do not operate fans or other machines which bring in air from outside. Fans that are part of a radon-reduction system or small exhaust fans operating only for short periods of time may run during the test. If you are doing a short-term test lasting just 2 or 3 days, be sure to close your windows and outside doors at least 12 hours before beginning the test, too. You should not conduct short-term tests lasting just 2 or 3 days during unusually severe storms or periods of unusually high winds. The test kit should be placed in the lowest lived-in level of the home (for example, the basement if it is frequently used, otherwise the first floor). It should be put in a room that is used regularly (like a living room, playroom, den or bedroom) but not your kitchen or bathroom. Place the kit at least 20 inches above the floor in a location where it won't be disturbed—away from drafts, high heat, high humidity, and exterior walls. Leave the kit in place for as long as the package says. Once you've finished the test, reseal the package and send it to the lab specified on the package right away for analysis. You should receive your test results within a few weeks.

EPA recommends the following testing steps:

Step 1. Take a short-term test. If your result is 4 pCi/L or higher (0.02 Working Levels [WL] or higher) take a follow-up test (Step 2) to be sure.

Step 2. Follow up with either a long-term test or a second short-term test:

For a better understanding of your year-round average radon level, take a long-term test.

If you need results quickly, take a second short-term test.

The higher your initial short-term test result, the more certain you can be that you should take a short-term rather than a long-term follow up test. If your first short-term test result is more than twice EPA's 4 pCi/L action level, you should take a second short-term test immediately.

Step 3. If you followed up with a long-term test: Fix your home if your long-term test result is 4 pCi/L or more (0.02 Working Levels [WL] or higher). If you followed up with a second short-term test: The higher your short-term results, the more certain you can be that you should fix your home. Consider fixing your home if the average of your first and second test is 4 pCi/L or higher (0.02 Working Levels [WL] or higher).

What Your Test Results Mean

The average indoor radon level is estimated to be about 1.3 pCi/L, and about 0.4 pCi/L of radon is normally found in the outside air. The U.S. Congress has set a long-term goal that indoor radon levels be no more than outdoor levels. While this goal is not yet technologically achievable in all cases, most homes today can be reduced to 2 pCi/L or below.

Sometimes short-term tests are less definitive about whether or not your home is above 4 pCi/L. This can happen when your results are close to 4 pCi/L. For example, if the average of your two short-term test results is 4.1 pCi/L, there is about a 50% chance that your year-round average is somewhat below 4 pCi/L. However, EPA believes that any radon exposure carries some risk—no level of radon is safe. Even radon levels below 4 pCi/L pose some risk, and you can reduce your risk of lung cancer by lowering your radon level.

If your living patterns change and you begin occupying a lower level of your home (such as a basement) you should retest your home on that level.

Even if your test result is below 4 pCi/L, you may want to test again sometime in the future.

Radon and Home Sales

More and more, home buyers and renters are asking about radon levels before they buy or rent a home. Because real estate sales happen quickly, there is often little time to deal with radon and other issues. The best thing to do is to test for radon now and save the results in case the buyer is interested in them. Fix a problem if it exists so it won't complicate your home sale. If you are planning to move, call your state radon office for EPA's pamphlet "Home Buyer's and Seller's Guide to Radon," which addresses some common questions. You can also use the results of two short-term tests done side-by-side (four inches apart) to decide whether to fix your home.

During home sales:

- Buyers often ask if a home has been tested, and if elevated levels were reduced.

- Buyers frequently want tests made by someone who is not involved in the home sale. Your state radon office can assist you in identifying a qualified tester.

- Buyers might want to know the radon levels in areas of the home (like a basement they plan to finish) that the seller might not otherwise test.

Today many homes are built to prevent radon from coming in. Your state or local area may require these radon-resistant construction features. Radon-resistant construction features usually keep radon levels in new homes below 2 pCi/L. If you are buying or renting a new home, ask the owner or builder if it has radon-resistant features. The EPA recommends building new homes with radon-resistant features in high radon potential (Zone 1) areas. For more information, refer to EPA's Map of Radon Zones and other useful EPA documents on radon-resistant new construction, or visit http://www.epa.gov/iaq/radon/index.html. Even if built radon-resistant, every new home should be tested for radon after occupancy. If you have a test result of 4 pCi/L or more, you can have a qualified mitigator easily add a vent fan to an existing passive system for about $300 and further reduce the radon level in your home.

Radon in Water

The radon in your home's indoor air can come from two sources, the soil or your water supply. Compared to radon entering the home through water, radon entering your home through the soil is usually a much larger risk.

The radon in your water supply poses an inhalation risk and an ingestion risk. Research has shown that your risk of lung cancer from breathing radon in air is much larger than your risk of stomach cancer from swallowing water with radon in it. Most of your risk from radon in water comes from radon released into the air when water is used for showering and other household purposes.

Radon in your home's water is not usually a problem when its source is surface water. A radon in water problem is more likely when its source is ground water, e.g. a private well or a public water supply system that uses ground water. Some public water systems treat their water to reduce radon levels before it is delivered to your home. If you are concerned that radon may be entering your home through the water and your water comes from a public water supply, contact your water supplier.

If you've tested your private well and have a radon in water problem, it can be easily fixed. Your home's water supply can be treated in two ways. Point-of-entry treatment can effectively remove radon from the water before it enters your home. Point-of-use treatment devices remove radon from your water at the tap, but only treat a small portion of the water you use and are not effective in reducing the risk from breathing radon released into the air from all water used in the home.

For more information, call EPA's Drinking Water Hotline at 800-426-4791 or visit http://www.epa.gov/safewater/radon.html If your water comes from a private well, you can also contact your state radon office.

How to Lower the Radon Level in Your Home

Since there is no known safe level of radon, there can always be some risk. But the risk can be reduced by lowering the radon level in your home.

A variety of methods are used to reduce radon in your home. In some cases, sealing cracks in floors and walls may help to reduce radon. In other cases, simple systems using pipes and fans may be used to reduce radon. Such systems, known as soil suction, do not require major changes to your home. These systems remove radon gas from below the concrete floor and the foundation before it can enter the home. Similar systems can also be installed in houses with crawl spaces. Radon contractors use other methods that may also work in your home. The right system depends on the design of your home and other factors.

Ways to reduce radon in your home are discussed in EPA's "Consumer's Guide to Radon Reduction." You can get a copy from your state radon office.

The cost of making repairs to reduce radon depends on how your home was built and the extent of the radon problem. Most homes can be fixed for about the same cost as other common home repairs like painting or having a new hot water heater installed. The average house costs about $1,200 for a contractor to fix, although this can range from about $800 to about $2,500. The cost is much less if a passive system was installed during construction.

Radon and Home Renovations

If you are planning any major structural renovation, such as converting an unfinished basement area into living space, it is especially important to test the area for radon before you begin the renovation. If your test results indicate a radon problem radon-resistant techniques can be inexpensively included as part of the renovation. Because major renovations can change the level of radon in any home, always test again after work is completed.

Lowering high radon levels requires technical knowledge and special skills. You should use a contractor who is trained to fix radon problems. A qualified contractor can study the radon problem in your home and help you pick the right treatment method.

Check with your state radon office for names of qualified or state certified radon contractors in your area. You can also contact private radon proficiency programs for lists of privately certified radon professionals in your area. For more information on private radon proficiency programs, visit http://www.epa.gov/iaq/radon/proficiency.html. Picking someone to fix your radon problem is much like choosing a contractor for other home repairs—you may want to get references and more than one estimate.

If you are considering fixing your home's radon problem yourself, you should first contact your state radon office for guidance and assistance.

You should also test your home again after it is fixed to be sure that radon levels have been reduced. Most soil suction radon reduction systems include a monitor that will indicate whether the system is operating properly. In addition, it's a good idea to retest your home every two years to be sure radon levels remain low.

The Risk of Living with Radon

Radon gas decays into radioactive particles that can get trapped in your lungs when you breathe. As they break down further, these particles release small bursts of energy. This can damage lung tissue and lead to lung cancer over the course of your lifetime. Not everyone exposed to elevated levels of radon will develop lung cancer. And the amount of time between exposure and the onset of the disease may be many years.

Like other environmental pollutants, there is some uncertainty about the magnitude of radon health risks. However, we know more about radon risks than risks from most other cancer-causing substances. This is because estimates of radon risks are based on studies of cancer in humans (underground miners).

Smoking combined with radon is an especially serious health risk. Stop smoking and lower your radon level to reduce your lung cancer risk.

Children have been reported to have greater risk than adults of certain types of cancer from radiation, but there are currently no conclusive data on whether children are at greater risk than adults from radon.

Your chances of getting lung cancer from radon depend mostly on:

- How much radon is in your home
- The amount of time you spend in your home
- Whether you are a smoker or have ever smoked

It's never too late to reduce your risk of lung cancer. Don't wait to test and fix a radon problem. If you are a smoker, stop smoking.

Some Common Myths about Radon

MYTH: Scientists are not sure that radon really is a problem.

FACT: Although some scientists dispute the precise number of deaths due to radon, all the major health organizations (like the Centers for Disease Control and Prevention, the American Lung Association and the American Medical Association) agree with estimates that radon causes thousands of preventable lung cancer deaths every year. This is especially true among smokers, since the risk to smokers is much greater than to non-smokers.

MYTH: Radon testing is difficult, time-consuming and expensive.

FACT: Radon testing is inexpensive and easy—it should take only a little of your time.

MYTH: Radon testing devices are not reliable and are difficult to find.

FACT: Reliable testing devices are available through the mail, in hardware stores and other retail outlets. Call your state radon office for a list of radon device companies or visit our radon proficiency program web site for information on two privately run national radon proficiency programs.

MYTH: Homes with radon problems can't be fixed.

FACT: There are solutions to radon problems in homes. Thousands of homeowners have already fixed radon problems in their homes. Radon levels can be readily lowered for $500 to $2,500. Call your state radon office or visit our radon proficiency program web site for information on how to acquire the services of a qualified professional.

MYTH: Radon affects only certain kinds of homes.

Table 42.1. Radon Risk If You Smoke

Radon Level	If 1,000 people who smoked were exposed to this level over a lifetime...	The risk of cancer from radon exposure compares to...	What to Do: Stop smoking and...
20 pCi/L	About 135 people could get lung cancer	100 times the risk of drowning	Fix your home
10 pCi/L	About 71 people could get lung cancer	100 times the risk of dying in a home fire	Fix your home
8 pCi/L	About 57 people could get lung cancer		Fix your home
4 pCi/L	About 29 people could get lung cancer	100 times the risk of dying in an airplane crash	Fix your home
2 pCi/L	About 15 people could get lung cancer	2 times the risk of dying in a car crash	Consider fixing between 2 and 4 pCi/L
1.3 pCi/L	About 9 people could get lung cancer	(Average indoor radon level)	(Reducing radon levels below 2 pCi/L is difficult.)
0.4 pCi/L	About 3 people could get lung cancer	(Average outdoor radon level)	(Reducing radon levels below 2 pCi/L is difficult.)

Note: If you are a former smoker, your risk may be lower.

FACT: House construction can affect radon levels. However, radon can be a problem in homes of all types: old homes, new homes, drafty homes, insulated homes, homes with basements and homes without basements.

MYTH: Radon is only a problem in certain parts of the country.

FACT: High radon levels have been found in every state. Radon problems do vary from area to area, but the only way to know the home's radon level is to test.

MYTH: A neighbor's test result is a good indication of whether your home has a problem.

FACT: It's not. Radon levels vary from home to home. The only way to know if your home has a radon problem is to test it.

Table 42.2. Radon Risk If You Have Never Smoked

Radon Level	If 1,000 people who never smoked were exposed to this level over a lifetime...	The risk of cancer from radon exposure compares to...	What to Do:
20 pCi/L	About 8 people could get lung cancer	The risk of being killed in a violent crime	Fix your home
10 pCi/L	About 4 people could get lung cancer		Fix your home
8 pCi/L	About 3 people could get lung cancer	10 times the risk of dying in an airplane crash	Fix your home
4 pCi/L	About 2 people could get lung cancer	The risk of drowning	Fix your home
2 pCi/L	About 1 person could get lung cancer	The risk of dying in a home fire	Consider fixing between 2 and 4 pCi/L
1.3 pCi/L	Less than 1 person could get lung cancer	(Average indoor radon level)	(Reducing radon levels below 2 pCi/L is difficult.)
0.4 pCi/L	Less than 1 person could get lung cancer	(Average outdoor radon level)	(Reducing radon levels below 2 pCi/L is difficult.)

Note: If you are a former smoker, your risk may be higher.

MYTH: Everyone should test their water for radon.

FACT: While radon gets into some homes through the water, it is important to first test the air in the home for radon. If you find high levels and your water comes from a well, call the Safe Drinking Water Hotline at 1-800-426-4791, or your state radon office for more information.

MYTH: It is difficult to sell homes where radon problems have been discovered.

FACT: Where radon problems have been fixed, home sales have not been blocked or frustrated. The added protection is some times a good selling point.

MYTH: I've lived in my home for so long, it doesn't make sense to take action now.

FACT: You will reduce your risk of lung cancer when you reduce radon levels, even if you've lived with a radon problem for a long time.

MYTH: Short-term tests cannot be used for making a decision about whether to fix your home.

FACT: A short-term test, followed by a second short-term test may be used to decide whether to fix your home. However, the closer the average of your two short-term tests is to 4 pCi/L, the less certain you can be about whether your year-round average is above or below that level. Keep in mind that radon levels below 4 pCi/L still pose some risk. Radon levels can be reduced in some homes to 2 pCi/L or below.

Surgeon General Health Advisory

"Indoor radon gas is a national health problem. Radon causes thousands of deaths each year. Millions of homes have elevated radon levels. Homes should be tested for radon. When elevated levels are confirmed, the problem should be corrected."

Chapter 43

Managing Radioactive Materials and Waste

Any activity that produces or uses radioactive materials generates radioactive waste. Mining, nuclear power generation, and various processes in industry, defense, medicine, and scientific research produce byproducts that include radioactive waste. Radioactive waste can be in gas, liquid or solid form, and its level of radioactivity can vary. The waste can remain radioactive for a few hours or several months or even hundreds of thousands of years.

Are There Different Kinds of Radioactive Waste?

Yes, radioactive waste sorts into six general categories:

- spent nuclear fuel from nuclear reactors,
- high-level radioactive waste from the reprocessing of spent nuclear fuel;
- transuranic radioactive waste, resulting mainly from manufacture of nuclear weapons;
- uranium mill tailings from the mining and milling of uranium ore;
- low-level radioactive waste, generally in the form of radioactively contaminated industrial or research waste; and
- naturally occurring radioactive material.

"Managing Radioactive Materials and Waste," an undated fact sheet produced by the U.S. Environmental Protection Agency (EPA). Available online at http://www.epa.gov/radiation/manage.htm. Cited February 2003.

Mixed waste contains both radioactive and chemical components. Mixed waste is not a category of nuclear waste because depending on the source and level of radioactivity, the waste may be categorized, for instance, as low-level versus high-level radioactive waste.

What about Disposing of Radioactive Waste?

Proper disposal is key to protecting the public's health and safety and the quality of the environment. However, because it can be so hazardous and can remain radioactive for so long, finding suitable disposal facilities for radioactive waste is difficult. Depending on the type of waste disposed, the disposal facility may need to contain radiation for a very long time.

Radioactive waste disposal practices have changed substantially since the 1970's. Evolving environmental protection considerations have provided the impetus to improve disposal technologies, and, in some cases, clean up facilities that are no longer in use. Designs for new disposal facilities and disposal methods must meet environmental protection and pollution prevention standards that are stricter than originally foreseen at the beginning of the atomic age.

How Is Radioactive Waste Disposal Regulated?

Disposal of radioactive waste is a complex issue, not only because of the nature of the waste, but also because of the complicated regulatory structure for managing it. There are a variety of stakeholders affected, and there are a number of regulatory entities involved. Federal government agencies involved in radioactive waste management include: the Environmental Protection Agency, the Nuclear Regulatory Commission, the Department of Energy, and the Department of Transportation. In addition, the states and affected Indian Tribes play a prominent role in protecting the public against the hazards of radioactive waste.

What Is EPA Doing about Radioactive Waste Management?

Generally speaking, EPA's role in radioactive waste management is to set (develop and issue) radiation protection standards and to provide technical expertise during radioactive site cleanup. EPA also works with and provides assistance to other federal agencies and state and local governments on radioactive waste issues.

Setting Standards

EPA sets generally applicable radiation protection standards for the safe management of radioactive waste. Federal, state, and other organizations implement EPA's standards in waste management regulations.

In some cases, such as the U.S. Department of Energy's (DOE) Waste Isolation Pilot Plant (WIPP) and Yucca Mountain repository, Congress has assigned EPA responsibility for setting site-specific standards. For WIPP, EPA also oversees DOE's activities and re-examines its certification of the facility's compliance with the standards every 5 years.

Chapter 44

Microwave Oven Radiation

Microwaves are used to detect speeding cars, to send telephone and television communications, and to treat muscle soreness. Industry uses microwaves to dry and cure plywood, to cure rubber and resins, to raise bread and doughnuts, and to cook potato chips. But the most common consumer use of microwave energy is in microwave ovens. That use has soared in the past decade.

The Food and Drug Administration (FDA) has regulated the manufacture of microwave ovens since 1971. On the basis of current knowledge about microwave radiation, the Agency believes that ovens that meet the FDA standard and are used according to the manufacturer's instructions are safe for use.

What Is Microwave Radiation?

Microwaves are a form of electromagnetic radiation; that is, they are waves of electrical and magnetic energy moving together through space. Electromagnetic radiation ranges from the energetic x-rays to the less energetic radio frequency waves used in broadcasting. Microwaves fall into the radio frequency band of electromagnetic radiation. Microwaves should not be confused with x-rays, which are more powerful.

"Microwave Oven Radiation," a fact sheet produced by the Center for Devices and Radiological Health (CDRH), U.S. Food and Drug Administration (FDA), 2000. Available online at http://www.fda.gov/cdrh/consumer/microwave.html.

Microwaves have three characteristics that allow them to be used in cooking: they are reflected by metal; they pass through glass, paper, plastic, and similar materials; and they are absorbed by foods.

Cooking with Microwaves

Microwaves are produced inside the oven by an electron tube called a magnetron. The microwaves bounce back and forth within the metal interior until they are absorbed by food. Microwaves cause the water molecules in food to vibrate, producing heat that cooks the food. That's why foods high in water content, like fresh vegetables, can be cooked more quickly than other foods. The microwave energy is changed to heat as soon as it is absorbed by food. Thus, it can not make food radioactive or contaminated.

Although heat is produced directly in the food, microwave ovens do not cook food from the inside out. When thick foods like roasts are cooked, the outer layers are heated and cooked primarily by microwaves while the inside is cooked mainly by the slower conduction of heat from the hot outer layers.

Microwave cooking can be more energy efficient than conventional cooking because foods cook faster and the energy heats only the food, not the oven compartment. Microwave cooking does not reduce the nutritional value of foods any more than conventional cooking. In fact, foods cooked in a microwave oven may keep more of their vitamins and minerals, because microwave ovens can cook more quickly and without adding water.

Glass, paper, ceramic, or plastic containers are used in microwave cooking because the microwaves pass through them. Although such containers can not be heated by microwaves, they can become hot from the heat of the food cooking inside. Some plastic containers should not be used in a microwave oven—they can be melted by the heat of the food inside. Generally, metal pans or aluminum foil should also not be used in a microwave oven, as the microwaves are reflected off these materials causing the food to cook unevenly and possibly damaging the oven. The instructions that come with each microwave oven indicate the kinds of containers to use. They also cover how to test containers to see whether or not they can be used in microwave ovens.

FDA recommends that microwave ovens not be used in home canning. It is believed that neither microwave ovens nor conventional ovens produce or maintain temperatures high enough to kill the harmful bacteria that occur in some foods while canning.

Microwave Oven Safety Standard

All microwave ovens made after October 1971 are covered by a radiation safety standard enforced by the FDA. The standard limits the amount of microwaves that can leak from an oven throughout its lifetime. The limit is 5 milliwatts of microwave radiation per square centimeter at approximately 2 inches from the oven surface. This is far below the level known to harm people. Furthermore, as you move away from an oven, the level of any leaking microwave radiation that might be reaching you decreases dramatically. For example, someone standing 20 inches from an oven would receive approximately one one-hundredth of the amount of microwaves received at 2 inches.

The standard also requires all ovens to have two independent interlock systems that stop the production of microwaves the moment the latch is released or the door opened. In addition, a monitoring system stops oven operation in case one or both of the interlock systems fail. The noise that many ovens continue to make after the door is open is usually the fan. The noise does not mean that microwaves are being produced. There is no residual radiation remaining after microwave production has stopped. In this regard a microwave oven is much like an electric light that stops glowing when it is turned off.

All ovens made since October 1971 must have a label stating that they meet the safety standard. In addition, FDA requires that all ovens made after October 1975 have a label explaining precautions for use. This requirement may be dropped if the manufacturer has proven that the oven will not exceed the allowable leakage limit even if used under the conditions cautioned against on the label.

To make sure the standard is met, FDA tests microwave ovens in commercial establishments, dealer and distributor premises, manufacturing plants, and its own laboratories. FDA also evaluates manufacturers' radiation testing and quality control programs. When FDA finds a radiation safety problem in a certain model or make of oven, it requires the manufacturer to correct all defective ovens at no cost to the consumer.

Although FDA believes the standard assures that microwave ovens do not present any radiation hazard, the Agency continues to reassess its adequacy as new information becomes available.

Microwave Ovens and Health

Much research is under way on microwaves and how they might affect the human body. It is known that microwave radiation can heat body tissue the same way it heats food. Exposure to high levels of microwaves can cause a painful burn. The lens of the eye is particularly sensitive to intense heat, and exposure to high levels of microwaves can cause cataracts. Likewise, the testes are very sensitive to changes in temperature. Accidental exposure to high levels of microwave energy can alter or kill sperm, producing temporary sterility. But these types of injuries—burns, cataracts, temporary sterility—can only be caused by exposure to large amounts of microwave radiation, much more than can leak from a microwave oven.

Less is known about what happens to people exposed to low levels of microwaves. To find out, large numbers of people who had been exposed to microwaves would have to be studied for many years. This information is not available. Much research has been done with experimental animals, but it is difficult to translate the effects of microwaves on animals to possible effects on humans. For one thing, there are differences in the way animals and humans absorb microwaves. For another, experimental conditions can't exactly simulate the conditions under which people use microwave ovens. However, these studies do help to better understand the possible effects of radiation.

One experiment, for example, showed that repeated exposure to low-level microwave radiation (less than 10 milliwatts per square centimeter) does not cause cataracts in rabbits. On the other hand, some animals display an avoidance reaction when exposed to low levels of microwaves—that is, they try to get away from the microwaves. Other effects noted in experimental animals include a decreased ability to perform certain tasks, genetic changes and an immune response (the body acts as if it were responding to protect itself from a disease). While these and similar effects have been observed in animals, their significance for human health remains unclear.

These kinds of findings, together with the fact that many scientific questions about exposure to low-levels of microwaves are not yet answered, point to the need for FDA to continue to enforce strict radiation controls. They also underscore the need for consumers to take certain common sense precautions.

Have Radiation Injuries Resulted from Microwave Ovens?

There have been allegations of radiation injury from microwave ovens. The injuries known to FDA, however, have been injuries that could have happened with any oven or cooking surface. For example, people have been burned by the hot food, splattering grease, or steam from food cooked in a microwave oven.

Ovens and Pacemakers

At one time there was concern that leakage from microwave ovens could interfere with certain electronic cardiac pacemakers. There was similar concern about pacemaker interference from electric shavers, auto ignition systems, and other electronic products. Because there are so many other products that also could cause this problem, FDA does not require microwave ovens to carry warnings for people with pacemakers. The problem has been largely resolved since pacemakers are now designed so they are shielded against such electrical interference. However, patients with pacemakers may wish to consult their physicians about this.

Checking Ovens for Leakage

There is little cause for concern about excess microwaves leaking from ovens unless the door hinges, latch, or seals are damaged, or if the oven was made before 1971. In FDA's experience, most ovens tested show little or no detectable microwave leakage. If there is some problem and you believe your oven might be leaking excessive microwaves, contact the oven manufacturer, a microwave oven service organization, your state health department, or the nearest FDA office. Some oven manufacturers will arrange for your oven to be checked. Many states have programs for inspecting ovens or they may be able to refer you to microwave oven servicing organizations that are equipped to test ovens for excessive emission. A limited number of ovens are also tested in homes by FDA as part of its overall program to make sure that ovens meet the safety standard.

A word of caution about the microwave testing devices being sold to consumers: FDA has tested a number of these devices and found them generally inaccurate and unreliable. If used, they should be relied on only for a very approximate reading. The sophisticated testing devices used by public health authorities to measure oven leakage are far more accurate and are periodically tested.

Tips on Safe Microwave Oven Operation

- Follow the manufacturer's instruction manual for recommended operating procedures and safety precautions for your oven model.

- Don't operate an oven if the door does not close firmly or is bent, warped, or otherwise damaged.

361

- Never operate an oven if you have reason to believe it will continue to operate with the door open.

- To add to the margin of safety already built into the oven, don't stand directly against an oven (and don't allow children to do this) for long periods of time while it is operating.

- Users should not heat water or liquids in the microwave oven for excessive amounts of time.

Erupted Hot Water Phenomena in Microwave Ovens

FDA has received reports of serious skin burns or scalding injuries around people's hands and faces as a result of hot water erupting out of a cup after it had been over-heated in a microwave oven. Over-heating of water in a cup can result in superheated water (past its boiling temperature) without appearing to boil.

This type of phenomena occurs if water is heated in a clean cup. If foreign materials such as instant coffee or sugar are added before heating, the risk is greatly reduced. If superheating has occurred, a slight disturbance or movement such as picking up the cup, or pouring in a spoon full of instant coffee, may result in a violent eruption with the boiling water exploding out of the cup.

What Can Consumers Do to Avoid Super-Heated Water?

Users should follow the precautions and recommendations found in the microwave oven instruction manuals, specifically the heating time. Users should not use excessive amounts of time when heating water or liquids in the microwave oven. Determine the best time setting to heat the water just to the desired temperature and use that time setting regularly.

Other Tips for Microwave Oven Use

- Some ovens should not be operated when empty. Refer to the instruction manual for your oven.

- Clean the oven cavity, the outer edge of the cavity, and the door with water and a mild detergent. A special microwave oven cleaner is not necessary. Do not use scouring pads, steel wool, or other abrasives.

Chapter 45

Smoke Detectors and Radiation

Smoke detectors and alarms are important home safety devices. Ionization chamber and photoelectric smoke detectors are the two most common types available commercially. Because these pages are most concerned with radiation protection, we will focus mainly on the ionization chamber technology.

Ionization chamber smoke detectors contain a small amount of radioactive material encapsulated in a metal chamber. They take advantage of the ions created by ionizing radiation to develop a low, but steady electrical current. Smoke particles entering the chamber disrupt the current and trigger the detector's alarm. Ionization chamber detectors react more quickly to fast flaming fires that give off little smoke.

How much radiation is in smoke detectors?

The radiation source in an ionization chamber detector is a very small disc, about 3 to 5 millimeters in diameter, weighing about 0.5 gram. It is a composite of americium-241 in a gold matrix. The average activity in a smoke detector source is about one microcurie, 1 millionth of a curie.

Americium emits alpha particles and low energy gamma rays. It has a half-life of about 432 years. The long half-life means that americium decays very slowly, emitting very little radiation. At the end

---

"Smoke Detectors and Radiation," an undated fact sheet produced by the U.S. Environmental Protection Agency (EPA). Available online at http://www.epa.gov/radiation/sources/smoke_alarm.htm. Cited February 2003.

of the 10-year useful life of the smoke detector, it retains essentially all its original activity.

How much radiation exposure will I get from a smoke detector?

As long as the radiation source stays in the detector, exposures would be negligible (less than about 1/100 of a millirem per year), since alpha particles cannot travel very far or penetrate even a single sheet of paper, and the gamma rays emitted by americium are relatively weak. If the source were removed, it would be very easy for a small child to swallow, but even then exposures would be very low because the source would pass through the body fairly rapidly (by contrast, the same amount of americium in a loose powdered form would give a significant dose if swallowed or inhaled). Still, it is not a good idea to separate the source from the detector apparatus.

Owning and Operating a Smoke Alarm

Regardless of the detection technology used in your smoke alarm, the product label, User's Manual or Warranty should state the expected useful life of the smoke detector. For example, smoke alarms with the UL label have been certified with an expected useful life of 10 years. The product label also will tell you whether this includes the useful life of the battery. If you do not have a lithium long life battery (10 years), fire officials recommend that you change your batteries at the same time you turn your clock back each year for the end of Daylight Saving Time. It's also important to make sure your smoke alarm is working properly. You should test the alarm periodically (there should be a button to press). But be very careful if you use a source of smoke to test the detector.

Smoke alarm and heat detector (which senses the heat from a fire to trigger an alarm or sprinkler system, but does not detect smoke) technologies are all relatively inexpensive for a homeowner. A smoke alarm can usually be purchased for $10 to $25. Many companies make separate products using either photoelectric or ionization technologies, or they combine the technologies in one product. Read the packaging and label material on the product. Smoke and heat detector technologies may also be combined with home break-in alarm equipment to provide a total home security system connected to your local fire and police services. Whether you choose an electrical or battery-operated model, you must follow the manufacturer's recommendations for installation, testing and maintenance to get maximum protection.

Chapter 46

Television Radiation

Putting Television Radiation in Perspective

Man cannot escape some radiation. We are surrounded by natural radioactivity in the earth and by cosmic rays from outer space. This is called background radiation and cannot be controlled. Manmade radiation, however, can and must be controlled.

Much of the manmade radiation people are exposed to comes from electronic products. These include diagnostic x-ray machines, television sets, microwave cooking ovens, radar devices, and lasers. In some cases, as with diagnostic x-rays, radiation from these devices is intended and serves a useful purpose. In others, as with TV sets, radiation is not intended and is not essential to the use of the product.

Why Do TV Receivers Give Off X-Rays?

X-rays may be produced when electrons, accelerated by high voltage, strike an obstacle while traveling in a vacuum, as in a TV tube. Since many of the components in television sets operate at thousands of volts, there is the potential for x-ray generation. These components

"We Want You to Know about Television Radiation," a fact sheet produced by the Center for Devices and Radiological Health (CDRH), U.S. Food and Drug Administration (FDA), 1999. Available online at http://www.fda.gov/cdrh/consumer/TVRad.html. Cited February 2003. Despite the older date of this document it will be helpful to those seeking information about the health effects of radiation emission from televisions.

may produce x-rays capable of escaping from the receiver cabinet or picture tube. It is this kind of radiation that can make TV sets a potential hazard. It should be emphasized, however, that most TV sets have been found not to give off any measurable level of radiation, and there is no evidence that radiation from TV sets has resulted in human injury.

Why Is the TV Radiation a Hazard?

Scientists are not yet certain what specific health effects may be expected from exposure to extremely low doses of low-level radiation over prolonged periods of time. The currently acceptable assumption is that there is no threshold of exposure below which x-radiation may not adversely affect human health. It is advisable, therefore, that x-radiation from TV sets, as well as other electronic products commonly used, be kept down to the lowest practicable level. It was for this purpose that Congress enacted the Radiation Control for Health and Safety Act of 1968.

Setting a Radiation Safety Standard

The Food and Drug Administration (FDA) has the responsibility for carrying out an electronic product radiation control program mandated by the Radiation Control for Health and Safety Act. Through it's Center for Devices and Radiological Health, FDA sets and enforces standards of performance for electronic products to assure that radiation emissions from them do not pose a hazard to public health.

A Federal standard limiting x-ray emissions from TV receivers to 0.5 milliroentgen per hour was issued on December 25, 1969. The standard was made applicable in three progressively more stringent phases, starting with sets manufactured after January 15, 1970. After the third phase had been reached, on June 1, 1971, the overall effect of the standard was to require that TV receivers must not emit x-radiation above the 0.5 milliroentgen per hour level under the most adverse operating conditions.

Assuring That TV Sets Meet the Standard

FDA has set up a special staff to assure that manufacturers are producing sets which comply with the Federal standard. All TV manufacturers must submit written reports to FDA outlining their plans for assuring that each set coming off the assembly line complies with the Federal x-ray limit. The manufacturers must provide test data to support their reports. They also must maintain records of test data and prepare an annual report to FDA summarizing these records. In addition, FDA representatives visit manufacturers' production facilities to obtain firsthand information on radiation control and record-keeping procedures and to measure x-ray leakage from randomly selected sets. TV sets also are tested in FDA's laboratories to determine compliance with the standard.

If a TV set is found to be emitting x-rays in excess of the limit, the manufacturer must take steps to correct it. If the manufacturer is unwilling to make required changes, legal action may be taken.

Television receivers which are offered for importation into the United States and which do not meet the standard are not allowed into the country and are destroyed if not exported in 90 days. Importers, however, may petition FDA for permission to correct the violations.

How Safe Are Home Sets Today?

X-radiation emissions from properly operated and serviced home television receivers manufactured since about the middle of 1968 are generally at levels too low to present a public health hazard. FDA occasionally finds some TV receivers which fail to comply with the standard, however, and it requires corrective action by the manufacturer.

What You Can Do

To assure that a new television receiver is as x-ray-free as is technically feasibly, purchasers should check the back of the set for a label or tag certifying that it meets the Federal standard on emissions. The label or tag must appear on all sets manufactured after January 15, 1970.

When the TV x-ray problem first became a public concern in 1966, the Surgeon General recommended that viewers sit at least six feet from an operating receiver to reduce the quite low potential of biological damage. Since that time, however, steps have been taken by both Government and industry to reduce further this exposure potential. There should now be no health hazard in watching TV at a distance at which the image quality is satisfactory to the viewer.

When your set needs servicing, call a qualified serviceman to assure that x-ray emissions are kept to a minimum. The primary cause of increased x-ray emission has been found to be adjustment of operating voltages to levels higher than recommended by manufacturers. Qualified servicemen have been trained in the proper adjustment of the voltage to reduce the possibility of x-ray production.

New TV x-ray detectors developed by FDA make it relatively easy for trained servicemen to identify sets with above maximum x-ray emissions. If excessive x-ray leakage is found and it cannot be corrected by the serviceman, the State or local health agency should be contacted for advice.

Caution should be exercised in trying to check a set with do-it-yourself devices. Even those devices based on sound scientific principles may be inadequate for detecting radiation from all portions of the set.

Chapter 47

Hazards of Electric and Magnetic Fields

Since the mid-twentieth century, electricity has been an essential part of our lives. Electricity powers our appliances, office equipment, and countless other devices that we use to make life safer, easier, and more interesting. Use of electric power is something we take for granted. However, some have wondered whether the electric and magnetic fields (EMF) produced through the generation, transmission, and use of electric power [power-frequency EMF, 50 or 60 hertz (Hz)] might adversely affect our health. Numerous research studies and scientific reviews have been conducted to address this question.

Unfortunately, initial studies of the health effects of EMF did not provide straightforward answers. The study of the possible health effects of EMF has been particularly complex and results have been reviewed by expert scientific panels in the United States and other countries. This chapter summarizes the results of these reviews. Although questions remain about the possibility of health effects related to EMF, recent reviews have substantially reduced the level of concern.

The largest evaluation to date was led by two U.S. government institutions, the National Institute of Environmental Health Sciences (NIEHS) of the National Institutes of Health and the Department of Energy (DOE), with input from a wide range of public and private agencies. This evaluation, known as the Electric and Magnetic Fields

Excerpted from "EMF: Electric and Magnetic Fields Associated with the Use of Electric Power, Questions and Answers," a brochure prepared by the National Institute of Environmental Health Sciences (NIEHS), 2002. Available online at http://www.niehs.nih.gov/emfrapid.

Research and Public Information Dissemination (EMF RAPID) Program, was a six-year project with the goal of providing scientific evidence to determine whether exposure to power-frequency EMF involves a potential risk to human health.

In 1999, at the conclusion of the EMF RAPID Program, the NIEHS reported to the U.S. Congress that the overall scientific evidence for human health risk from EMF exposure is weak. No consistent pattern of biological effects from exposure to EMF had emerged from laboratory studies with animals or with cells. However, epidemiological studies (studies of disease incidence in human populations) had shown a fairly consistent pattern that associated potential EMF exposure with a small increased risk for leukemia in children and chronic lymphocytic leukemia in adults. Since 1999, several other assessments have been completed that support an association between childhood leukemia and exposure to power-frequency EMF.

These more recent reviews, however, do not support a link between EMF exposures and adult leukemias. For both childhood and adult leukemias, interpretation of the epidemiological findings has been difficult due to the absence of supporting laboratory evidence or a scientific explanation linking EMF exposures with leukemia.

EMF exposures are complex and exist in the home and workplace as a result of all types of electrical equipment and building wiring as well as a result of nearby power lines.

EMF Basics

What Are Electric and Magnetic Fields?

Electric and magnetic fields (EMF) are invisible lines of force that surround any electrical device. Power lines, electrical wiring, and electrical equipment all produce EMF. There are many other sources of EMF as well. The focus of this chapter is on power-frequency EMF—that is, EMF associated with the generation, transmission, and use of electric power.

Electric fields are produced by voltage and increase in strength as the voltage increases. The electric field strength is measured in units of volts per meter (V/m). Magnetic fields result from the flow of current through wires or electrical devices and increase in strength as the current increases. Magnetic fields are measured in units of gauss (G) or tesla (T).

Most electrical equipment has to be turned on, i.e., current must be flowing, for a magnetic field to be produced. Electric fields are often present even when the equipment is switched off, as long as it remains connected to the source of electric power. Brief bursts of EMF (sometimes called transients) can also occur when electrical devices are turned on or off.

Electric fields are shielded or weakened by materials that conduct electricity—even materials that conduct poorly, including trees, buildings, and human skin. Magnetic fields, however, pass through most materials and are therefore more difficult to shield. Both electric fields and magnetic fields decrease rapidly as the distance from the source increases.

Even though electrical equipment, appliances, and power lines produce both electric and magnetic fields, most recent research has focused on potential health effects of magnetic field exposure. This is because some epidemiological studies have reported an increased cancer risk associated with estimates of magnetic field exposure. No similar associations have been reported for electric fields; many of the studies examining biological effects of electric fields were essentially negative.

Characteristics of Electric and Magnetic Fields

Electric fields and magnetic fields can be characterized by their wavelength, frequency, and amplitude (strength). The direction of the field alternates from one polarity to the opposite and back to the first polarity in a period of time called one cycle. Wavelength describes the distance between a peak on the wave and the next peak of the same polarity. The frequency of the field, measured in hertz (Hz), describes the number of cycles that occur in one second. Electricity in North America alternates through 60 cycles per second, or 60 Hz. In many other parts of the world, the frequency of electric power is 50 Hz.

The term EMF usually refers to electric and magnetic fields at extremely low frequencies such as those associated with the use of electric power. The term EMF can be used in a much broader sense as well, encompassing electromagnetic fields with low or high frequencies.

When we use EMF in this chapter, we mean extremely low frequency (ELF) electric and magnetic fields, ranging from 3 to 3,000 Hz. This range includes power-frequency (50 or 60 Hz) fields. In the ELF range, electric and magnetic fields are not coupled or interrelated in the same way that they are at higher frequencies. So, it is more useful to refer to them as electric and magnetic fields rather than electromagnetic fields. In the popular press, however, you will see both terms used, abbreviated as EMF.

How Are Power-Frequency EMF Different from Other Types of Electromagnetic Energy?

X-rays, visible light, microwaves, radio waves, and EMF are all forms of electromagnetic energy. One property that distinguishes different forms of electromagnetic energy is the frequency, expressed in hertz (Hz). Power-frequency EMF, 50 or 60 Hz, carries very little energy, has no ionizing effects, and usually has no thermal effects. Just as various chemicals affect our bodies in different ways, various forms of electromagnetic energy can have very different biological effects.

Some types of equipment or operations simultaneously produce electromagnetic energy of different frequencies. Welding operations, for example, can produce electromagnetic energy in the ultraviolet, visible, infrared, and radio-frequency ranges, in addition to power-frequency EMF. Microwave ovens produce 60-Hz fields of several hundred milligauss, but they also create microwave energy inside the oven that is at a much higher frequency (about 2.45 billion Hz). We are shielded from the higher frequency fields inside the oven by its casing, but we are not shielded from the 60-Hz fields.

Cellular telephones communicate by emitting high-frequency electric and magnetic fields similar to those used for radio and television broadcasts. These radio-frequency and microwave fields are quite different from the extremely low frequency EMF produced by power lines and most appliances.

How Are Alternating Current Sources of EMF Different from Direct Current Sources?

Some equipment can run on either alternating current (AC) or direct current (DC). In most parts of the United States, if the equipment is plugged into a household wall socket, it is using AC electric current that reverses direction in the electrical wiring—or alternates—60 times per second, or at 60 hertz (Hz). If the equipment uses batteries, then electric current flows in one direction only. This produces a static or stationary magnetic field, also called a direct current field. Some battery-operated equipment can produce time-varying magnetic fields as part of its normal operation.

What Happens When I Am Exposed to EMF?

In most practical situations, DC electric power does not induce electric currents in humans. Strong DC magnetic fields are present in some industrial environments, can induce significant currents when a person moves, and may be of concern for other reasons, such as potential effects on implanted medical devices.

AC electric power produces electric and magnetic fields that create weak electric currents in humans. These are called induced currents. Much of the research on how EMF may affect human health has focused on AC-induced currents.

Electric Fields

A person standing directly under a high-voltage transmission line may feel a mild shock when touching something that conducts electricity. These sensations are caused by the strong electric fields from the high-voltage electricity in the lines. They occur only at close range because the electric fields rapidly become weaker as the distance from the line increases. Electric fields may be shielded and further weakened by buildings, trees, and other objects that conduct electricity.

Magnetic Fields

Alternating magnetic fields produced by AC electricity can induce the flow of weak electric currents in the body. However, such currents are estimated to be smaller than the measured electric currents produced naturally by the brain, nerves, and heart.

Doesn't the Earth Produce EMF?

Yes. The earth produces EMF, mainly in the form of static fields, similar to the fields generated by DC electricity. Electric fields are produced by air turbulence and other atmospheric activity. The earth's magnetic field of about 500 mG is thought to be produced by electric currents flowing deep within the earth's core. Because these fields are static rather than alternating, they do not induce currents in stationary objects as do fields associated with alternating current. Such static fields can induce currents in moving and rotating objects.

Evaluating Potential Health Effects

How Do We Evaluate Whether EMF Exposures Cause Health Effects?

Animal experiments, laboratory studies of cells, clinical studies, computer simulations, and human population (epidemiological) studies all provide valuable information. When evaluating evidence that certain exposures cause disease, scientists consider results from studies in various disciplines. No single study or type of study is definitive.

Laboratory Studies

Laboratory studies with cells and animals can provide evidence to help determine if an agent such as EMF causes disease. Cellular studies can increase our understanding of the biological mechanisms by which disease occurs. Experiments with animals provide a means to observe effects of specific agents under carefully controlled conditions. Neither cellular nor animal studies, however, can recreate the complex nature of the whole human organism and its environment.

Therefore, we must use caution in applying the results of cellular or animal studies directly to humans or concluding that a lack of an effect in laboratory studies proves that an agent is safe. Even with these limitations, cellular and animal studies have proven very useful over the years for identifying and understanding the toxicity of numerous chemicals and physical agents.

Very specific laboratory conditions are needed for researchers to be able to detect EMF effects, and experimental exposures are not easily comparable to human exposures. In most cases, it is not clear how EMF actually produces the effects observed in some experiments. Without understanding how the effects occur, it is difficult to evaluate how laboratory results relate to human health effects.

Some laboratory studies have reported that EMF exposure can produce biological effects, including changes in functions of cells and tissues and subtle changes in hormone levels in animals. It is important to distinguish between a biological effect and a health effect. Many biological effects are within the normal range of variation and are not necessarily harmful. For example, bright light has a biological effect on our eyes, causing the pupils to constrict, which is a normal response.

Clinical Studies

In clinical studies, researchers use sensitive instruments to monitor human physiology during controlled exposure to environmental agents. In EMF studies, volunteers are exposed to electric or magnetic fields at higher levels than those commonly encountered in everyday life. Researchers measure heart rate, brain activity, hormonal levels, and other factors in exposed and unexposed groups to look for differences resulting from EMF exposure.

Epidemiology

A valuable tool to identify human health risks is to study a human population that has experienced the exposure. This type of research is called epidemiology.

The epidemiologist observes and compares groups of people who have had or have not had certain diseases and exposures to see if the risk of disease is different between the exposed and unexposed groups. The epidemiologist does not control the exposure and cannot experimentally control all the factors that might affect the risk of disease.

How Do We Characterize EMF Exposure?

No one knows which aspect of EMF exposure, if any, affects human health. Because of this uncertainty, in addition to the field strength, we must ask how long an exposure lasts, how it varies, and at what time of day or night it occurs. House wiring, for example, is often a significant source of EMF exposure for an individual, but the magnetic fields produced by the wiring depend on the amount of current flowing. As heating, lighting, and appliance use varies during the day, magnetic field exposure will also vary.

For many studies, researchers describe EMF exposures by estimating the average field strength. Some scientists believe that average exposure may not be the best measurement of EMF exposure and that other parameters, such as peak exposure or time of exposure, may be important.

Results of EMF Research

Is There a Link between EMF Exposure and Childhood Leukemia?

Despite more than two decades of research to determine whether elevated EMF exposure, principally to magnetic fields, is related to an increased risk of childhood leukemia, there is still no definitive answer. Much progress has been made, however, with some lines of research leading to reasonably clear answers and others remaining unresolved. The best available evidence at this time leads to the following answers to specific questions about the link between EMF exposure and childhood leukemia:

Is There An Association between Power Line Configurations (Wire Codes) and Childhood Leukemia?

No.

Is There An Association between Measured Fields and Childhood Leukemia?

Yes, but the association is weak, and it is not clear whether it represents a cause-and-effect relationship.

What Is the Epidemiological Evidence for Evaluating a Link between EMF Exposure and Childhood Leukemia?

The initial studies, starting with the pioneering research of Dr. Nancy Wertheimer and Ed Leeper in 1979 in Denver, Colorado, focused on power line configurations near homes. Power lines were systematically evaluated and coded for their presumed ability to produce elevated magnetic fields in homes and classified into groups with higher and lower predicted magnetic field levels.

Although the first study and two that followed in Denver and Los Angeles showed an association between wire codes indicative of elevated magnetic fields and childhood leukemia, larger, more recent studies in the central part of the United States and in several provinces of Canada did not find such an association. In fact, combining the evidence from all the studies, we can conclude with some confidence that wire codes are not associated with a measurable increase in the risk of childhood leukemia.

The other approach to assessing EMF exposure in homes focused on the measurements of magnetic fields. Unlike wire codes, which are only applicable in North America due to the nature of the electric power distribution system, measured fields have been studied in relation to childhood leukemia in research conducted around the world, including Sweden, England, Germany, New Zealand, and Taiwan. Large, detailed studies have recently been completed in the United States, Canada, and the United Kingdom that provide the most evidence for making an evaluation. These studies have produced variable findings, some reporting small associations, others finding no associations.

After reviewing all the data, the U.S. National Institute of Environmental Health Sciences (NIEHS) concluded in 1999 that the evidence was weak, but that it was still sufficient to warrant limited concern. The NIEHS rationale was that no individual epidemiological study provided convincing evidence linking magnetic field exposure with childhood leukemia, but the overall pattern of results for some methods of measuring exposure suggested a weak association between increasing exposure to EMF and increasing risk of childhood leukemia. The small number of cases in these studies made it impossible to firmly demonstrate this association. However, the fact that similar results had been observed in studies of different populations using a variety of study designs supported this observation.

A major challenge has been to determine whether the most highly elevated, but rarely encountered, levels of magnetic fields are associated with an increased risk of leukemia. Early reports focused on the risk associated with exposures above 2 or 3 milligauss, but the more recent studies have been large enough to also provide some information on levels above 3 or 4 milligauss. It is estimated that 4.5% of homes in the United States have magnetic fields above 3 milligauss, and 2.5% of homes have levels above 4 milligauss.

To determine what the integrated information from all the studies says about magnetic fields and childhood leukemia, two groups have conducted pooled analyses in which the original data from relevant studies were integrated and analyzed. One report (Greenland et al., 2000) combined 12 relevant studies with magnetic field measurements, and the other considered 9 such studies (Ahlbom et al., 2000). The details of the two-pooled analyses are different, but their findings are similar. There is weak evidence for an association (relative risk of approximately 2) at exposures above 3 mG. However, few individuals had high exposures in these studies; therefore, even combining all studies, there is uncertainty about the strength of the association.

Is There a Link between EMF Exposure and Childhood Brain Cancer or Other Forms of Cancer in Children?

Although the earliest studies suggested an association between EMF exposure and all forms of childhood cancer, those initial findings have not been confirmed by other studies. At present, the available series of studies indicates no association between EMF exposure and childhood cancers other than leukemia. Far fewer of these studies have been conducted than studies of childhood leukemia.

Is There a Link between Residential EMF Exposure and Cancer in Adults?

The few studies that have been conducted to address EMF and adult cancer do not provide strong evidence for an association. Thus, a link has not been established between residential EMF exposure and adult cancers, including leukemia, brain cancer, and breast cancer.

Have Clusters of Cancer or Other Adverse Health Effects Been Linked to EMF Exposure?

An unusually large number of cancers, miscarriages, or other adverse health effects that occur in one area or over one period of time is called a cluster. Sometimes clusters provide an early warning of a health hazard. But most of the time the reason for the cluster is not known. There have been no proven instances of cancer clusters linked with EMF exposure.

If EMF Does Cause or Promote Cancer, Shouldn't Cancer Rates Have Increased Along with the Increased Use of Electricity?

Not necessarily. Although the use of electricity has increased greatly over the years, EMF exposures may not have increased. Changes in building wiring codes and in the design of electrical appliances have in some cases resulted in lower magnetic field levels. Rates for various types of cancer have shown both increases and decreases through the years, due in part to improved prevention, diagnosis, reporting, and treatment.

Is There a Link between EMF Exposure in Electrical Occupations and Cancer?

For almost as long as we have been concerned with residential exposure to EMF and childhood cancers, researchers have been studying workplace exposure to EMF and adult cancers, focusing on leukemia and brain cancer. This research began with surveys of job titles and cancer risks, but has progressed to include very large, detailed studies of the health of workers, especially electric utility workers, in the United States, Canada, France, England, and several Northern European countries. Some studies have found evidence that suggests a link between EMF exposure and both leukemia and brain cancer, whereas other studies of similar size and quality have not found such associations.

Efforts have also been made to pool the findings across several of the above studies to produce more accurate estimates of the association between EMF and cancer (Kheifets et al., 1999). The combined summary statistics across studies provide insufficient evidence for an association between EMF exposure in the workplace and either leukemia or brain cancer.

Have Studies of Workers in Other Industries Suggested a Link between EMF Exposure and Cancer?

One of the largest studies to report an association between cancer and magnetic field exposure in a broad range of industries was conducted in Sweden (1993). The study included an assessment of EMF exposure in 1,015 different workplaces and involved more than 1,600 people in 169 different occupations. An association was reported between estimated EMF exposure and increased risk for chronic lymphocytic leukemia. An association was also reported between exposure to magnetic fields and brain cancer, but there was no dose-response relationship.

Another Swedish study (1994) found an excess risk of lymphocytic leukemia among railway engine drivers and conductors. However, the total cancer incidence (all tumors included) for this group of workers was lower than in the general Swedish population. A study of Norwegian railway workers found no evidence for an association between EMF exposure and leukemia or brain cancer. Although both positive and negative effects of EMF exposure have been reported, the majority of studies show no effects.

Is There a Link between EMF Exposure and Breast Cancer?

Researchers have been interested in the possibility that EMF exposure might cause breast cancer, in part because breast cancer is such a common disease in adult women. Early studies identified a few electrical workers with male breast cancer, a very rare disease. A link between EMF exposure and alterations in the hormone melatonin was considered a possible hypothesis. This idea provided motivation to conduct research addressing a possible link between EMF exposure and breast cancer.

Overall, the published epidemiological studies have not shown such an association.

What Have We Learned from Clinical Studies?

Laboratory studies with human volunteers have attempted to answer questions such as:

- Does EMF exposure alter normal brain and heart function?
- Does EMF exposure at night affect sleep patterns?
- Does EMF exposure affect the immune system?
- Does EMF exposure affect hormones?

The following kinds of biological effects have been reported. Keep in mind that a biological effect is simply a measurable change in some biological response. It may or may not have any bearing on health.

Heart rate. An inconsistent effect on heart rate by EMF exposure has been reported. When observed, the biological response is small (on average, a slowing of about three to five beats per minute), and the response does not persist once exposure has ended. Two laboratories, one in the United States and one in Australia, have reported effects of EMF on heart rate variability. Exposures used in these experiments were relatively high (about 300 mG), and lower exposures failed to produce the effect. Effects have not been observed consistently in repeated experiments.

Sleep electrophysiology. A laboratory report suggested that overnight exposure to 60-Hz magnetic fields may disrupt brain electrical activity (EEG) during night sleep. In this study subjects were exposed to either continuous or intermittent magnetic fields of 283 mG. Individuals exposed to the intermittent magnetic fields showed alterations in traditional EEG sleep parameters indicative of a pattern of poor and disrupted sleep. Several studies have reported no effect with continuous exposure.

Hormones, immune system, and blood chemistry. Several clinical studies with human volunteers have evaluated the effects of power-frequency EMF exposure on hormones, the immune system, and blood chemistry. These studies provide little evidence for any consistent effect.

Melatonin. The hormone melatonin is secreted mainly at night and primarily by the pineal gland, a small gland attached to the brain. Some laboratory experiments with cells and animals have shown that melatonin can slow the growth of cancer cells, including breast cancer cells. Suppressed nocturnal melatonin levels have been observed in some studies of laboratory animals exposed to both electric and magnetic fields. These observations led to the hypothesis that EMF exposure might reduce melatonin and thereby weaken one of the body's defenses against cancer.

Many clinical studies with human volunteers have now examined whether various levels and types of magnetic field exposure affect blood levels of melatonin. Exposure of human volunteers at night to power-frequency EMF under controlled laboratory conditions has no apparent effect on melatonin. Some studies of people exposed to EMF at work or at home do report evidence for a small suppression of melatonin. It is not clear whether the decreases in melatonin reported under environmental conditions are related to the presence of EMF exposure or to other factors.

What Effects of EMF Have Been Reported in Laboratory Studies of Cells?

Over the years, scientists have conducted more than 1,000 laboratory studies to investigate potential biological effects of EMF exposure. Most have been in vitro studies; that is, studies carried out on cells isolated from animals and plants, or on cell components such as cell membranes. Other studies involved animals, mainly rats and mice. In general, these studies do not demonstrate a consistent effect of EMF exposure.

Most in vitro studies have used magnetic fields of 1,000 mG (100 μT) or higher, exposures that far exceed daily human exposures. In most incidences, when one laboratory has reported effects of EMF exposure on cells, other laboratories have not been able to reproduce the findings. For such research results to be widely accepted by scientists as valid they must be replicated—that is, scientists in other laboratories should be able to repeat the experiment and get similar results. Cellular studies have investigated potential EMF effects on cell proliferation and differentiation, gene expression, enzyme activity, melatonin, and DNA. Scientists reviewing the EMF research literature find overall that the cellular studies provide little convincing evidence of EMF effects at environmental levels.

Have Effects of EMF Been Reported in Laboratory Studies in Animals?

Researchers have published more than 30 detailed reports on both long-term and short-term studies of EMF exposures in laboratory animals (bioassays). Long-term animal bioassays constitute an important group of studies in EMF research. Such studies have a proven record for predicting the carcinogenicity of chemicals, physical agents, and other suspected cancer-causing agents. In the EMF studies, large groups of mice or rats were continuously exposed to EMF for two years or longer and were then evaluated for cancer. The U.S. National Toxicology Program has an extensive historical database for hundreds of different chemical and physical agents evaluated using this model. EMF long-term bioassays examined leukemia, brain cancer, and breast cancer—the diseases some epidemiological studies have associated with EMF exposure.

Several different approaches have been used to evaluate effects of EMF exposure in animal bioassays. To investigate whether EMF could promote cancer after genetic damage had occurred, some long-term studies used cancer initiators such as ultraviolet light, radiation, or certain chemicals that are known to cause genetic damage. Researchers compared groups of animals treated with cancer initiators to groups treated with cancer initiators and then exposed to EMF, to see if EMF exposure promoted the cancer growth (initiation-promotion model). Other studies tested the cancer promotion potential of EMF using mice that were predisposed to cancer because they had defects in the genes that control cancer.

Can EMF Exposure Damage DNA?

Studies have attempted to determine whether EMF has genotoxic potential; that is, whether EMF exposure can alter the genetic material of living organisms. This question is important because genotoxic agents often also cause cancer or birth defects. Studies of genotoxicity have included tests on bacteria, fruit flies, and some tests on rats and mice. Nearly 100 studies on EMF genotoxicity have been reported. Most evidence suggests that EMF exposure is not genotoxic. Based on experiments with cells, some researchers have suggested that EMF exposure may inhibit the cell's ability to repair normal DNA damage, but this idea remains speculative because of the lack of genotoxicity observed in EMF animal studies.

Your EMF Environment

How Do We Define EMF Exposure?

Scientists are still uncertain about the best way to define exposure because experiments have yet to show which aspect of the field, if any, may be relevant to reported biological effects. Important aspects of exposure could be the highest intensity, the average intensity, or the amount of time spent above a certain baseline level. The most widely used measure of EMF exposure has been the time-weighted average magnetic field level.

How Is EMF Exposure Measured?

Several kinds of personal exposure meters are now available. These automatically record the magnetic field as it varies over time. To determine a person's EMF exposure, the personal exposure meter is usually worn at the waist or is placed as close as possible to the person during the course of a work shift or day.

EMF can also be measured using survey meters, sometimes called gauss-meters. These measure the EMF levels in a given location at a given time. Such measurements do not necessarily reflect personal EMF exposure because they are not always taken at the distance from the EMF source that the person would typically be from the source. Measurements are not always made in a location for the same amount of time that a person spends there. Such spot measurements also fail to capture variations of the field over time, which can be significant.

What Levels of EMF are Found in Common Environments?

Magnetic field exposures can vary greatly from site to site for any type of environment. The data shown in the Table 47.1 are median measurements taken at four different sites for each environment category.

What EMF Field Levels Are Encountered in the Home?

Electric fields. Electric fields in the home, on average, range from 0 to 10 volts per meter. They can be hundreds, thousands, or even millions of times weaker than those encountered outdoors near power lines. Electric fields directly beneath power lines may vary from a few volts per meter for some overhead distribution lines to several thousands of volts per meter for extra high voltage power lines. Electric fields from power lines rapidly become weaker with distance and can be greatly reduced by walls and roofs of buildings.

Magnetic fields. Magnetic fields are not blocked by most materials. Magnetic fields encountered in homes vary greatly. Magnetic fields rapidly become weaker with distance from the source.

Table 47.1. EMF Exposures in Common Environments

Magnetic fields measured in milligauss (mG)

Environment	Median* Exposure	Top 5th Percentile
Office Building		
Support staff	0.6	3.7
Professional	0.5	2.6
Maintenance	0.6	3.8
Visitor	0.6	2.1
School		
Teacher	0.6	3.3
Student	0.5	2.9
Custodian	1.0	4.9
Administrative staff	1.3	6.9
Hospital		
Patient	0.6	3.6
Medical staff	0.8	5.6
Visitor	0.6	2.4
Maintenance	0.6	5.9
Machine Shop		
Machinist	0.4	6.0
Welder	1.1	24.6
Engineer	1.0	5.1
Assembler	0.5	6.4
Office staff	0.7	4.7
Grocery Store		
Cashier	2.7	11.9
Butcher	2.4	12.8
Office staff	2.1	7.1
Customer	1.1	7.7

*The median of four measurements. For this table, the median is the average of the two middle measurements.

Source: National Institute for Occupational Safety and Health (NIOSH).

What Are EMF Levels Close to Electrical Appliances?

Magnetic fields close to electrical appliances are often much stronger than those from other sources, including magnetic fields directly under power lines. Appliance fields decrease in strength with distance more quickly than do power line fields. Magnetic field strength (magnitude) does not depend on how large, complex, powerful, or noisy the appliance is. Magnetic fields near large appliances are often weaker than those near small devices.

What EMF Levels Are Found near Power Lines?

Power transmission lines bring power from a generating station to an electrical substation. Power distribution lines bring power from the substation to your home. Transmission and distribution lines can be either overhead or underground. Overhead lines produce both electric fields and magnetic fields. Underground lines do not produce electric fields above ground but may produce magnetic fields above ground.

Power transmission lines. At a distance of 300 feet and at times of average electricity demand, the magnetic fields from many lines can be similar to typical background levels found in most homes. The distance at which the magnetic field from the line becomes indistinguishable from typical background levels differs for different types of lines.

Power distribution lines. Typical voltage for power distribution lines in North America ranges from 4 to 24 kilovolts (kV). Electric field levels directly beneath overhead distribution lines may vary from a few volts per meter to 100 or 200 volts per meter. Magnetic fields directly beneath overhead distribution lines typically range from 10 to 20 mG for main feeders and less than 10 mG for laterals. Such levels are also typical directly above underground lines. Peak EMF levels, however, can vary considerably depending on the amount of current carried by the line. Peak magnetic field levels as high as 70 mG have been measured directly below overhead distribution lines and as high as 40 mG above underground lines.

How Strong Is the EMF from Electric Power Substations?

In general, the strongest EMF around the outside of a substation comes from the power lines entering and leaving the substation. The strength of the EMF from equipment within the substations, such as transformers, reactors, and capacitor banks, decreases rapidly with increasing distance. Beyond the substation fence or wall, the EMF produced by the substation equipment is typically indistinguishable from background levels.

Do Electrical Workers Have Higher EMF Exposure Than Other Workers?

Most of the information we have about occupational EMF exposure comes from studies of electric utility workers. It is therefore difficult to compare electrical workers' EMF exposures with those of other workers because there is less information about EMF exposures in work environments other than electric utilities.

Early studies did not include actual measurements of EMF exposure on the job but used job titles as an estimate of EMF exposure among electrical workers. Recent studies, however, have included extensive EMF exposure assessments. A report published in 1994 provides some information about estimated EMF exposures of workers in Los Angeles in a number of electrical jobs in electric utilities and other industries. Electrical workers had higher average EMF exposures (9.6 mG) than did workers in other jobs (1.7 mG). For this study, the category electrical workers included electrical engineering technicians, electrical engineers, electricians, power line workers, power station operators, telephone line workers, TV repairers, and welders.

What EMF Exposure Occurs during Travel?

Inside a car or bus, the main sources of magnetic field exposure are those you pass by (or under) as you drive, such as power lines. Car batteries involve direct current (DC) rather than alternating current (AC). Alternators can create EMF, but at frequencies other than 60 Hz. The rotation of steel-belted tires is also a source of EMF.

Most trains in the United States are diesel powered. Some electrically powered trains operate on AC, such as the passenger trains between Washington, D.C. and New Haven, Connecticut. Measurements taken on these trains using personal exposure monitors have suggested that average 60-Hz magnetic field exposures for passengers and conductors may exceed 50 mG.

A U.S. government-sponsored exposure assessment study of electric rail systems found average 60-Hz magnetic field levels in train operator compartments that ranged from 0.4 mG (Boston high speed trolley) to 31.1 mG (North Jersey transit).

Workers who maintain the tracks on electric rail lines, primarily in the northeastern United States, also have elevated magnetic field exposures at both 25 Hz and 60 Hz. Measurements taken by the National Institute for Occupational Safety and Health show that typical average daily exposures range from 3 to 18 mG, depending on how often trains pass the work site. Rapid transit and light rail systems in the United States, such as the Washington D.C. Metro and the San Francisco Bay Area Rapid Transit, run on DC electricity. These DC-powered trains contain equipment that produces AC fields. For example, areas of strong AC magnetic fields have been measured on the Washington Metro close to the floor, during braking and acceleration, presumably near equipment located underneath the subway cars.

How Can I Find Out How Strong the EMF Is Where I Live and Work?

For specific information about EMF from a particular power line, contact the utility that operates the line. Some will perform home EMF measurements. You can take your own EMF measurements with a magnetic field meter. For a spot measurement to provide a useful estimate of your EMF exposure, it should be taken at a time of day and location when and where you are typically near the equipment. Keep in mind that the strength of a magnetic field drops off quickly with distance.

Independent technicians will conduct EMF measurements for a fee. Search the Internet under "EMF meters" or "EMF measurement." You should investigate the experience and qualifications of commercial firms, since governments do not standardize EMF measurements or certify measurement contractors.

How Much Do Computers Contribute to My EMF Exposure?

Personal computers themselves produce very little EMF. However, the video display terminal (VDT) or monitor provides some magnetic field exposure unless it is of the new flat-panel design. Conventional VDTs containing cathode ray tubes use magnetic fields to produce the image on the screen, and some emission of those magnetic fields is unavoidable.

Unlike most other appliances which produce predominantly 60-Hz magnetic fields, VDTs emit magnetic fields in both the extremely low frequency (ELF) and very low frequency (VLF) frequency ranges. Many newer VDTs have been designed to minimize magnetic field emissions, and those identified as "TCO'99 compliant" meet a standard for low emissions.

Does EMF Affect People with Pacemakers or Other Medical Devices?

According to the U.S. Food and Drug Administration (FDA), interference from EMF can affect various medical devices including cardiac pacemakers and implantable defibrillators. Most current research in this area focuses on higher frequency sources such as cellular phones, citizens band radios, wireless computer links, microwave signals, radio and television transmitters, and paging transmitters.

Sources such as welding equipment, power lines at electric generating plants, and rail transportation equipment can produce lower frequency EMF strong enough to interfere with some models of pacemakers and defibrillators. The occupational exposure guidelines developed by the American Conference of Governmental Industrial Hygienists (ACGIH) state that workers with cardiac pacemakers should not be exposed to a 60-Hz magnetic field greater than 1 gauss (1,000 mG) or a 60-Hz electric field greater than 1 kilovolt per meter (1,000 V/m). Workers who are concerned about EMF exposure effects on pacemakers, implantable defibrillators, or other implanted electronic medical devices should consult their doctors or industrial hygienists.

What about Products Advertised as Producing Low or Reduced Magnetic Fields?

Virtually all electrical appliances and devices emit electric and magnetic fields. The strengths of the fields vary appreciably both between types of devices and among manufacturers and models of the same type of device. Some appliance manufacturers are designing new models that, in general, have lower EMF than older models. As a result, the words low field or reduced field may be relative to older models and not necessarily relative to other manufacturers or devices. At this time, there are no domestic or international standards or guidelines limiting the EMF emissions of appliances.

The U.S. government has set no standards for magnetic fields from computer monitors or video display terminals (VDTs). The Swedish Confederation of Professional Employees (TCO) established in 1992 a standard recommending strict limits on the EMF emissions of computer monitors. The VDTs should produce magnetic fields of no more than 2 mG at a distance of 30 cm (about 1 ft) from the front surface of the monitor and 50 cm (about 1 ft 8 in) from the sides and back of the monitor. The TCO'92 standard has become a de facto standard in the VDT industry worldwide. A 1999 standard, promulgated by the Swedish TCO (known as the TCO'99 standard), provides for international and environmental labeling of personal computers. Many computer monitors marketed in the U.S. are certified as compliant with TCO'99 and are thereby assured to produce low magnetic fields.

Beware of advertisements claiming that the federal government has certified that the advertised equipment produces little or no EMF. The federal government has no such general certification program for the emissions of low-frequency EMF. The U.S. Food and Drug Administration's Center for Devices and Radiological Health (CDRH) does certify medical equipment and equipment producing high levels of ionizing radiation or microwave radiation. Information about certain devices as well as general information about EMF is available from the CDRH at 888-463-6332.

Are Cellular Telephones and Towers Sources of EMF Exposure?

Cellular telephones and towers involve radio-frequency and microwave-frequency electromagnetic fields. These are in a much higher frequency range than are the power-frequency electric and magnetic fields associated with the transmission and use of electricity. The U.S. Federal Communications Commission (FCC) licenses communications systems that use radio-frequency and microwave electromagnetic fields and ensures that licensed facilities comply with exposure standards. Public information on this topic is published on two FCC Internet sites: http://www.fcc.gov/oet/info/documents/bulletins/#56 and http://www.fcc.gov/oet/rfsafety/.

The U.S. Food and Drug Administration also provides information about cellular telephones on its web site (http://www.fda.gov/cdrh/ocd/mobilphone.html).

What Can Be Done to Limit EMF Exposure?

Personal exposure to EMF depends on three things: the strength of the magnetic field sources in your environment, your distance from those sources, and the time you spend in the field. If you are concerned about EMF exposure, your first step should be to find out where the major EMF sources are and move away from them or limit the time you spend near them. Magnetic fields from appliances decrease dramatically about an arm's length away from the source. In many cases, rearranging a bed, a chair, or a work area to increase your distance from an electrical panel or some other EMF source can reduce your EMF exposure.

Another way to reduce EMF exposure is to use equipment designed to have relatively low EMF emissions. Sometimes electrical wiring in a house or a building can be the source of strong magnetic field exposure. Incorrect wiring is a common source of higher-than-usual magnetic fields. Wiring problems are also worth correcting for safety reasons.

In its 1999 report to Congress, the National Institute of Environmental Health Sciences suggested that the power industry continue its current practice of siting power lines to reduce EMF exposures.

There are more costly actions, such as burying power lines, moving out of a home, or restricting the use of office space that may reduce exposures. Because scientists are still debating whether EMF is a hazard to health, it is not clear that the costs of such measures are warranted. Some EMF reduction measures may create other problems. For instance, compacting power lines reduces EMF but increases the danger of accidental electrocution for line workers.

We are not sure which aspects of the magnetic field exposure, if any, to reduce. Future research may reveal that EMF reduction measures based on today's limited understanding are inadequate or irrelevant. No action should be taken to reduce EMF exposure if it increases the risk of a known safety hazard.

Chapter 48

Cell Phones and Wireless Phones: Are They Safe?

Do wireless phones pose a health hazard?

The available scientific evidence does not show that any health problems are associated with using wireless phones. There is no proof, however, that wireless phones are absolutely safe. Wireless phones emit low levels of radio-frequency energy (RF) in the microwave range while being used. They also emit very low levels of RF when in the stand-by mode. Whereas high levels of RF can produce health effects (by heating tissue), exposure to low level RF that does not produce heating effects causes no known adverse health effects. Many studies of low level RF exposures have not found any biological effects. Some studies have suggested that some biological effects may occur, but such findings have not been confirmed by additional research. In some cases, other researchers have had difficulty in reproducing those studies, or in determining the reasons for inconsistent results.

What is radio-frequency energy (RF)?

Radio-frequency (RF) energy is another name for radio waves. It is one form of electromagnetic energy that makes up the electromagnetic spectrum. Some of the other forms of energy in the electromagnetic spectrum are gamma rays, x-rays and light. Electromagnetic energy (or electromagnetic radiation) consists of waves of electric and

"Cell Phone Facts: Consumer Information on Wireless Phones, Questions and Answers," a fact sheet produced by the U.S. Food and Drug Administration (FDA), 2002. Available online at http://www.fda.gov/cellphones/qa.html.

magnetic energy moving together (radiating) through space. The area where these waves are found is called an electromagnetic field.

Radio waves are created due to the movement of electrical charges in antennas. As they are created, these waves radiate away from the antenna. All electromagnetic waves travel at the speed of light. The major differences between the different types of waves are the distances covered by one cycle of the wave and the number of waves that pass a certain point during a set time period. The wavelength is the distance covered by one cycle of a wave. The frequency is the number of waves passing a given point in one second. For any electromagnetic wave, the wavelength multiplied by the frequency equals the speed of light. The frequency of an RF signal is usually expressed in units called hertz (Hz). One Hz equals one wave per second. One kilohertz (kHz) equals one thousand waves per second, one megahertz (MHz) equals one million waves per second, and one gigahertz (GHz) equals one billion waves per second.

RF energy includes waves with frequencies ranging from about 3000 waves per second (3 kHz) to 300 billion waves per second (300 GHz). Microwaves are a subset of radio waves that have frequencies ranging from around 300 million waves per second (300 MHz) to three billion waves per second (3 GHz).

What biological effects can be caused by RF energy?

The biological effects of radio-frequency energy should not be confused with the effects from other types of electromagnetic energy. Very high levels of electromagnetic energy, such as is found in x-rays and gamma rays can ionize biological tissues. Ionization is a process where electrons are stripped away from their normal locations in atoms and molecules. It can permanently damage biological tissues including DNA, the genetic material. Ionization only occurs with very high levels of electromagnetic energy such as x-rays and gamma rays. Often the term radiation is used when discussing ionizing radiation (such as that associated with nuclear power plants).

The energy levels associated with radio-frequency energy, including both radio waves and microwaves, are not great enough to cause the ionization of atoms and molecules. Therefore, RF energy is a type of non-ionizing radiation. Other types of non-ionizing radiation include visible light, infrared radiation (heat) and other forms of electromagnetic radiation with relatively low frequencies.

Large amounts of RF energy can heat tissue. This can damage tissues and increase body temperatures. Two areas of the body, the eyes and the testes, are particularly vulnerable to RF heating because there is relatively little blood flow in them to carry away excess heat.

The amount of RF radiation routinely encountered by the general public is too low to produce significant heating or increased body temperature. Still, some people have questions about the possible health effects of low levels of RF energy. It is generally agreed that further research is needed to determine what effects actually occur and whether they are dangerous to people. In the meantime, standards-setting organizations and government agencies are continuing to monitor the latest scientific findings to determine whether changes in safety limits are needed to protect human health.

FDA, EPA and other U.S. government agencies responsible for public health and safety have worked together and in connection with WHO to monitor developments and identify research needs related to RF biological effects.

What levels of RF energy are considered safe?

Various organizations and countries have developed standards for exposure to radio-frequency energy. These standards recommend safe levels of exposure for both the general public and for workers. In the United States, the FCC has used safety guidelines for RF environmental exposure since 1985.

The FCC guidelines for human exposure to RF electromagnetic fields are derived from the recommendations of two expert organizations, the National Council on Radiation Protection and Measurements (NCRP) and the Institute of Electrical and Electronics Engineers (IEEE). In both cases, the recommendations were developed by scientific and engineering experts drawn from industry, government, and academia after extensive reviews of the scientific literature related to the biological effects of RF energy.

Many countries in Europe and elsewhere use exposure guidelines developed by the International Commission on Non-Ionizing Radiation Protection (ICNIRP). The ICNIRP safety limits are generally similar to those of the NCRP and IEEE, with a few exceptions. For example, ICNIRP recommends different exposure levels in the lower and upper frequency ranges and for localized exposure from certain products such as hand-held wireless telephones. Currently, the World Health Organization is working to provide a framework for international harmonization of RF safety standards.

The NCRP, IEEE, and ICNIRP all have identified a whole-body Specific Absorption Rate (SAR) value of 4 watts per kilogram (4 W/kg) as a threshold level of exposure at which harmful biological effects may occur. Exposure guidelines in terms of field strength, power density and localized SAR were then derived from this threshold value. In addition, the NCRP, IEEE, and ICNIRP guidelines vary depending on the frequency of the RF exposure. This is due to the finding that whole-body human absorption of RF energy varies with the frequency of the RF signal. The most restrictive limits on whole-body exposure are in the frequency range of 30-300 MHz where the human body absorbs RF energy most efficiently. For products that only expose part of the body, such as wireless phones, exposure limits in terms of SAR only are specified.

The exposure limits used by the FCC are expressed in terms of SAR, electric and magnetic field strength, and power density for transmitters operating at frequencies from 300 kHz to 100 GHz.

Why has the FCC adopted guidelines for RF exposure?

The FCC authorizes and licenses products, transmitters, and facilities that generate RF and microwave radiation. It has jurisdiction over all transmitting services in the U.S. except those specifically operated by the Federal Government. While the FCC does not have the expertise to determine radiation exposure guidelines on its own, it does have the expertise and authority to recognize and adopt technically sound standards promulgated by other expert agencies and organizations, and has done so. (Our joint efforts with the FDA in developing this website is illustrative of the kind of inter-agency efforts and consultation we engage in regarding this health and safety issue.)

Under the National Environmental Policy Act of 1969 (NEPA), the FCC has certain responsibilities to consider whether its actions will significantly affect the quality of the human environment. Therefore, FCC approval and licensing of transmitters and facilities must be evaluated for significant impact on the environment. Human exposure to RF radiation emitted by FCC-regulated transmitters is one of several factors that must be considered in such environmental evaluations. In 1996, the FCC revised its guidelines for RF exposure as a result of a multi-year proceeding and as required by the Telecommunications Act of 1996.

Radio and television broadcast stations, satellite-earth stations, experimental radio stations and certain wireless communication facilities are required to undergo routine evaluation for RF compliance when they submit an application to the FCC for construction or modification of a transmitting facility or renewal of a license. Failure to comply with the FCC's RF exposure guidelines could lead to the preparation of a formal Environmental Assessment, possible Environmental Impact Statement and eventual rejection of an application. Technical guidelines for evaluating compliance with the FCC RF safety requirements can be found in the FCC's Office of Engineering and Technology (OET) Bulletin 65. http://www.fcc.gov/oet/info/documents/bulletins/#65.

Low-powered, intermittent, or inaccessible RF transmitters and facilities are normally excluded from the requirement for routine evaluation for RF exposure. These exclusions are based on standard calculations and measurement data indicating that a transmitting station or equipment operating under the conditions prescribed is unlikely to cause exposures in excess of the guidelines under normal conditions of use. Such exclusions are not exclusions from compliance, but, rather, exclusions from routine evaluation. The FCC's policies on RF exposure and categorical exclusion can be found in Section 1.1307(b) of the FCC's Rules and Regulations [(47 CFR 1.1307(b)].

How can I obtain the specific absorption rate (SAR) value for my wireless phone?

The FCC requires that wireless phones sold in the United States demonstrate compliance with human exposure limits adopted by the FCC in 1996. The relative amount of RF energy absorbed in the head of a wireless telephone-user is given by the Specific Absorption Rate (SAR), as explained above. The FCC requires wireless phones to comply with a safety limit of 1.6 watts per kilogram (1.6 W/kg) in terms of SAR.

Information on SAR for a specific phone model can be obtained for many recently manufactured phones using the FCC identification (ID) number for that model. The FCC ID number is usually printed somewhere on the case of the phone. Sometimes it may be necessary to remove the battery pack to find the number. Once you have the ID number, go to the following Web address: http://www.fcc.gov/oet/fccid. Type the FCC ID number exactly as requested (the Grantee Code is the first three characters, the Equipment Product Code is the rest of the FCC ID number). Then click on "Start Search." The "Grant of Equipment Authorization" for your telephone should appear. Read through the grant for the section on "SAR Compliance," "Certification of Compliance with FCC Rules for RF Exposure" or similar language. This section should contain the value(s) for typical or maximum SAR for your phone.

Phones and other products authorized since June 2, 2000, should have the maximum SAR levels noted directly on the "Grant of Equipment Authorization." For phones and products authorized between about mid-1998 and June 2000, detailed information on SAR levels is typically found in the exhibits associated with the grant. Once a grant is accessed, the exhibits can be viewed by clicking on "View Exhibit." Grants authorized prior to 1998 are not part of the electronic database but, rather, have been documented in the form of paper records.

The FCC database does not list phones by model number. However, consumers may find SAR information from other sources as well. Some wireless phone manufacturers make SAR information available on their own Web sites. In addition, some non-government Web sites provide SARs for specific models of wireless phones. However, the FCC has not reviewed these sites and makes no guarantees of their accuracy. Finally, phones certified by the Cellular Telecommunications and Internet Association (CTIA) are required to provide SAR information to consumers in the instructional materials that come with the phones.

Do hands-free kits for wireless phones reduce risks from exposure to RF emissions?

Since there are no known risks from exposure to RF emissions from wireless phones, there is no reason to believe that hands-free kits reduce risks. Hands-free kits can be used with wireless phones for convenience and comfort. These systems reduce the absorption of RF energy in the head because the phone, which is the source of the RF emissions, will not be placed against the head. On the other hand, if the phone is mounted against the waist or other part of the body during use, then that part of the body will absorb more RF energy. Wireless phones marketed in the U.S. are required to meet safety requirements regardless of whether they are used against the head or against the body. Either configuration should result in compliance with the safety limit.

Do wireless phone accessories that claim to shield the head from RF radiation work?

Since there are no known risks from exposure to RF emissions from wireless phones, there is no reason to believe that accessories that claim to shield the head from those emissions reduce risks. Some products that claim to shield the user from RF absorption use special phone cases, while others involve nothing more than a metallic accessory attached to the phone. Studies have shown that these products generally do not work as advertised. Unlike hand-free kits, these so-called shields may interfere with proper operation of the phone. The phone may be forced to boost its power to compensate, leading to an increase in RF absorption. In February 2002, the Federal trade Commission (FTC) charged two companies that sold devices that claimed to protect wireless phone users from radiation with making false and unsubstantiated claims. According to FTC, these defendants lacked a reasonable basis to substantiate their claim.

What are wireless telephone base stations?

Fixed antennas used for wireless telecommunications are referred to as cellular base stations, cell stations, PCS (Personal Communications Service) stations or telephone transmission towers. These base stations consist of antennas and electronic equipment. Because the antennas need to be high in the air, they are often located on towers, poles, water tanks, or rooftops. Typical heights for freestanding base station towers are 50-200 feet.

Some base stations use antennas that look like poles, 10 to 15 feet in length, that are referred to as omni-directional antennas. These types of antennas are usually found in rural areas. In urban and suburban areas, wireless providers now more commonly use panel or sector antennas for their base stations. These antennas consist of rectangular panels, about 1 by 4 feet in dimension. The antennas are usually arranged in three groups of three antennas each. One antenna in each group is used to transmit signals to wireless phones, and the other two antennas in each group are used to receive signals from wireless phones.

At any base station site, the amount of RF energy produced depends on the number of radio channels (transmitters) per antenna and the power of each transmitter. Typically, 21 channels per antenna sector are available. For a typical cell site using sector antennas, each of the three transmitting antennas could be connected to up to 21 transmitters for a total of 63 transmitters. However, it is unlikely that all of the transmitters would be transmitting at the same time. When omni-directional antennas are used, a cellular base station could theoretically use up to 96 transmitters, but this would be very unusual, and, once again, it is unlikely that all transmitters would be in operation simultaneously. Base stations used for PCS communications generally require fewer transmitters than those used for cellular radio transmissions, since PCS carriers usually have a higher density of base station antenna sites.

Are wireless telephone base stations safe?

The electromagnetic RF signals transmitted from base station antennas stations travel toward the horizon in relatively narrow paths. For example, the radiation pattern for an antenna array mounted on a tower can be likened to a thin pancake centered around the antenna system. The individual pattern for a single array of sector antennas is wedge-shaped, like a piece of pie. As with all forms of electromagnetic energy, the power decreases rapidly as one moves away from the antenna. Therefore, RF exposure on the ground is much less than exposure very close to the antenna and in the path of the transmitted radio signal. In fact, ground-level exposure from such antennas is typically thousands of times less than the exposure levels recommended as safe by expert organizations. So exposure to nearby residents would be well within safety margins.

Cellular and PCS base stations in the United States are required to comply with limits for exposure recommended by expert organizations and endorsed by government agencies responsible for health and safety. Measurements made near cellular and PCS base station antennas mounted on towers have confirmed that ground-level exposures are typically thousands of times less than the exposure limits adopted by the FCC. In fact, in order to be exposed to levels at or near the FCC limits for cellular or PCS frequencies an individual would essentially have to remain in the main transmitted radio signal (at the height of the antenna) and within a few feet from the antenna. This is, of course, very unlikely to occur.

When cellular and PCS antennas are mounted on rooftops, RF levels on that roof or on others near by would probably be greater than those typically encountered on the ground. However, exposure levels approaching or exceeding safety guidelines should be encountered only very close to or directly in front of the antennas. In addition, for sector-type antennas, typically used for such rooftop base stations, RF levels to the side and in back of these antennas are insignificant. General guidelines on antenna installations and circumstances that might give rise to a concern about an facility's conformance with FCC regulations can be found in *A Local Government Official's Guide to Transmitting Antenna RF Emission Safety: Rules, Procedures, and Practical Guidance.* This Guide can be accessed at: http://www.fcc.gov/oet/rfsafety.

Does the FCC maintain a database that includes information on the location and technical parameters of all the transmitting towers it regulates?

Each of the FCC Bureaus maintains its own licensing database system for the service(s) it regulates (e.g., television, cellular service, satellite earth stations.) The FCC issues two types of licenses: site specific and market based. In the case of site specific licensed facilities, technical operating information is collected from the licensee as part of the licensing process. However, in the case of market based licensing (e.g., PCS, cellular), the licensee is granted the authority to operate a radio communications system in a geographic area using as many facilities as are required, and the licensee is not required to provide the FCC with specific location and operating parameters of these facilities.

Information on site specific licensed facilities can be found the "General Menu Reports" (GenMen) at http://gullfoss2.fcc.gov/cgi-bin/ws.exe/genmen/index.hts. The various FCC Bureaus also publish on at least a weekly basis, bulk extracts of their licensing databases. Each licensing database has its own unique file structure. These extracts consist of multiple, very large files. The FCC's Office of Engineering and Technology (OET) maintains an index to these databases at http://www.fcc.gov/oet/info/database/fadb.html. Entry points into the various databases include frequency, state/county, latitude/longitude, call-sign and licensee name.

What is FDA's role concerning the safety of wireless phones?

Under the law, FDA does not review the safety of radiation-emitting consumer products such as wireless phones before they can be sold, as it does with new drugs or medical devices. However, the agency has authority to take action if wireless phones are shown to emit radiofrequency energy (RF) at a level that is hazardous to the user. In such a case, FDA could require the manufacturers of wireless phones to notify users of the health hazard and to repair, replace or recall the phones so that the hazard no longer exists.

Although the existing scientific data do not justify FDA regulatory actions, FDA has urged the wireless phone industry to take a number of steps, including the following:

• Support needed research into possible biological effects of RF of the type emitted by wireless phones;

- Design wireless phones in a way that minimizes any RF exposure to the user that is not necessary for device function; and

- Cooperate in providing users of wireless phones with the best possible information on possible effects of wireless phone use on human health.

FDA belongs to an interagency working group of the federal agencies that have responsibility for different aspects of RF safety to ensure coordinated efforts at the federal level. The following agencies belong to this working group:

- National Institute for Occupational Safety and Health

- Environmental Protection Agency

- Federal Communications Commission

- Occupational Safety and Health Administration

- National Telecommunications and Information Administration

The National Institutes of Health participates in some interagency working group activities, as well. FDA shares regulatory responsibilities for wireless phones with the Federal Communications Commission (FCC). All phones that are sold in the United States must comply with FCC safety guidelines that limit RF exposure. FCC relies on FDA and other health agencies for safety questions about wireless phones.

FCC also regulates the base stations that the wireless phone networks rely upon. While these base stations operate at higher power than do the wireless phones themselves, the RF exposures that people get from these base stations are typically thousands of times lower than those they can get from wireless phones. Base stations are thus not the primary subject of the safety questions discussed in this chapter.

What kinds of phones are the subject of this update?

The term wireless phone refers here to hand-held wireless phones with built-in antennas, often called cell, mobile, or PCS phones. These types of wireless phones can expose the user to measurable radiofrequency energy (RF) because of the short distance between the phone and the user's head. These RF exposures are limited by Federal Communications Commission safety guidelines that were developed with the advice of FDA and other federal health and safety agencies. When the phone is located at greater distances from the user, the exposure to RF is drastically lower because a person's RF exposure decreases rapidly with increasing distance from the source. The so-called cordless phones, which have a base unit connected to the telephone wiring in a house, typically operate at far lower power levels, and thus produce RF exposures well within the FCC's compliance limits.

What are the results of the research done already?

The research done thus far has produced conflicting results, and many studies have suffered from flaws in their research methods. Animal experiments investigating the effects of radio-frequency energy (RF) exposures characteristic of wireless phones have yielded conflicting results that often cannot be repeated in other laboratories. A few animal studies, however, have suggested that low levels of RF could accelerate the development of cancer in laboratory animals. However, many of the studies that showed increased tumor development used animals that had been genetically engineered or treated with cancer-causing chemicals so as to be pre-disposed to develop cancer in the absence of RF exposure. Other studies exposed the animals to RF for up to 22 hours per day. These conditions are not similar to the conditions under which people use wireless phones, so we don't know with certainty what the results of such studies mean for human health.

Three large epidemiology studies have been published since December 2000. Between them, the studies investigated any possible association between the use of wireless phones and primary brain cancer, glioma, meningioma, or acoustic neuroma, tumors of the brain or salivary gland, leukemia, or other cancers. None of the studies demonstrated the existence of any harmful health effects from wireless phone RF exposures. However, none of the studies can answer questions about long-term exposures, since the average period of phone use in these studies was around three years.

What research is needed to decide whether RF exposure from wireless phones poses a health risk?

A combination of laboratory studies and epidemiological studies of people actually using wireless phones would provide some of the data that are needed. Lifetime animal exposure studies could be completed in a few years. However, very large numbers of animals would be needed to provide reliable proof of a cancer promoting effect if one exists. Epidemiological studies can provide data that is directly applicable to human populations, but 10 or more years' follow-up may be needed to provide answers about some health effects, such as cancer. This is because the interval between the time of exposure to a cancer-causing agent and the time tumors develop—if they do—may be many, many years. The interpretation of epidemiological studies is hampered by difficulties in measuring actual RF exposure during day-to-day use of wireless phones. Many factors affect this measurement, such as the angle at which the phone is held, or which model of phone is used.

What is FDA doing to find out more about the possible health effects of wireless phone RF?

FDA is working with the U.S. National Toxicology Program and with groups of investigators around the world to ensure that high priority animal studies are conducted to address important questions about the effects of exposure to radio-frequency energy (RF).

FDA has been a leading participant in the World Health Organization International Electromagnetic Fields (EMF) Project since its inception in 1996. An influential result of this work has been the development of a detailed agenda of research needs that has driven the establishment of new research programs around the world. The Project has also helped develop a series of public information documents on EMF issues.

FDA and the Cellular Telecommunications & Internet Association (CTIA) have a formal Cooperative Research and Development Agreement (CRADA) to do research on wireless phone safety. FDA provides the scientific oversight, obtaining input from experts in government, industry, and academic organizations. CTIA-funded research is conducted through contracts to independent investigators. The initial research will include both laboratory studies and studies of wireless phone users. The CRADA will also include a broad assessment of additional research needs in the context of the latest research developments around the world.

What steps can I take to reduce my exposure to radio-frequency energy from my wireless phone?

If there is a risk from these products—and at this point we do not know that there is—it is probably very small. But if you are concerned about avoiding even potential risks, you can take a few simple steps to minimize your exposure to radio-frequency energy (RF). Since time is a key factor in how much exposure a person receives, reducing the amount of time spent using a wireless phone will reduce RF exposure.

If you must conduct extended conversations by wireless phone every day, you could place more distance between your body and the source of the RF, since the exposure level drops off dramatically with distance. For example, you could use a headset and carry the wireless phone away from your body or use a wireless phone connected to a remote antenna.

Again, the scientific data do not demonstrate that wireless phones are harmful. But if you are concerned about the RF exposure from these products, you can use measures like those described previously to reduce your RF exposure from wireless phone use.

What about children using wireless phones?

The scientific evidence does not show a danger to users of wireless phones, including children and teenagers. If you want to take steps to lower exposure to radio-frequency energy (RF), the measures described above would apply to children and teenagers using wireless phones. Reducing the time of wireless phone use and increasing the distance between the user and the RF source will reduce RF exposure.

Some groups sponsored by other national governments have advised that children be discouraged from using wireless phones at all. For example, the government in the United Kingdom distributed leaflets containing such a recommendation in December 2000. They noted that no evidence exists that using a wireless phone causes brain tumors or other ill effects. Their recommendation to limit wireless phone use by children was strictly precautionary; it was not based on scientific evidence that any health hazard exists.

What about wireless phone interference with medical equipment?

Radio-frequency energy (RF) from wireless phones can interact with some electronic devices. For this reason, FDA helped develop a detailed test method to measure electromagnetic interference (EMI) of implanted cardiac pacemakers and defibrillators from wireless telephones. This test method is now part of a standard sponsored by the Association for the Advancement of Medical instrumentation (AAMI).

The final draft, a joint effort by FDA, medical device manufacturers, and many other groups, was completed in late 2000. This standard will allow manufacturers to ensure that cardiac pacemakers and defibrillators are safe from wireless phone EMI.

FDA has tested hearing aids for interference from handheld wireless phones and helped develop a voluntary standard sponsored by the Institute of Electrical and Electronic Engineers (IEEE). This standard specifies test methods and performance requirements for hearing aids and wireless phones so that that no interference occurs when a person uses a compatible phone and a compatible hearing aid at the same time. This standard was approved by the IEEE in 2000.

FDA continues to monitor the use of wireless phones for possible interactions with other medical devices. Should harmful interference be found to occur, FDA will conduct testing to assess the interference and work to resolve the problem.

Which other federal agencies have responsibilities related to potential RF health effects?

Certain agencies in the Federal Government have been involved in monitoring, researching or regulating issues related to human exposure to RF radiation. These agencies include the Food and Drug Administration (FDA), the Environmental Protection Agency (EPA), the Occupational Safety and Health Administration (OSHA), the National Institute for Occupational Safety and Health (NIOSH), the National Telecommunications and Information Administration (NTIA) and the Department of Defense (DOD).

By authority of the Radiation Control for Health and Safety Act of 1968, the Center for Devices and Radiological Health (CDRH) of the FDA develops performance standards for the emission of radiation from electronic products including x-ray equipment, other medical devices, television sets, microwave ovens, laser products and sunlamps. The CDRH established a product performance standard for microwave ovens in 1971 limiting the amount of RF leakage from ovens. However, the CDRH has not adopted performance standards for other RF-emitting products. The FDA is, however, the lead federal health agency in monitoring the latest research developments and advising other agencies with respect to the safety of RF-emitting products used by the public, such as cellular and PCS phones.

The EPA has, in the past, considered developing federal guidelines for public exposure to RF radiation. However, EPA activities related to RF safety and health are presently limited to advisory functions.

For example, the EPA now chairs an Inter-agency Radio-frequency Working Group, which coordinates RF health-related activities among the various federal agencies with health or regulatory responsibilities in this area.

OSHA is responsible for protecting workers from exposure to hazardous chemical and physical agents. In 1971, OSHA issued a protection guide for exposure of workers to RF radiation [29 CFR 1910.97]. However, this guide was later ruled to be only advisory and not mandatory. Moreover, it was based on an earlier RF exposure standard that has now been revised. At the present time, OSHA uses the IEEE and/or FCC exposure guidelines for enforcement purposes under OSHA's "general duty clause" (for more information see: http://www.osha-slc.gov/SLTC/radio-frequencyradiation/index.html.

NIOSH is part of the U.S. Department of Health and Human Services. It conducts research and investigations into issues related to occupational exposure to chemical and physical agents. NIOSH has, in the past, undertaken to develop RF exposure guidelines for workers, but final guidelines were never adopted by the agency. NIOSH conducts safety-related RF studies through its Physical Agents Effects Branch in Cincinnati, Ohio.

The NTIA is an agency of the U.S. Department of Commerce and is responsible for authorizing Federal Government use of the RF electromagnetic spectrum. Like the FCC, the NTIA also has NEPA responsibilities and has considered adopting guidelines for evaluating RF exposure from U.S. Government transmitters such as radar and military facilities.

The Department of Defense (DOD) has conducted research on the biological effects of RF energy for a number of years. This research is now conducted primarily at the U.S. Air Force Research Laboratory located at Brooks Air Force Base, Texas.

Who funds and carries out research on the biological effects of RF energy?

Research into possible biological effects of RF energy is carried out in laboratories in the United States and around the world. In the U.S., most research has been funded by the Department of Defense, due to the extensive military use of RF equipment such as radar and high-powered radio transmitters. In addition, some federal agencies responsible for health and safety, such as the Environmental Protection Agency (EPA) and the U.S. Food and Drug Administration (FDA), have sponsored and conducted research in this area. At the present time, most of the non-military research on biological effects of RF energy in the U.S. is being funded by industry organizations. More research is being carried out overseas, particularly in Europe.

In 1996, the World Health Organization (WHO) established the International EMF Project to review the scientific literature and work towards resolution of health concerns over the use of RF technology. WHO maintains a Web site that provides extensive information on this project and about RF biological effects and research (http://www.who.ch/peh-emf).

FDA, EPA and other U.S. government agencies responsible for public health and safety have worked together and in connection with WHO to monitor developments and identify research needs related to RF biological effects.

Part Six

Biological Hazards

Chapter 49

Anthrax

Bacillus anthracis, the etiologic agent of anthrax, is a large, gram-positive, non-motile, spore-forming bacterial rod. The three virulence factors of *B. anthracis* are edema toxin, lethal toxin and a capsular antigen. Human anthrax has three major clinical forms: cutaneous, inhalation, and gastrointestinal. If left untreated, anthrax in all forms can lead to septicemia and death.

A confirmed case of anthrax is defined as:

1. A clinically compatible case of cutaneous, inhalational, or gastrointestinal illness that is laboratory-confirmed by isolation of *B. anthracis* from an affected tissue or site, or

2. A clinically compatible case of cutaneous, inhalational, or gastrointestinal disease with other laboratory evidence of *B. anthracis* infection based on at least two supportive laboratory tests.

The last case of inhalational anthrax in the United States, before 2001, was in 1976 in California. A home craftsman, who worked with yarn, died. *Bacillus anthracis* was isolated from some of the imported yarns used by the patient.

"FAQs about Anthrax," a fact sheet produced by Public Health Emergency Preparedness and Response (PHEPR), Centers for Disease Control and Prevention (CDC), 2002. Available online at http://www.bt.cdc.gov/documentsapp/faqanthrax.asp.

The last case of cutaneous anthrax, before 2001, occurred in North Dakota, in 2000. It was the only case since 1992.

Before October 2001, the last cases of anthrax, all cutaneous, were Florida—1973, South Carolina—1974, and North Carolina—1987.

Signs and Symptoms

Cutaneous anthrax is the most common naturally occurring type of infection (>95%) and usually occurs after skin contact with contaminated meat, wool, hides, or leather from infected animals. The incubation period ranges from 1-12 days. The skin infection begins as a small papule, progresses to a vesicle in 1-2 days followed by a necrotic ulcer. The lesion is usually painless, but patients also may have fever, malaise, headache, and regional lymphadenopathy. Most (about 95%) anthrax infections occur when the bacterium enters a cut of abrasion on the skin. Skin infection begins as a raised bump that resembles a spider bite, but (within 1-2 days) it develops into a vesicle and then a painless ulcer, usually 1-3 cm in diameter, with a characteristic black necrotic (dying) area in the center. Lymph glands in the adjacent area may swell. About 20% of untreated cases of cutaneous anthrax will result in death. Deaths are rare if patients are given appropriate antimicrobial therapy.

Inhalational anthrax is the most lethal form of anthrax. Anthrax spores must be aerosolized in order to cause inhalational anthrax. The number of spores that cause human infection is unknown. The incubation period of inhalational anthrax among humans is unclear, but it is reported to range from 1 to 7 days, possibly ranging up to 60 days. It resembles a viral respiratory illness and initial symptoms include sore throat, mild fever, muscle aches and malaise. These symptoms may progress to respiratory failure and shock with meningitis frequently developing.

Gastrointestinal anthrax usually follows the consumption of raw or undercooked contaminated meat and has an incubation period of 1-7 days. It is associated with severe abdominal distress followed by fever and signs of septicemia. The disease can take an oropharyngeal or abdominal form. Involvement of the pharynx is usually characterized by lesions at the base of the tongue, sore throat, dysphagia, fever, and regional lymphadenopathy. Lower bowel inflammation usually causes nausea, loss of appetite, vomiting and fever, followed by abdominal pain, vomiting blood, and bloody diarrhea.

People should watch for the following symptoms:

- Fever (temperature greater than 100 degrees F). The fever may be accompanied by chills or night sweats.

- Flu-like symptoms. Cough, usually a non-productive cough, chest discomfort, shortness of breath, fatigue, muscle aches. Sore throat, followed by difficulty swallowing, enlarged lymph nodes, headache, nausea, loss of appetite, abdominal distress, vomiting, or diarrhea.

- A sore, especially on your face, arms or hands, that starts as a raised bump and develops into a painless ulcer with a black area in the center.

Questions and Answers about Anthrax

Is anthrax contagious?

No. Anthrax is not contagious; the illness cannot be transmitted from person to person.

What are the case fatality rates for the various forms of anthrax?

Early treatment of cutaneous anthrax is usually curative, and early treatment of all forms is important for recovery. Patients with cutaneous anthrax have reported case fatality rates of 20% without antibiotic treatment and less than 1% with it. Although case-fatality estimates for inhalational anthrax are based on incomplete information, the rate is extremely high, approximately 75%, even with all possible supportive care including appropriate antibiotics. Estimates of the impact of the delay in post-exposure prophylaxis or treatment on survival are not known. For gastrointestinal anthrax, the case-fatality rate is estimated to be 25%-60% and the effect of early antibiotic treatment on that case-fatality rate is not defined.

Can the presence of Bacillus anthracis spores be detected by a characteristic appearance, odor, or taste?

Bacillus anthracis spores do not have a characteristic appearance (e.g., color), smell, or taste. Spores themselves are too small to be seen by the naked eye, but have been mixed with powder to transport them. The U.S. Postal Service advises that individuals be suspicious of letters or packages with any powdery substance on them, regardless of color.

What would be the approximate size of enough Bacillus anthracis spores to cause infection?

They could not be seen by the naked eye but could be seen under a microscope.

How can I know my cold or flu this season is not anthrax?

Many human illnesses begin with what are commonly referred to as flu-like symptoms, such as fever and muscle aches. However, in most cases anthrax can be distinguished from the flu because the flu has additional symptoms. In previous reports of anthrax cases, early symptoms usually did not include a runny nose, which is typical of the flu and common cold.

If I have the flu, can I still get anthrax?

Yes, a person could theoretically get both the flu and anthrax, either at the same time or at different times.

Exposure

A person can be said to be exposed to anthrax when that person comes in contact with the anthrax bacteria and a culture taken from that person is positive for anthrax. A person can be exposed without having disease. A person who might have come in contact with anthrax, but without a positive culture would be said to be potentially exposed. Disease caused by anthrax occurs when there is some sign of illness, such as the skin lesion that occurs with cutaneous anthrax.

A person who is exposed to anthrax but is given appropriate antibiotics can avoid developing disease.

What kind of mail should be considered suspicious?

Some characteristics of suspicious packages and envelopes include the following:

- Inappropriate or unusual labeling

    Excessive postage

    Handwritten or poorly typed addresses

    Misspellings of common words

Strange return address or no return address

Incorrect titles or title without a name

Not addressed to a specific person

Marked with restrictions, such as "Personal," "Confidential," or "Do not x-ray"

Marked with any threatening language

Postmarked from a city or state that does not match the return address

- Appearance

    Powdery substance felt through or appearing on the package or envelope

    Oily stains, discolorations, or odor

    Lopsided or uneven envelope

    Excessive packaging material such as masking tape, string, etc.

- Other suspicious signs

    Excessive weight

    Ticking sound

    Protruding wires or aluminum foil

If a package or envelope appears suspicious, DO NOT OPEN IT.

What should people do who get a letter of package with powder?

- Do not shake or empty the contents of any suspicious package or envelope.

- Do not carry the package or envelope, show it to others or allow others to examine it.

- Put the package or envelope down on a stable surface; do not sniff, touch, taste, or look closely at it or at any contents which may have spilled.

- Alert others in the area about the suspicious package or envelope. Leave the area, close any doors, and take actions to prevent others from entering the area. If possible, shut off the ventilation system.

- WASH hands with soap and water to prevent spreading potentially infectious material to face or skin. Seek additional instructions for exposed or potentially exposed persons.

- If at work, notify a supervisor, a security officer, or a law enforcement official. If at home, contact the local law enforcement agency.

- If possible, create a list of persons who were in the room or area when this suspicious letter or package was recognized and a list of persons who also may have handled this package or letter.

Give this list to both the local public health authorities and law enforcement officials. These recommendations were published on October 26, 2001, in "Update: Investigation of bioterrorism-related anthrax and interim guidelines for exposure management and antimicrobial therapy." (*MMWR* 2001;50:909-919)

What should I do to protect my family and myself if a dangerous chemical agent were released in my community?

Emergency management teams would lead efforts in the event of a chemical attack and would let you know if you need to evacuate the area or seek some type of shelter.

CDC does not recommend purchasing gas masks. The likelihood that you would be involved in a chemical attack is low, and your protection is the responsibility of state and federal law enforcement officials. They are on high alert to ensure that such an event does not happen. In addition, CDC believes that purchasing a gas mask causes a false sense of security and can do more harm than good. Masks that aren't used properly or that do not fit well will not give you adequate protection.

Are nasal swabs sufficient for diagnosing anthrax?

No. Nasal swabs should not be used to diagnose cases of anthrax or to evaluate whether a person has been exposed to *B. anthracis*. The results of nasal swabs are not a predictor for disease, and the ability of this method to correctly identify those who have been exposed has not been quantified. At best, a positive result may be interpreted only to indicate exposure; at worst, a negative result is not useful in any way. Nasal swab screening of potentially exposed persons may be used in conjunction with environmental sampling during an epidemiologic investigation in order to determine the extent of exposure in a given area.

When is the collection of nasal swabs useful?

Nasal swabs may be useful as part of an epidemiologic investigation to help define an area exposed to aerosolized *B. anthracis*. When a possible anthrax exposure occurs at a known time, nasal swabs are quickly performed as one of the environmental tests to determine where airborne spores may have traveled.

A positive nasal swab suggests that you were recently in the vicinity of airborne anthrax spores—it does not necessarily mean that you received enough bacteria to make you sick. A negative nasal swab does not provide any information—it does not rule out the possibility that you were exposed to airborne anthrax if there was a release into the environment near you. Therefore, the nasal swab is, at best, a relatively crude test that tells us something in the positive but nothing in the negative.

When is the collection of nasal swabs not useful or recommended?

The collection of nasal swabs for culture should not be done to diagnose anthrax, to determine someone's risk of exposure, or to determine someone's need for prophylactic antibiotics. Nasal swabs should not be used to determine whether someone should stop prophylactic antibiotic treatment. Nasal swabs are not considered useful for diagnostic purposes.

Why are environmental scans done even when nasal swab cultures are no longer considered useful?

Unlike the human body, equipment does not have a self-cleaning mechanism. Equipment and surfaces may still be contaminated with anthrax spores for a period of time after an exposure has occurred. For this reason, it still makes sense to swab tables long after it no longer makes sense to swab noses.

Laboratory Testing

Can I get screened or tested to find out whether I have been exposed to anthrax?

There is no screening test for anthrax; there is no test that a doctor can do for you that says you've been exposed to or carry it. The only way exposure can be determined is through a public health investigation. The tests that you hear or read about, such as nasal swabs and environmental tests, are not tests to determine whether an individual should be treated. These kinds of tests are used only to determine the extent of exposure in a given building or workplace.

If the patient is suspected of being exposed to anthrax, should he/she be quarantined or should other family members be tested?

Direct person-to-person spread of anthrax is extremely unlikely and anthrax is not contagious. Therefore, there is no need to quarantine individuals suspected of being exposed to anthrax or to immunize or treat contacts of persons ill with anthrax, such as household contacts, friends, or coworkers, unless they also were also exposed to the same source of infection.

When an area is tested for the presence of Bacillus anthracis, *how long does it take to get the results?*

Before testing can begin, samples must be collected in a form suitable for testing. The length of time it takes to get test results depends on both the kind of test to be performed and the laboratory's workload. Some tests may take only a short time to perform, but confirmation takes longer. It may take many days to get the test results.

Testing is a two-step process. The first test, a screening test, may be positive within 2 hours if the sample is large and contains a lot of *Bacillus anthracis*, the organism that causes the disease anthrax. However, a positive reading on this first test must be confirmed with a second, more accurate test. This confirmation test, conducted by a more sophisticated laboratory, takes much longer. The length of time needed depends in part on how fast the bacteria grow, but results are usually available 1 to 3 days after the sample is received in the laboratory.

Does CDC recommend the use of home test kits for anthrax?

Hand-held assays (sometimes referred to as Smart Tickets) are sold commercially for the rapid detection of *Bacillus anthracis*. These assays are intended only for the screening of environmental samples. First responder and law enforcement communities are using these as instant screening devices and should forward any positive samples to authorities for more sensitive and specialized confirmatory testing. The results of these assays should not be used to make decisions about patient management or prophylaxis. The utility and validity of these assays are unknown.

At this time, CDC does not have enough scientific data to recommend the use of these assays. The analytical sensitivity of these assays is limited by the technology, and data provided by manufacturers indicate that a minimum of 10,000 spores is required to generate a positive signal. This number of spores would suggest a heavy contamination of the area (sample). Therefore a negative result does not rule out a lower level of contamination. Data collected from field use also indicate specificity problems with some of these assays. Some positive results have been obtained with spores of the non-anthrax *Bacillus* bacteria that may be found in the environment.

For these reasons, CDC has been asked to evaluate the sensitivity and specificity of the commercially available rapid, hand-held assays for *B. anthracis*. When this study is completed, results will be made available. Conclusions from this study are not expected in the near future.

How effective and reliable are anthrax tests?

There are many kinds of tests, and the reliability of each has not been determined. In general, findings from culturing environmental samples are specific; that is, a positive result reflects the true presence of *Bacillus anthracis*, and a negative result likely means that no *B. anthracis* is present.

What is the turnaround time for an anthrax test of an environmental sample?

Before testing can begin, samples must be collected and arrive in a form suitable for testing. The length of time necessary to get results of tests depends on transportation to the laboratory and the specific tests to be done. Testing is a two-step process. Initial screening tests (such as Gram stain) may be positive within two hours if the sample is large and the concentration of bacteria is high. These tests are used to narrow the definition of the sample. The confirmation tests take much longer, depending in part on how fast the bacteria grow, but are usually available 24–48 hours after the sample is received by the laboratory.

Diagnosis

Anthrax is diagnosed by isolating *B. anthracis* from the blood, skin lesions, or respiratory secretions or by measuring specific antibodies in the blood of persons with suspected cases. In patients with symptoms compatible with anthrax, providers should confirm the diagnosis by obtaining the appropriate laboratory specimens based on the clinical form of anthrax that is suspected (i.e., cutaneous, inhalational, or gastrointestinal).

Preventive Therapy

Ciprofloxacin, or Cipro as it is commonly known, is a broad-spectrum, synthetic antimicrobial agent active against several microorganisms. The use of ciprofloxacin is warranted only under the strict supervision of a physician.

Antibiotics, just like all medicines, have expiration dates. If you received your ciprofloxacin through a pharmacist, the expiration date should be listed on the bottle. If you can't find it or have questions about the expiration date, contact your pharmacist directly.

Adverse health effects include vomiting, diarrhea, headaches, dizziness, sun sensitivity, and rash. Hypertension, blurred vision, and other central nervous system effects occur in <1% of patients and may be accentuated by caffeine or medications containing theophylline.

Considerations for choosing an antimicrobial agent include effectiveness, resistance, side effects, and cost. As a measure to preserve the effectiveness of ciprofloxacin against anthrax and other infections, use of doxycycline for preventive therapy may be preferable. As always, the selection of the antimicrobial agent for an individual patient should be based on side-effect profiles, history of reactions, and the clinical setting.

There is no need to buy or store antibiotics, and indeed, it can be detrimental to both the individual and to the community. First, only people who are exposed to anthrax should take antibiotics, and health authorities must make that determination. Second, individuals may not stockpile or store the correct antibiotics. Third, under emergency plans, the Federal government can ship appropriate antibiotics from its stockpile to wherever they are needed.

CDC does not recommend using antibiotics unless a specific disease has been identified. There are several different agents that could be used for bioterrorism, such as bacteria, viruses, and toxins. Not a single antibiotic (or vaccine) works for all of these agents. Antibiotics only kill bacteria, not viruses or other agents that could also be used in a bioterrorist event. Antibiotics are not harmless drugs. They can cause serious side effects and drug interactions. National and state public health officials have large supplies of needed drugs and vaccines if a bioterrorism event should occur. These supplies can be sent anywhere in the United States within 12 hours.

Ciprofloxacin and doxycycline are FDA approved for postexposure prophylaxis, and ciprofloxacin, doxycycline, and amoxicillin are FDA approved for treatment. In the current situation of intentional anthrax distribution, doxycycline and ciprofloxacin are the recommended drugs for prophylaxis.

People at risk for inhalational anthrax should receive 60 days of antibiotics. These people include the following:

- People who have been exposed to an air space known to have been contaminated with aerosolized *B. anthracis*.

- People who share the air space within a facility where others have acquired inhalational anthrax.

- People who have been along the transit pathway of an envelope (or other vehicle) containing *B. anthracis* that may have been aerosolized.

- Unvaccinated laboratory workers who have handled powder that has tested positive for *B. anthracis* and who may not have used appropriate biosafety precautions.

People who are unsure if they are at risk should discuss any concerns with their healthcare provider or local/state public health department.

People who are determined not to be at risk for inhalational anthrax do not need to take the 60-day course of prophylactic antibiotics. Prophylactic antibiotics are not indicated for the prevention of cutaneous anthrax, for hospital personnel caring for patients with anthrax, or for persons who routinely open or handle mail if there has not been a credible threat.

Treatment

Treatment protocols for cases of inhalational and cutaneous anthrax associated with this bioterrorist attack are found in the *MMWR*, 10/26/2001; 50(42), 909-919.

If you develop side effects from the antibiotic, call your health care provider immediately. Depending on the type of side effects, you may be able to continue taking the medicine, or may be switched to an alternative antibiotic. If necessary, your physician may contact your State Department of Health for consultation on possible alternate antibiotics.

Risks of using tetracyclines and fluoroquinolones in children must be weighed carefully against the risk for developing a life-threatening disease due to *B. anthracis*. Both agents can have adverse health reactions in children. If adverse reactions are suspected, therapy may be changed to amoxicillin or penicillin.

As with all antibiotics, take the medication according to the schedule you were instructed, and even if you begin to feel better, continue taking it for the full number of days. If you need an extension of the antibiotic at the end of your prescribed number of days, local emergency healthcare workers or your healthcare provider will inform and tell you how to get more medicine. They may also tell you to discontinue the antibiotic, or will change the type of antibiotic, depending on results of laboratory tests.

Side effects which sometimes occur including nausea, mild diarrhea, stomach pain, headache and dizziness. Talk with your doctor if you have any of these problems while you are taking the antibiotic. Certain foods and medications should not be taken with ciprofloxacin; this should be discussed at the time the antibiotic is prescribed, so that side effects will not occur from the combinations. Ciprofloxacin also can cause sun sensitivity which increases the chances of sunburn.

More serious side effects include central nervous system side effects such as confusion, tremors, hallucinations, depression, and increased risk of seizures. High blood pressure and blurred vision are also possible. Allergic reactions could cause difficulty breathing; closing of the throat; swelling of the lips, tongue, or face; hives or severe diarrhea. Pain, inflammation, or rupture of a tendon are possible and also severe tissue inflammation of the colon could occur. Call your doctor or seek medical advice right away if you are having any of these side effects. This list is NOT a complete list of side effects reported with ciprofloxacin. Your health care provider can discuss with you a more complete list of side effects.

Less serious side effects include diarrhea, upset stomach, nausea, sore mouth or throat, sensitivity to sunlight, vaginal yeast infection or itching of the mouth lasting more than 2 days. You should talk with your doctor if you have any of these problems while taking doxycycline. Certain foods and medications should not be taken with doxycycline, and this should be discussed with your healthcare provider at the time the antibiotic is prescribed, so that side effects will not occur from the combinations. Doxycycline also causes sun sensitivity which increases the chances of sunburn. Serious side effects of doxycycline that are possible but uncommon include: life-threatening allergic reaction (symptoms are trouble breathing; closing of the throat; swelling of the lips, tongue, or face; hives), blood problems (symptoms are unusual bleeding or bruising), liver damage (symptoms are yellowing of the skin or eyes, dark urine, nausea, vomiting, loss of appetite, abdominal pain), irritation of the esophagus. Call your doctor or seek medical attention right away if you are having any of these side effects. This list is NOT a complete list of side effects reported with doxycycline. Your health care provider can discuss with you a more complete list of side effects.

Both doxycycline and ciprofloxacin are effective in treating *Bacillus anthracis* that we are dealing with in these investigations. Although CDC first recommended the use of either drug for post-exposure prophylaxis for the prevention of inhalational anthrax, we are now recommending doxycycline in order to prevent other bacteria from developing resistance to ciprofloxacin. Ciprofloxacin is part of the fluoroquinolone family of drugs, a relatively new class of antibiotics used to treat infections caused by organisms for which doctors do not have information about antimicrobial susceptibility. This kind of treatment is known as empiric therapy. Ciprofloxacin and other fluoroquinolones are used for empiric treatment for a variety of serious and common infections in the United States, including pneumonia, gastrointestinal infections, and urinary tract infections.

The number of people who have been exposed to *B. anthracis* and need antibiotics has increased dramatically since CDC first issued guidelines for treatment. If all those people take ciprofloxacin, other bacteria they carry in their bodies may develop resistance to fluoroquinolones, potentially limiting the usefulness of these drugs as empiric therapy. Doxycycline is less frequently used for empiric treatment than ciprofloxacin; therefore, we have fewer concerns regarding this drug and the emergence of new resistant bacteria.

There are different strains of *Bacillus anthracis*. Some strains of *B. anthracis* may be naturally resistant to certain antibiotics and not others. In addition, there may be biologically mutant strains that are engineered to be resistant to various antibiotics. A laboratory analysis can help to define which strain of *B. anthracis* is present and which antibiotic would be the most effective in treating the resulting anthrax.

Although FDA does not regulate the practice of medicine, the agency is strongly recommending that physicians not prescribe ciprofloxacin for individual patients to have on hand for possible use against inhaled anthrax. Indiscriminate and widespread use of ciprofloxacin could hasten the development of drug-resistant organisms and lessen the effects of these agents against many infections.

Other fluoroquinolones, such as ofloxacin and levofloxacin, are not specifically recommended as alternatives to ciprofloxacin because of a lack of sufficient data on their efficacy. However, if first-line drugs were not available, these other fluoroquinolones may be effective.

Anthrax spores grow like plant seeds. If you plant seeds and give them sun and water, they will grow into plants. If you give anthrax spores the right environment, such as the human body, they can grow into the harmful form of the bacteria that can cause anthrax disease. It takes anthrax spores an average of 7 days to grow into the harmful form of the bacteria, but it can take longer. For this reason, you must continue taking preventive antibiotics for the full 60 days.

Side Effects

Taking your antibiotic with food may help reduce nausea. Ciprofloxacin and doxycycline should not be taken within 2 hours of taking antacids. Ciprofloxacin and doxycycline should not be taken with dairy or calcium-fortified products (such as ice cream or calcium-fortified orange juice).

Antibiotics may disrupt bacteria in the gastrointestinal tract, causing diarrhea. Food may help relieve the diarrhea. If the diarrhea does not go away, your doctor may recommend another antibiotic. If you develop severe, long-lasting diarrhea, you may have a serious condition and should consult your doctor.

Occasionally, women develop yeast infections while taking amoxicillin. You may treat the infection with over-the-counter medicines such as clotrimazole. If the symptoms do not go away, you should consult your doctor.

Any side effect that forces you not to take your medicine is serious enough that you should consult or see your doctor. Serious side effects of ciprofloxacin include seizures, mental confusion, rash that does not go away, or excessive diarrhea. If you have any of these effects, call your doctor. Serious side effects of doxycycline include jaundice (yellow eyes or skin), rash that does not go away, or excessive diarrhea. If you have any of these effects, call your doctor.

Any reaction that causes a rapid swelling of the lips and face, shortness of breath, or hives is a medical emergency. You should call 911. These types of reactions are extremely rare.

Vaccine

A vaccine has been developed for anthrax that is protective against invasive disease, but it is currently only recommended for high-risk populations. CDC and academic partners are continuing to support the development of the next generation of anthrax vaccines.

The Advisory Committee on Immunization Practices (ACIP) has recommend anthrax vaccination for the following groups:

- Persons who work directly with the organism in the laboratory.

- Persons who work with imported animal hides or furs in areas where standards are insufficient to prevent exposure to anthrax spores.

- Persons who handle potentially infected animal products in high-incidence areas; while incidence is low in the United States, veterinarians who travel to work in other countries where incidence is higher should consider being vaccinated.

- Military personnel deployed to areas with high risk for exposure to the organism.

The immunization consists of three subcutaneous injections given 2 weeks apart, followed by three additional subcutaneous injections given at 6, 12, and 18 months. Annual booster injections of the vaccine are recommended thereafter.

Mild local reactions occur in 30% of recipients and consist of slight tenderness and redness at the injection site. Severe local reactions are infrequent and consist of extensive swelling of the forearm in addition to the local reaction. Systemic reactions occur in fewer than 0.2% of recipients.

Chapter 50

Botulism

Botulism is a rare but serious paralytic illness caused by a nerve toxin that is produced by the bacterium *Clostridium botulinum*. There are three main kinds of botulism. Foodborne botulism is caused by eating foods that contain the botulism toxin. Wound botulism is caused by toxin produced from a wound infected with *Clostridium botulinum*. Infant botulism is caused by consuming the spores of the botulinum bacteria, which then grow in the intestines and release toxin. All forms of botulism can be fatal and are considered medical emergencies. Foodborne botulism can be especially dangerous because many people can be poisoned by eating a contaminated food.

What kind of germ is Clostridium botulinum*?*

Clostridium botulinum is the name of a group of bacteria commonly found in soil. These rod-shaped organisms grow best in low oxygen conditions. The bacteria form spores which allow them to survive in a dormant state until exposed to conditions that can support their growth. There are seven types of botulism toxin designated by the letters A through G; only types A, B, E and F cause illness in humans.

"Botulism," a fact sheet produced by the Centers for Disease Control and Prevention (CDC), 2001. Available online at http://www.cdc.gov/ncidod/dbmd/diseaseinfo/botulism_g.htm.

How common is botulism?

In the United States an average of 110 cases of botulism are reported each year. Of these, approximately 25% are foodborne, 72% are infant botulism, and the rest are wound botulism. Outbreaks of foodborne botulism involving two or more persons occur most years and usually caused by eating contaminated home-canned foods. The number of cases of foodborne and infant botulism has changed little in recent years, but wound botulism has increased because of the use of black-tar heroin, especially in California.

What are the symptoms of botulism?

The classic symptoms of botulism include double vision, blurred vision, drooping eyelids, slurred speech, difficulty swallowing, dry mouth, and muscle weakness. Infants with botulism appear lethargic, feed poorly, are constipated, and have a weak cry and poor muscle tone. These are all symptoms of the muscle paralysis caused by the bacterial toxin. If untreated, these symptoms may progress to cause paralysis of the arms, legs, trunk and respiratory muscles. In foodborne botulism, symptoms generally begin 18 to 36 hours after eating a contaminated food, but they can occur as early as 6 hours or as late as 10 days.

How is botulism diagnosed?

Physicians may consider the diagnosis if the patient's history and physical examination suggest botulism. However, these clues are usually not enough to allow a diagnosis of botulism. Other diseases such as Guillain-Barré syndrome, stroke, and myasthenia gravis can appear similar to botulism, and special tests may be needed to exclude these other conditions. These tests may include a brain scan, spinal fluid examination, nerve conduction test (electromyography, or EMG), and a Tensilon test for myasthenia gravis. The most direct way to confirm the diagnosis is to demonstrate the botulism toxin in the patient's serum or stool by injecting serum or stool into mice and looking for signs of botulism. The bacteria can also be isolated from the stool of persons with foodborne and infant botulism. These tests can be performed at some state health department laboratories and at CDC.

How can botulism be treated?

The respiratory failure and paralysis that occur with severe botulism may require a patient to be on a breathing machine (ventilator) for weeks, plus intensive medical and nursing care. After several weeks, the paralysis slowly improves. If diagnosed early, foodborne and wound botulism can be treated with an antitoxin which blocks the action of toxin circulating in the blood. This can prevent patients from worsening, but recovery still takes many weeks. Physicians may try to remove contaminated food still in the gut by inducing vomiting or by using enemas. Wounds should be treated, usually surgically, to remove the source of the toxin-producing bacteria. Good supportive care in a hospital is the mainstay of therapy for all forms of botulism. Currently, antitoxin is not routinely given for treatment of infant botulism.

Are there complications from botulism?

Botulism can result in death due to respiratory failure. However, in the past 50 years the proportion of patients with botulism who die has fallen from about 50% to 8%. A patient with severe botulism may require a breathing machine as well as intensive medical and nursing care for several months. Patients who survive an episode of botulism poisoning may have fatigue and shortness of breath for years and long-term therapy may be needed to aid recovery.

How can botulism be prevented?

Botulism can be prevented. Foodborne botulism has often been from home-canned foods with low acid content, such as asparagus, green beans, beets and corn. However, outbreaks of botulism from more unusual sources such as chopped garlic in oil, chile peppers, tomatoes, improperly handled baked potatoes wrapped in aluminum foil, and home-canned or fermented fish. Persons who do home canning should follow strict hygienic procedures to reduce contamination of foods. Oils infused with garlic or herbs should be refrigerated. Potatoes which have been baked while wrapped in aluminum foil should be kept hot until served or refrigerated. Because the botulism toxin is destroyed by high temperatures, persons who eat home-canned foods should consider boiling the food for 10 minutes before eating it to ensure safety. Instructions on safe home canning can be obtained from county extension services or from the U.S. Department of Agriculture.

Because honey can contain spores of *Clostridium botulinum* and this has been a source of infection for infants, children less than 12 months old should not be fed honey. Honey is safe for persons 1 year of age and older. Wound botulism can be prevented by promptly seeking medical care for infected wounds and by not using injectable street drugs.

What are public health agencies doing to prevent or control botulism?

Public education about botulism prevention is an ongoing activity. Information about safe canning is widely available for consumers. State health departments and CDC have persons knowledgeable about botulism available to consult with physicians 24 hours a day. If antitoxin is needed to treat a patient, it can be quickly delivered to a physician anywhere in the country. Suspected outbreaks of botulism are quickly investigated, and if they involve a commercial product, the appropriate control measures are coordinated among public health and regulatory agencies. Physicians should report suspected cases of botulism to a state health department.

Chapter 51

Brucellosis

Brucellosis is an infectious disease caused by the bacteria of the genus *Brucella*. These bacteria are primarily passed among animals, and they cause disease in many different vertebrates. Various *Brucella* species affect sheep, goats, cattle, deer, elk, pigs, dogs, and several other animals. Humans become infected by coming in contact with animals or animal products that are contaminated with these bacteria. In humans brucellosis can cause a range of symptoms that are similar to the flu and may include fever, sweats, headaches, back pains, and physical weakness. Sever infections of the central nervous systems or lining of the heart may occur. Brucellosis can also cause long-lasting or chronic symptoms that include recurrent fevers, joint pain, and fatigue.

How common is brucellosis?

Brucellosis is not very common in the United States, where 100 to 200 cases occur each year. But brucellosis can be very common in countries where animal disease control programs have not reduced the amount of disease among animals.

Where is brucellosis usually found?

Although brucellosis can be found worldwide, it is more common in countries that do not have good standardized and effective public

---

"Brucellosis," a fact sheet produced by the Division of Bacterial and Mycotic Diseases, Centers for Disease Control and Prevention (CDC), 2001. Available online at http://www.cdc.gov/ncidod/dbmd/diseaseinfo/brucellosis_g.htm.

health and domestic animal health programs. Areas currently listed as high risk are the Mediterranean Basin (Portugal, Spain, Southern France, Italy, Greece, Turkey, North Africa), South and Central America, Eastern Europe, Asia, Africa, the Caribbean, and the Middle East. Unpasteurized cheeses, sometimes called village cheeses, from these areas may represent a particular risk for tourists.

How is brucellosis transmitted to humans, and who is likely to become infected?

Humans are generally infected in one of three ways: eating or drinking something that is contaminated with *Brucella*, breathing in the organism (inhalation), or having the bacteria enter the body through skin wounds. The most common way to be infected is by eating or drinking contaminated milk products. When sheep, goats, cows, or camels are infected, their milk is contaminated with the bacteria. If the milk is not pasteurized, these bacteria can be transmitted to persons who drink the milk or eat cheeses made it. Inhalation of *Brucella* organisms is not a common route of infection, but it can be a significant hazard for people in certain occupations, such as those working in laboratories where the organism is cultured. Inhalation is often responsible for a significant percentage of cases in abattoir employees. Contamination of skin wounds may be a problem for persons working in slaughterhouses or meat packing plants or for veterinarians. Hunters may be infected through skin wounds or by accidentally ingesting the bacteria after cleaning deer, elk, moose, or wild pigs that they have killed.

Can brucellosis be spread from person to person?

Direct person-to-person spread of brucellosis is extremely rare. Mothers who are breast-feeding may transmit the infection to their infants. Sexual transmission has also been reported. For both sexual and breast-feeding transmission, if the infant or person at risk is treated for brucellosis, their risk of becoming infected will probably be eliminated within 3 days. Although uncommon, transmission may also occur via contaminated tissue transplantation.

Is there a way to prevent infection?

Yes. Do not consume unpasteurized milk, cheese, or ice cream while traveling. If you are not sure that the dairy product is pasteurized, don't eat it. Hunters and animal herdsman should use rubber gloves when handling viscera of animals. There is no vaccine available for humans.

My dog has been diagnosed with brucellosis. Is that a risk for me?

B. canis is the species of *Brucella* species that can infect dogs. This species has occasionally been transmitted to humans, but the vast majority of dog infections do not result in human illness. Although veterinarians exposed to blood of infected animals are at risk, pet owners are not considered to be at risk for infection. This is partly because it is unlikely that they will come in contact with blood, semen, or placenta of the dog. The bacteria may be cleared from the animal within a few days of treatment; however re-infection is common and some animal body fluids may be infectious for weeks. Immunocompromised persons (cancer patients, HIV-infected individuals, or transplantation patients) should not handle dogs known to be infected with *B. canis*.

How is brucellosis diagnosed?

Brucellosis is diagnosed in a laboratory by finding *Brucella* organisms in samples of blood or bone marrow. Also, blood tests can be done to detect antibodies against the bacteria. If this method is used, two blood samples should be collected 2 weeks apart.

Is there a treatment for brucellosis?

Yes, but treatment can be difficult. Doctors can prescribe effective antibiotics. Usually, doxycycline and rifampin are used in combination for 6 weeks to prevent reoccurring infection. Depending on the timing of treatment and severity of illness, recovery may take a few weeks to several months. Mortality is low (<2%), and is usually associated with endocarditis.

I am a veterinarian, and I recently accidentally jabbed myself with the animal vaccine (RB-51 or B-19, or REV-1) while I was vaccinating cows (or sheep, goats). What do I need to do?

These are live vaccines, and B-19 is known to cause disease in humans. Although we know less about the other vaccines, the recommendations are the same. You should see a health care provider. A

431

baseline blood sample should be collected for testing for antibodies. We recommend that you take antibiotics (doxycycline and rifampin for B-19 and REV-1, or doxycycline alone for RB-51) for 3 weeks. At the end of that time you should be rechecked and a second blood sample should be collected. (The sample can also be collected at 2 weeks.) The same recommendations hold true for spraying vaccine in the eyes (6 weeks of treatment in this case) or spraying onto open wounds on the skin.

Chapter 52

Pneumonic Plague

Facts about Pneumonic Plague

Plague is an infectious disease that affects animals and humans. It is caused by the bacterium *Yersinia pestis*. This bacterium is found in rodents and their fleas and occurs in many areas of the world, including the United States.

Y. pestis is easily destroyed by sunlight and drying. Even so, when released into air, the bacterium will survive for up to one hour, although this could vary depending on conditions.

Pneumonic plague is one of several forms of plague. Depending on circumstances, these forms may occur separately or in combination:

- Pneumonic plague occurs when *Y. pestis* infects the lungs. This type of plague can spread from person to person through the air. Transmission can take place if someone breathes in aerosolized bacteria, which could happen in a bioterrorist attack. Pneumonic plague is also spread by breathing in *Y. pestis* suspended in respiratory droplets from a person (or animal) with pneumonic plague. Becoming infected in this way usually requires direct and close contact with the ill person or animal. Pneumonic plague may

---

Text in this chapter is from "Facts about Pneumonic Plague," a fact sheet produced by the Centers for Disease Control and Prevention (CDC), 2001, available online at http://www.bt.cdc.gov/documentsapp/FactSheet/Plague/About.asp; and "Frequently Asked Questions (FAQ) about Plague," a fact sheet produced by the CDC, 2002, available online at http://www.bt.cdc.gov/agent/plague/faq.asp.

also occur if a person with bubonic or septicemic plague is un-treated and the bacteria spread to the lungs.

- Bubonic plague is the most common form of plague. This occurs when an infected flea bites a person or when materials contami-nated with *Y. pestis* enter through a break in a person's skin. Patients develop swollen, tender lymph glands (called buboes) and fever, headache, chills, and weakness. Bubonic plague does not spread from person to person.

- Septicemic plague occurs when plague bacteria multiply in the blood. It can be a complication of pneumonic or bubonic plague or it can occur by itself. When it occurs alone, it is caused in the same ways as bubonic plague; however, buboes do not develop. Patients have fever, chills, prostration, abdominal pain, shock, and bleeding into skin and other organs. Septicemic plague does not spread from person to person.

Symptoms and Treatment

With pneumonic plague, the first signs of illness are fever, head-ache, weakness, and rapidly developing pneumonia with shortness of breath, chest pain, cough, and sometimes bloody or watery sputum. The pneumonia progresses for 2 to 4 days and may cause respiratory failure and shock. Without early treatment, patients may die.

Early treatment of pneumonic plague is essential. To reduce the chance of death, antibiotics must be given within 24 hours of first symptoms. Streptomycin, gentamicin, the tetracyclines, and chloram-phenicol are all effective against pneumonic plague.

Antibiotic treatment for 7 days will protect people who have had direct, close contact with infected patients. Wearing a close-fitting surgical mask also protects against infection.

A plague vaccine is not currently available for use in the United States.

Frequently Asked Questions (FAQ) about Plague

Why are we concerned about pneumonic plague as a bioweapon?

Yersinia pestis used in an aerosol attack could cause cases of the pneumonic form of plague. One to six days after becoming infected with the bacteria, people would develop pneumonic plague. Once people have the disease, the bacteria can spread to others who have close contact with them. Because of the delay between being exposed to the bacteria and becoming sick, people could travel over a large area before becoming contagious and possibly infecting others. Controlling the disease would then be more difficult. A bioweapon carrying *Y. pestis* is possible because the bacterium occurs in nature and could be isolated and grown in quantity in a laboratory. Even so, manufacturing an effective weapon using *Y. pestis* would require advanced knowledge and technology.

Is pneumonic plague different from bubonic plague?

Yes. Both are caused by *Yersinia pestis*, but they are transmitted differently and their symptoms differ. Pneumonic plague can be transmitted from person to person; bubonic plague cannot. Pneumonic plague affects the lungs and is transmitted when a person breathes in *Y. pestis* particles in the air. Bubonic plague is transmitted through the bite of an infected flea or exposure to infected material through a break in the skin. Symptoms include swollen, tender lymph glands called buboes. Buboes are not present in pneumonic plague. If bubonic plague is not treated, however, the bacteria can spread through the bloodstream and infect the lungs, causing a secondary case of pneumonic plague.

What are the signs and symptoms of pneumonic plague?

Patients usually have fever, weakness, and rapidly developing pneumonia with shortness of breath, chest pain, cough, and sometimes bloody or watery sputum. Nausea, vomiting, and abdominal pain may also occur. Without early treatment, pneumonic plague usually leads to respiratory failure, shock, and rapid death.

How do people become infected with pneumonic plague?

Pneumonic plague occurs when *Yersinia pestis* infects the lungs. Transmission can take place if someone breathes in *Y. pestis* particles, which could happen in an aerosol release during a bioterrorism attack. Pneumonic plague is also transmitted by breathing in *Y. pestis* suspended in respiratory droplets from a person (or animal) with pneumonic plague. Respiratory droplets are spread most readily by coughing or sneezing. Becoming infected in this way usually requires direct and close (within 6 feet) contact with the ill person or animal. Pneumonic plague may also occur if a person with bubonic or septicemic plague is untreated and the bacteria spread to the lungs.

Does plague occur naturally?

Yes. The World Health Organization reports 1,000 to 3,000 cases of plague worldwide every year. An average of 5 to 15 cases occur each year in the western United States. These cases are usually scattered and occur in rural to semi-rural areas. Most cases are of the bubonic form of the disease. Naturally occurring pneumonic plague is uncommon, although small outbreaks do occur. Both types of plague are readily controlled by standard public health response measures.

Can a person exposed to pneumonic plague avoid becoming sick?

Yes. People who have had close contact with an infected person can greatly reduce the chance of becoming sick if they begin treatment within 7 days of their exposure. Treatment consists of taking antibiotics for at least 7 days.

How quickly would someone get sick if exposed to plague bacteria through the air?

Someone exposed to *Yersinia pestis* through the air—either from an intentional aerosol release or from close and direct exposure to someone with plague pneumonia—would become ill within 1 to 6 days.

Can pneumonic plague be treated?

Yes. To prevent a high risk of death, antibiotics should be given within 24 hours of the first symptoms. Several types of antibiotics are effective for curing the disease and for preventing it. Available oral medications are a tetracycline (such as doxycycline) or a fluoroquinolone (such as ciprofloxacin). For injection or intravenous use, streptomycin or gentamicin antibiotics are used. Early in the response to a bioterrorism attack, these drugs would be tested to determine which is most effective against the particular weapon that was used.

Would enough medication be available in the event of a bioterrorism attack involving pneumonic plague?

National and state public health officials have large supplies of drugs needed in the event of a bioterrorism attack. These supplies can be sent anywhere in the United States within 12 hours.

What should someone do if they suspect they or others have been exposed to plague?

Get immediate medical attention: To prevent illness, a person who has been exposed to pneumonic plague must receive antibiotic treatment without delay. If an exposed person becomes ill, antibiotics must be administered within 24 hours of their first symptoms to reduce the risk of death.

Notify authorities: Immediately notify local or state health departments so they can begin to investigate and control the problem right away. If bioterrorism is suspected, the health departments will notify the CDC, FBI, and other appropriate authorities.

How can someone reduce the risk of getting pneumonic plague from another person or giving it to someone else?

People having direct and close contact with someone with pneumonic plague should wear tightly fitting disposable surgical masks. Patients with the disease should be isolated and medically supervised for at least the first 48 hours of antibiotic treatment. People who have been exposed to a contagious person can be protected from developing plague by receiving prompt antibiotic treatment.

How is plague diagnosed?

The first step is evaluation by a health worker. If the health worker suspects pneumonic plague, samples of the patient's blood, sputum, or lymph node aspirate are sent to a laboratory for testing. Once the laboratory receives the sample, preliminary results can be ready in less than two hours. Confirmation will take longer, usually 24 to 48 hours.

How long can plague bacteria exist in the environment?

Yersinia pestis is easily destroyed by sunlight and drying. Even so, when released into air, the bacterium will survive for up to one hour, depending on conditions.

Is a vaccine available to prevent pneumonic plague?

Currently, no plague vaccine is available in the United States. Research is in progress, but we are not likely to have vaccines for several years or more.

Chapter 53

Smallpox

Smallpox Overview

Smallpox is a serious, contagious, and sometimes fatal infectious disease. There is no specific treatment for smallpox disease, and the only prevention is vaccination. The name smallpox is derived from the Latin word for spotted and refers to the raised bumps that appear on the face and body of an infected person.

There are two clinical forms of smallpox. *Variola* major is the severe and most common form of smallpox, with a more extensive rash and higher fever. There are four types of *variola* major smallpox: ordinary (the most frequent type, accounting for 90% or more of cases); modified (mild and occurring in previously vaccinated persons); flat; and hemorrhagic (both rare and very severe).

Historically, *variola* major has an overall fatality rate of about 30%; however, flat and hemorrhagic smallpox usually are fatal. *Variola* minor is a less common presentation of smallpox, and a much less severe disease, with death rates historically of 1% or less.

Smallpox outbreaks have occurred from time to time for thousands of years, but the disease is now eradicated after a successful worldwide vaccination program. The last case of smallpox in the United States was in 1949. The last naturally occurring case in the world was

Text in this chapter is from "Smallpox Fact Sheet: Smallpox Overview," and "Smallpox Fact Sheet: Vaccine Overview," produced by the Centers for Disease Control and Prevention (CDC), 2002. Available online at http://www.bt.cdc.gov/agent/smallpox.

in Somalia in 1977. After the disease was eliminated from the world, routine vaccination against smallpox among the general public was stopped because it was no longer necessary for prevention.

Where Smallpox Comes from

Smallpox is caused by the *variola* virus that emerged in human populations thousands of years ago. Except for laboratory stockpiles, the *variola* virus has been eliminated. However, in the aftermath of the events of September and October, 2001, there is heightened concern that the *variola* virus might be used as an agent of bioterrorism. For this reason, the U.S. government is taking precautions for dealing with a smallpox outbreak.

Transmission

Generally, direct and fairly prolonged face-to-face contact is required to spread smallpox from one person to another. Smallpox also can be spread through direct contact with infected bodily fluids or contaminated objects such as bedding or clothing. Rarely, smallpox has been spread by virus carried in the air in enclosed settings such as buildings, buses, and trains. Humans are the only natural hosts of *variola*. Smallpox is not known to be transmitted by insects or animals.

A person with smallpox is sometimes contagious with onset of fever (prodrome phase), but the person becomes most contagious with the onset of rash. At this stage the infected person is usually very sick and not able to move around in the community. The infected person is contagious until the last smallpox scab falls off.

Smallpox Disease

Incubation Period: (Duration: 7 to 17 days) Not contagious.

Exposure to the virus is followed by an incubation period during which people do not have any symptoms and may feel fine. This incubation period averages about 12 to 14 days but can range from 7 to 17 days. During this time, people are not contagious.

Initial Symptoms (Prodrome): (Duration: 2 to 4 days) Sometimes contagious.*

The first symptoms of smallpox include fever, malaise, head and body aches, and sometimes vomiting. The fever is usually high, in the range

440

of 101 to 104 degrees Fahrenheit. At this time, people are usually too sick to carry on their normal activities. This is called the prodrome phase and may last for 2 to 4 days.

Early Rash: (Duration: about 4 days) Most contagious.

A rash emerges first as small red spots on the tongue and in the mouth. These spots develop into sores that break open and spread large amounts of the virus into the mouth and throat. At this time, the person becomes most contagious.

Around the time the sores in the mouth break down, a rash appears on the skin, starting on the face and spreading to the arms and legs and then to the hands and feet. Usually the rash spreads to all parts of the body within 24 hours. As the rash appears, the fever usually falls and the person may start to feel better.

By the third day of the rash, the rash becomes raised bumps.

By the fourth day, the bumps fill with a thick, opaque fluid and often have a depression in the center that looks like a bellybutton. (This is a major distinguishing characteristic of smallpox.)

Fever often will rise again at this time and remain high until scabs form over the bumps.

Pustular Rash: (Duration: about 5 days) Contagious.

The bumps become pustules—sharply raised, usually round and firm to the touch as if there's a small round object under the skin. People often say the bumps feel like BB pellets embedded in the skin.

Pustules and Scabs: (Duration: about 5 days) Contagious.

The pustules begin to form a crust and then scab. By the end of the second week after the rash appears, most of the sores have scabbed over.

Resolving Scabs: (Duration: about 6 days) Contagious.

The scabs begin to fall off, leaving marks on the skin that eventually become pitted scars. Most scabs will have fallen off three weeks after the rash appears. The person is contagious to others until all of the scabs have fallen off.

Scabs resolved: Not contagious.

Scabs have fallen off. Person is no longer contagious.

*Smallpox may be contagious during the prodrome phase, but is most infectious during the first 7 to 10 days following rash onset.

Vaccine Overview

The smallpox vaccine helps the body develop immunity to smallpox. The vaccine is made from a virus called *vaccinia* which is a pox-type virus related to smallpox. The smallpox vaccine contains the live *vaccinia* virus—not dead virus like many other vaccines. For that reason, the vaccination site must be cared for carefully to prevent the virus from spreading. Also, the vaccine can have side effects. The vaccine does not contain the smallpox virus and cannot give you smallpox.

Currently, the United States has a big enough stockpile of smallpox vaccine to vaccinate everyone in the country who might need it in the event of an emergency. Production of new vaccine is underway.

Length of Protection

Smallpox vaccination provides high level immunity for 3 to 5 years and decreasing immunity thereafter. If a person is vaccinated again later, immunity lasts even longer. Historically, the vaccine has been effective in preventing smallpox infection in 95% of those vaccinated. In addition, the vaccine was proven to prevent or substantially lessen infection when given within a few days of exposure. It is important to note, however, that at the time when the smallpox vaccine was used to eradicate the disease, testing was not as advanced or precise as it is today, so there may still be things to learn about the vaccine and its effectiveness and length of protection.

Receiving the Vaccine

The smallpox vaccine is not given with a hypodermic needle. It is not a shot as most people have experienced. The vaccine is given using a bifurcated (two-pronged) needle that is dipped into the vaccine solution. When removed, the needle retains a droplet of the vaccine. The needle is used to prick the skin a number of times in a few seconds. The pricking is not deep, but it will cause a sore spot and one or two droplets of blood to form. The vaccine usually is given in the upper arm.

If the vaccination is successful, a red and itchy bump develops at the vaccine site in three or four days. In the first week, the bump becomes a large blister, fills with pus, and begins to drain. During the second week, the blister begins to dry up and a scab forms. The scab falls off in the third week, leaving a small scar. People who are being vaccinated for the first time have a stronger reaction than those who are being revaccinated. The following pictures show the progression of the site where the vaccine is given.

Post-Vaccination Care

After vaccination, it is important to follow care instructions for the site of the vaccine. Because the virus is live, it can spread to other parts of the body, or to other people. The *vaccinia* virus (the live virus in the smallpox vaccine) may cause rash, fever, and head and body aches. In certain groups of people, complications from the *vaccinia* virus can be severe.

Benefit of Vaccine Following Exposure

Vaccination within 3 days of exposure will prevent or significantly lessen the severity of smallpox symptoms in the vast majority of people. Vaccination 4 to 7 days after exposure likely offers some protection from disease or may modify the severity of disease.

Smallpox Vaccine Safety

The smallpox vaccine is the best protection you can get if you are exposed to the smallpox virus. Anyone directly exposed to smallpox, regardless of health status, would be offered the smallpox vaccine because the risks associated with smallpox disease are far greater than those posed by the vaccine.

There are side effects and risks associated with the smallpox vaccine. Most people experience normal, usually mild reactions that include a sore arm, fever, and body aches. However, other people experience reactions ranging from serious to life threatening. People most likely to have serious side effects are: people who have had, even once, skin conditions (especially eczema or atopic dermatitis) and people with weakened immune systems, such as those who have received a transplant, are HIV positive, are receiving treatment for cancer, or are currently taking medications (like steroids) that suppress the immune system. In addition, pregnant women should not get the vaccine because of the risk it poses to the fetus. Women who are breastfeeding should not get the vaccine. Children younger than 12 months of age should not get the vaccine. Also, the Advisory Committee on Immunization Practices (ACIP) advises against non-emergency use of smallpox vaccine in children younger than 18 years of age. In addition, those allergic to the vaccine or any of its components should not receive the vaccine.

In the past, about 1,000 people for every 1 million people vaccinated for the first time experienced reactions that, while not life-threatening, were serious. These reactions included a toxic or allergic reaction at the site of the vaccination (*erythema multiforme*), spread of the *vaccinia* virus to other parts of the body and to other individuals (inadvertent inoculation), and spread of the *vaccinia* virus to other parts of the body through the blood (generalized *vaccinia*). These types of reactions may require medical attention. In the past, between 14 and 52 people out of every 1 million people vaccinated for the first time experienced potentially life-threatening reactions to the vaccine. Based on past experience, it is estimated that 1 or 2 people in 1 million who receive the vaccine may die as a result. Careful screening of potential vaccine recipients is essential to ensure that those at increased risk do not receive the vaccine.

Smallpox Vaccine Availability

Routine smallpox vaccination among the American public stopped in 1972 after the disease was eradicated in the United States. Until recently, the U.S. government provided the vaccine only to a few hundred scientists and medical professionals working with smallpox and similar viruses in a research setting.

After the events of September and October, 2001, however, the U.S. government took further actions to improve its level of preparedness against terrorism. One of many such measures—designed specifically to prepare for an intentional release of the smallpox virus—included updating and releasing a smallpox response plan. In addition, the U.S. government ordered production of enough smallpox vaccine to immunize the American public in the event of a smallpox outbreak.

Right now, the U.S. government has access to enough smallpox vaccine to effectively respond to a smallpox outbreak in the United States.

Chapter 54

Tularemia

Facts about Tularemia

Tularemia is an infectious disease caused by a hardy bacterium, *Francisella tularensis*, found in animals (especially rodents, rabbits, and hares).

People can get tularemia many different ways, such as through the bite of an infected insect or other arthropod (usually a tick or deerfly), handling infected animal carcasses, eating or drinking contaminated food or water, or breathing in *F. tularensis*.

Symptoms of tularemia could include sudden fever, chills, headaches, muscle aches, joint pain, dry cough, progressive weakness, and pneumonia. Persons with pneumonia can develop chest pain and bloody spit and can have trouble breathing or can sometimes stop breathing. Other symptoms of tularemia depend on how a person was exposed to the tularemia bacteria. These symptoms can include ulcers on the skin or mouth, swollen and painful lymph glands, swollen and painful eyes, and a sore throat. Symptoms usually appear 3 to 5 days after exposure to the bacteria, but can take as long as 14 days.

Tularemia is not known to be spread from person to person, so people who have tularemia do not need to be isolated. People who have been exposed to *F. tularensis* should be treated as soon as possible. The disease can be fatal if it is not treated with the appropriate antibiotics.

Text in this chapter is from "Facts about Tularemia," and "Frequently Asked Questions (FAQ) about Tularemia," fact sheets produced by the Centers for Disease Control and Prevention (CDC), 2002. Available online at http://www. bt.cdc.gov/documentsapp/FactSheet/tularemia.

A vaccine for tularemia is under review by the Food and Drug Administration and is not currently available in the United States.

Frequently Asked Questions about Tularemia

Does tularemia occur naturally in the United States?

Yes. It is a widespread disease of animals. Approximately 200 cases of tularemia in humans are reported annually in the United States, mostly in persons living in the south-central and western states. Nearly all cases occur in rural areas and are associated with the bites of infective ticks and biting flies or with the handling of infected rodents, rabbits, or hares. Occasional cases result from inhaling infectious aerosols and from laboratory accidents.

Why are we concerned about tularemia as a bioweapon?

Francisella tularensis is highly infectious: a small number of bacteria (10-50 organisms) can cause disease. If *F. tularensis* were used as a bioweapon, the bacteria would likely be made airborne for exposure by inhalation. Persons who inhale an infectious aerosol would generally experience severe respiratory illness, including life-threatening pneumonia and systemic infection, if they were not treated. The bacteria that cause tularemia occur widely in nature and could be isolated and grown in quantity in a laboratory, although manufacturing an effective aerosol weapon would require considerable sophistication.

Can someone become infected with the tularemia bacteria from another person?

No. People have not been known to transmit the infection to others, so infected persons do not need to be isolated.

How quickly would someone become sick if they were exposed to the tularemia bacteria?

The incubation period for tularemia is typically 3 to 5 days, with a range of 1 to 14 days.

What are the signs and symptoms of tularemia?

Depending on the route of exposure, the tularemia bacteria may cause skin ulcers, swollen and painful lymph glands, inflamed eyes, sore throat, oral ulcers, or pneumonia. If the bacteria were inhaled, symptoms would include the abrupt onset of fever, chills, headache, muscle aches, joint pain, dry cough, and progressive weakness. Persons with pneumonia can develop chest pain, difficulty breathing, bloody sputum, and respiratory failure. 40% or more of persons with the lung and systemic forms of the disease may die if they are not treated with appropriate antibiotics.

What should someone do if they suspect they or others have been exposed to the tularemia bacteria?

Seek prompt medical attention. If a person has been exposed to *Francisella tularensis*, treatment with tetracycline antibiotics for 14 days after exposure may be recommended.

Local and state health departments should be immediately notified so an investigation and control activities can begin quickly. If the exposure is thought to be due to criminal activity (bioterrorism), local and state health departments will notify CDC, the FBI, and other appropriate authorities.

How is tularemia diagnosed?

When tularemia is clinically suspected, the healthcare worker will collect specimens, such as blood or sputum, from the patient for testing in a diagnostic or reference laboratory. Laboratory test results for tularemia may be presumptive or confirmatory.

Presumptive (preliminary) identification may take less than 2 hours, but confirmatory testing will take longer, usually 24 to 48 hours.

Can tularemia be effectively treated with antibiotics?

Yes. After potential exposure or diagnosis, early treatment is recommended with an antibiotic from the tetracycline (such as doxycycline) or fluoroquinolone (such as ciprofloxacin) class, which are taken orally, or the antibiotics streptomycin or gentamicin, which are given intramuscularly or intravenously. Sensitivity testing of the tularemia bacterium can be done in the early stages of a response to determine which antibiotics would be most effective.

How long can **Francisella tularensis** *exist in the environment?*

Francisella tularensis can remain alive for weeks in water and soil.

Is there a vaccine available for tularemia?

In the past, a vaccine for tularemia has been used to protect laboratory workers, but it is currently under review by the Food and Drug Administration.

Chapter 55

Viral Hemorrhagic Fevers

Viral hemorrhagic fevers (VHFs) refer to a group of illnesses that are caused by several distinct families of viruses. In general, the term viral hemorrhagic fever is used to describe a severe multisystem syndrome (multisystem in that multiple organ systems in the body are affected). Characteristically, the overall vascular system is damaged, and the body's ability to regulate itself is impaired. These symptoms are often accompanied by hemorrhage (bleeding); however, the bleeding is itself rarely life-threatening. While some types of hemorrhagic fever viruses can cause relatively mild illnesses, many of these viruses cause severe, life-threatening disease.

The Special Pathogens Branch (SPB) primarily works with hemorrhagic fever viruses that are classified as biosafety level four (BSL-4) pathogens. The Division of Vector-Borne Infectious Diseases, also in the National Center for Infectious Diseases, works with the non-BSL-4 viruses that cause two other hemorrhagic fevers, dengue hemorrhagic fever and yellow fever.

How are hemorrhagic fever viruses grouped?

VHFs are caused by viruses of four distinct families: arenaviruses, filoviruses, bunyaviruses, and flaviviruses. Each of these families share a number of features:

"Viral Hemorrhagic Fevers," a fact sheet produced by the Centers for Disease Control and Prevention (CDC), 2002. Available online at http://www.cdc.gov/ncidod/dvrd/spb/mnpages/dispages/vhf.htm.

449

- They are all RNA viruses, and all are covered, or enveloped, in a fatty (lipid) coating.

- Their survival is dependent on an animal or insect host, called the natural reservoir.

- The viruses are geographically restricted to the areas where their host species live.

- Humans are not the natural reservoir for any of these viruses. Humans are infected when they come into contact with infected hosts. However, with some viruses, after the accidental transmission from the host, humans can transmit the virus to one another.

- Human cases or outbreaks of hemorrhagic fevers caused by these viruses occur sporadically and irregularly. The occurrence of outbreaks cannot be easily predicted.

- With a few noteworthy exceptions, there is no cure or established drug treatment for VHFs.

In rare cases, other viral and bacterial infections can cause a hemorrhagic fever; scrub typhus is a good example.

What carries viruses that cause viral hemorrhagic fevers?

Viruses associated with most VHFs are zoonotic. This means that these viruses naturally reside in an animal reservoir host or arthropod vector. They are totally dependent on their hosts for replication and overall survival. For the most part, rodents and arthropods are the main reservoirs for viruses causing VHFs. The multimammate rat, cotton rat, deer mouse, house mouse, and other field rodents are examples of reservoir hosts. Arthropod ticks and mosquitoes serve as vectors for some of the illnesses. However, the hosts of some viruses remain unknown—Ebola and Marburg viruses are well-known examples.

Where are cases of viral hemorrhagic fever found?

Taken together, the viruses that cause VHFs are distributed over much of the globe. However, because each virus is associated with one or more particular host species, the virus and the disease it causes are usually seen only where the host species live(s). Some hosts, such as the rodent species carrying several of the New World arenaviruses, live in geographically restricted areas. Therefore, the risk of getting VHFs caused by these viruses is restricted to those areas. Other hosts range over continents, such as the rodents that carry viruses which cause various forms of hantavirus pulmonary syndrome (HPS) in North and South America, or the different set of rodents that carry viruses which cause hemorrhagic fever with renal syndrome (HFRS) in Europe and Asia. A few hosts are distributed nearly worldwide, such as the common rat. It can carry Seoul virus, a cause of HFRS; therefore, humans can get HFRS anywhere where the common rat is found.

While people usually become infected only in areas where the host lives, occasionally people become infected by a host that has been exported from its native habitat. For example, the first outbreaks of Marburg hemorrhagic fever, in Marburg and Frankfurt, Germany, and in Yugoslavia, occurred when laboratory workers handled imported monkeys infected with Marburg virus. Occasionally, a person becomes infected in an area where the virus occurs naturally and then travels elsewhere. If the virus is a type that can be transmitted further by person-to-person contact, the traveler could infect other people. For instance, in 1996, a medical professional treating patients with Ebola hemorrhagic fever (Ebola HF) in Gabon unknowingly became infected. When he later traveled to South Africa and was treated for Ebola HF in a hospital, the virus was transmitted to a nurse. She became ill and died. Because more and more people travel each year, outbreaks of these diseases are becoming an increasing threat in places where they rarely, if ever, have been seen before.

How are hemorrhagic fever viruses transmitted?

Viruses causing hemorrhagic fever are initially transmitted to humans when the activities of infected reservoir hosts or vectors and humans overlap. The viruses carried in rodent reservoirs are transmitted when humans have contact with urine, fecal matter, saliva, or other body excretions from infected rodents. The viruses associated with arthropod vectors are spread most often when the vector mosquito or tick bites a human, or when a human crushes a tick. However, some of these vectors may spread virus to animals, livestock, for example. Humans then become infected when they care for or slaughter the animals.

Some viruses that cause hemorrhagic fever can spread from one person to another, once an initial person has become infected. Ebola, Marburg, Lassa and Crimean-Congo hemorrhagic fever viruses are examples. This type of secondary transmission of the virus can occur directly, through close contact with infected people or their body fluids. It can also occur indirectly, through contact with objects contaminated with infected body fluids. For example, contaminated syringes and needles have played an important role in spreading infection in outbreaks of Ebola hemorrhagic fever and Lassa fever.

What are the symptoms of viral hemorrhagic fever illnesses?

Specific signs and symptoms vary by the type of VHF, but initial signs and symptoms often include marked fever, fatigue, dizziness, muscle aches, loss of strength, and exhaustion. Patients with severe cases of VHF often show signs of bleeding under the skin, in internal organs, or from body orifices like the mouth, eyes, or ears. However, although they may bleed from many sites around the body, patients rarely die because of blood loss. Severely ill patient cases may also show shock, nervous system malfunction, coma, delirium, and seizures. Some types of VHF are associated with renal (kidney) failure.

How are patients with viral hemorrhagic fever treated?

Patients receive supportive therapy, but generally speaking, there is no other treatment or established cure for VHFs. Ribavirin, an antiviral drug, has been effective in treating some individuals with Lassa fever or HFRS. Treatment with convalescent-phase plasma has been used with success in some patients with Argentine hemorrhagic fever.

How can cases of viral hemorrhagic fever be prevented and controlled?

With the exception of yellow fever and Argentine hemorrhagic fever, for which vaccines have been developed, no vaccines exist that can protect against these diseases. Therefore, prevention efforts must concentrate on avoiding contact with host species. If prevention methods fail and a case of VHF does occur, efforts should focus on preventing further transmission from person to person, if the virus can be transmitted in this way. Because many of the hosts that carry hemorrhagic fever viruses are rodents, disease prevention efforts include:

- controlling rodent populations;
- discouraging rodents from entering or living in homes or workplaces;

• encouraging safe cleanup of rodent nests and droppings.

For hemorrhagic fever viruses spread by arthropod vectors, prevention efforts often focus on community-wide insect and arthropod control. In addition, people are encouraged to use insect repellant, proper clothing, bed nets, window screens, and other insect barriers to avoid being bitten.

For those hemorrhagic fever viruses that can be transmitted from one person to another, avoiding close physical contact with infected people and their body fluids is the most important way of controlling the spread of disease. Barrier nursing or infection control techniques include isolating infected individuals and wearing protective clothing. Other infection control recommendations include proper use, disinfection, and disposal of instruments and equipment used in treating or caring for patients with VHF, such as needles and thermometers.

In conjunction with the World Health Organization, CDC has developed practical, hospital-based guidelines, titled *Infection Control for Viral Hemorrhagic Fevers In the African Health Care Setting*. The manual can help health-care facilities recognize cases and prevent further hospital-based disease transmission using locally available materials and few financial resources.

What needs to be done to address the threat of viral hemorrhagic fevers?

Scientists and researchers are challenged with developing containment, treatment, and vaccine strategies for these diseases. Another goal is to develop immunologic and molecular tools for more rapid disease diagnosis, and to study how the viruses are transmitted and exactly how the disease affects the body (pathogenesis). A third goal is to understand the ecology of these viruses and their hosts in order to offer preventive public health advice for avoiding infection.

Part Eight

Foodborne Hazards

Chapter 56

Preventing Foodborne Illness

"It must be something I ate," is often the explanation people give for a bout of home-grown "Montezuma's Revenge" (acute diarrhea) or some other unwelcome gastrointestinal upset.

Despite the fact that America's food supply is the safest in the world, the unappetizing truth is that what we eat can very well be the vehicle for foodborne illnesses that can cause a variety of unpleasant symptoms and may be life-threatening to the less healthy among us. Seventy-six of million cases of foodborne diarrheal disease occur in the United States every year.

The Food and Drug Administration has given high priority to combating microbial contamination of the food supply. But the agency can't do the job alone. Consumers have a part to play, especially when it comes to following safe food-handling practices in the home.

The prime causes of foodborne illness are bacteria, viruses and parasites. Bacteria causing foodborne illness include *Escherichia coli O157:H7*, *Campylobacter jejuni*, *Salmonella*, *Staphylococcus aureus*, *Listeria monocytogenes*, *Clostridium perfringens*, *Vibrio parahaemolyticus*, *Vibrio vulnificus*, and *Shigella*. Viruses, such as hepatitis A virus, and Norwalk and Norwalk-like virus, can also cause foodborne illness. Parasites are another origin of this type of illness and include *Giardia lamblia*, *Cyclospora cayetanensis*, and *Cryptosporidium parvum*.

"The Unwelcome Dinner Guest: Preventing Foodborne Illness," from *FDA Consumer,* magazine, January-February 1991; Updated June 2002. U.S. Food and Drug Administration (FDA). Publication Number (FDA) 00-2244. Available online at http://www.cfsan.fda.gov/~dms/fdunwelc.html.

These organisms can become unwelcome guests at the dinner table. They're in a wide range of foods, including meat, milk and other dairy products, spices, chocolate, seafood, and even water. Specific foods that have been implicated in foodborne illnesses are unpasteurized fruit and vegetable juices and ciders; raw or undercooked eggs or foods containing undercooked eggs; chicken, tuna, potato and macaroni salads; cream-filled pastries and fresh produce.

Poultry is the food most often contaminated with disease-causing organisms. It's been estimated that 60 percent or more of raw poultry sold at retail probably carries some disease-causing bacteria.

Bacteria such as *Listeria monocytogenes*, *Vibrio vulnificus*, *Vibrio parahaemolyticus* and *Salmonella* have been found in raw seafood. Oysters, clams, mussels, scallops, and cockles may be contaminated with hepatitis A virus.

Careless food handling sets the stage for the growth of disease-causing bugs. For example, hot or cold foods left standing too long at room temperature provide an ideal climate for bacteria to grow. Improper cooking also plays a role in foodborne illness.

Foods may be cross-contaminated when cutting boards and kitchen tools that have been used to prepare a contaminated food, such as raw chicken, are not cleaned before being used for another food, such as vegetables.

Symptoms

Common symptoms of foodborne illness include diarrhea, abdominal cramping, fever, headache, vomiting, severe exhaustion, and sometimes blood or pus in the stools. However, symptoms will vary according to the type of bacteria and by the amount of contaminants eaten.

In rare instances, symptoms may come on as early as a half hour after eating the contaminated food but they typically do not develop for several days or weeks. Symptoms of viral or parasitic illnesses may not appear for several weeks after exposure. Symptoms usually last only a day or two, but in some cases can persist a week to 10 days. For most healthy people, foodborne illnesses are neither long-lasting nor life-threatening. However, they can be severe in the very young, the very old, and people with certain diseases and conditions.

These conditions include:

• liver disease, either from excessive alcohol use, viral hepatitis, or other causes

- hemochromatosis, an iron disorder

- diabetes

- stomach problems, including previous stomach surgery and low stomach acid (for example, from antacid use)

- cancer

- immune disorders, including HIV infection

- long-term steroid use, as for asthma and arthritis.

When symptoms are severe, the victim should see a doctor or get emergency help. This is especially important for those who are most vulnerable. For mild cases of foodborne illness, the individual should drink plenty of liquids to replace fluids lost through vomiting and diarrhea.

Prevention Tips

The idea that the food on the dinner table can make someone sick may be disturbing, but there are many steps you can take to protect your families and dinner guests. It's just a matter of following basic rules of food safety.

- Prevention of foodborne illness starts with your trip to the supermarket. Pick up your packaged and canned foods first. Don't buy food in cans that are bulging or dented or in jars that are cracked or have loose or bulging lids. Look for any expiration dates on the labels and never buy outdated food. Likewise, check the use by or sell by date on dairy products such as cottage cheese, cream cheese, yogurt, and sour cream and pick the ones that will stay fresh longest in your refrigerator.

- If you have a health problem, especially one that may have impaired your immune system, don't eat raw shellfish and use only pasteurized milk and cheese, and pasteurized or concentrated ciders and juices.

- Choose eggs that are refrigerated in the store. Before putting them in your cart, open the carton and make sure that the eggs are clean and none are cracked.

- Select frozen foods and perishables such as meat, poultry or fish last. Always put these products in separate plastic bags so that drippings don't contaminate other foods in your shopping cart.

- Don't buy frozen seafood if the packages are open, torn or crushed on the edges. Avoid packages that are above the frost line in the store's freezer. If the package cover is transparent, look for signs of frost or ice crystals. This could mean that the fish has either been stored for a long time or thawed and refrozen.

- Check for cleanliness at the meat or fish counter and the salad bar. For instance, cooked shrimp lying on the same bed of ice as raw fish could become contaminated.

- When shopping for shellfish, buy from markets that get their supplies from state-approved sources; stay clear of vendors who sell shellfish from roadside stands or the back of a truck. And if you're planning to harvest your own shellfish, heed posted warnings about the safety of the water.

- Take an ice chest along to keep frozen and perishable foods cold if it will take more than an hour to get your groceries home.

Safe Storage

The first rule of food storage in the home is to refrigerate or freeze perishables right away. The refrigerator temperature should be 5 degrees Celsius (about 40° Fahrenheit), and the freezer should be -18° C (0° F). Check both fridge and freezer periodically with a good thermometer.

Poultry and meat heading for the refrigerator may be stored as purchased in the plastic wrap for a day or two. If only part of the meat or poultry is going to be used right away, it can be wrapped loosely for refrigerator storage. Just make sure juices can't escape to contaminate other foods. Wrap tightly foods destined for the freezer. Leftovers should be stored in tight containers. Store eggs in their carton in the refrigerator itself rather than on the door, where the temperature is warmer.

Seafood should always be kept in the refrigerator or freezer until preparation time.

Don't crowd the refrigerator or freezer so tightly that air can't circulate. Check the leftovers in covered dishes and storage bags daily for spoilage. Anything that looks or smells suspicious should be thrown out.

A sure sign of spoilage is the presence of mold, which can grow even under refrigeration. While not a major health threat, mold can make food unappetizing. Most moldy foods should be thrown out. But you might be able to save molding hard cheeses, salami, and firm fruits and vegetables if you cut out not only the mold but a large area around it. Cutting the larger area around the mold is important because much of the mold growth is below the surface of the food.

Many items besides fresh meats, vegetables, and dairy products need to be kept cold. For instance, mayonnaise and ketchup should go in the refrigerator after opening. Always check the labels on cans or jars to determine how the contents should be stored. If you've neglected to refrigerate items, it's usually best to throw them out.

For foods that can be stored at room temperature, some precautions will help make sure they remain safe. Potatoes and onions should not be stored under the sink, because leakage from the pipes can damage the food. Potatoes don't belong in the refrigerator either. Store them in a cool, dry place. Don't store foods near household cleaning products and chemicals.

Check canned goods to see whether any are sticky on the outside. This may indicate a leak. Newly purchased cans that appear to be leaking should be returned to the store, which should notify FDA.

Keep It Clean

The first cardinal rule of safe food preparation in the home is: Keep everything clean. The cleanliness rule applies to the areas where food is prepared and, most importantly, to the cook. Wash hands with warm water and soap for at least 20 seconds before starting to prepare a meal and after handling raw meat or poultry. Cover long hair with a net or scarf, and be sure that any open sores or cuts on the hands are completely covered. If the sore or cut is infected, stay out of the kitchen.

Keep the work area clean and uncluttered. Wash countertops with a solution of 5 milliliters (1 teaspoon) of chlorine bleach to about 1 liter (1 quart) of water or with a commercial kitchen cleaning agent diluted according to product directions. They're the most effective at getting rid of bacteria.

Also, be sure to keep dishcloths and sponges clean because, when wet, these materials harbor bacteria and may promote their growth. Wash dishcloths and sponges weekly in hot water in the washing machine.

While you're at it, sanitize the kitchen sink drain periodically by pouring down the sink a solution of 5 milliliters of bleach to 1 liter of water or a commercial kitchen cleaning agent. Food particles get trapped in the drain and disposal and, along with moistness, create an ideal environment for bacterial growth.

Use smooth cutting boards made of hard maple or plastic and free of cracks and crevices. Avoid boards made of soft, porous materials. Wash cutting boards with hot water, soap, and a scrub brush. Then, sanitize them in an automatic dishwasher or by rinsing with a solution of 5 milliliters of chlorine bleach to about 1 liter of water.

Always wash and sanitize cutting boards after using them for raw foods, such as seafood or chicken, and before using them for ready-to-eat foods. Consider using one cutting board only for foods that will be cooked, such as raw fish, and another only for ready-to-eat foods, such as bread, fresh fruit, and cooked fish.

Always use clean utensils and wash them between cutting different foods.

Wash the lids of canned foods before opening to keep dirt from getting into the food. Also, clean the blade of the can opener after each use. Food processors and meat grinders should be taken apart and cleaned as soon as possible after they are used.

Do not put cooked meat on an unwashed plate or platter that has held raw meat.

Wash fresh fruits and vegetables thoroughly, rinsing in warm water. Don't use soap or other detergents. If necessary—and appropriate—use a small scrub brush to remove surface dirt.

Keep Temperature Right

The second cardinal rule of safe home food preparation is: Keep hot foods hot and cold foods cold.

Use a thermometer with a small-diameter stem to ensure that meats are completely cooked. Insert the thermometer 1 to 2 inches into the center of the food and wait 30 seconds to ensure an accurate measurement. Beef (including ground beef), lamb, and pork should be cooked to at least 71° C (160° F); whole poultry and thighs to 82° C (180° F); poultry breasts to 77° C (170° F); and ground chicken or turkey to 74° C (165° F). Don't eat poultry that is pink inside.

Eggs should be cooked until the white and the yolk are firm. Avoid foods containing raw eggs, such as homemade ice cream, mayonnaise, eggnog, cookie dough, and cake batter, because they carry a *Salmonella* risk. Their commercial counterparts usually don't because they're made with pasteurized eggs. Cooking the egg-containing product to an internal temperature of at least 71° C (160° F) will kill the bacteria.

Table 56.1. How Long Will It Keep?

Following is a rundown of storage guidelines for some of the foods that are regulars on America's dinner tables.

	Storage Period	
Product	***In Refrigerator*** *5 degrees Celsius* *(about 40° Fahrenheit)*	***In Freezer*** *-18° C* *(0° F)*
Fresh Meat:		
Beef: Ground	1-2 days	3-4 months
Steaks and Roasts	3-5 days	6-12 months
Pork:		
chops	3-5 days	4-6 months
Ground	1-2 days	3-4 months
Roasts	3-5 days	4-6 months
Cured meats:		
Lunch meat	3-5 days	1-2 months
Sausage	1-2 days	1-2 months
Gravy	1-2 days	2-3 months
Fish:		
lean (such as cod)	1-2 days	up to 6 months
fatty (such as blue, perch, salmon)	1-2 days	2-3 months
Chicken:		
whole	1-2 days	12 months
parts	1-2 days	9 months
giblets	1-2 days	3-4 months
Dairy Products:		
Swiss, brick, processed cheese	3-4 weeks	*
Milk	5 days	1 month
Eggs:		
fresh in shell	3 weeks	-
hard-boiled	1 week	-

* Cheese can be frozen, but freezing will affect the texture and taste.

(Sources: Food Marketing Institute for fish and dairy products, USDA for all other foods.)

Seafood should be thoroughly cooked. FDA's 1999 Food Code recommends cooking most seafood to an internal temperature of 63° C (145° F) for 15 seconds. If you don't have a meat thermometer, look for other signs of doneness. For example:

• Fish is done when the thickest part becomes opaque and the fish flakes easily when poked with a fork.

• Shrimp can be simmered three to five minutes or until the shells turn red.

• Clams and mussels are steamed over boiling water until the shells open (five to 10 minutes). Then boil three to five minutes longer.

• Oysters should be sautéed, baked or boiled until plump, about five minutes.

Protect food from cross-contamination after cooking, and eat it promptly.

Cooked foods should not be left standing on the table or kitchen counter for more than two hours. Disease-causing bacteria grow in temperatures between 4° and 60° C (40° and 140° F). Cooked foods that have been in this temperature range for more than two hours should not be eaten.

If a dish is to be served hot, get it from the stove to the table as quickly as possible. Reheated foods should be brought to a temperature of at least 74° C (165° F). Keep cold foods in the refrigerator or on a bed of ice until serving. This rule is particularly important to remember in the summer months.

After the meal, leftovers should be refrigerated as soon as possible. (Never mind that scintillating dinner table conversation.) Meats should be cut in slices of three inches or less and all foods should be stored in small, shallow containers to hasten cooling. Be sure to remove all the stuffing from roast turkey or chicken and store it separately. Giblets should also be stored separately. Leftovers should be used within three days.

And here are just a few more parting tips to keep your favorite dishes safe. Don't thaw meat and other frozen foods at room temperature. Instead, move them from the freezer to the refrigerator for a day or two; or defrost submerged in cold water flowing fast enough to break up and float off loose particles in an overflow. You can also defrost in the microwave oven, or during the cooking process. Never taste any

food that looks or smells off, or comes out of leaking, bulging or severely damaged cans or jars with leaky lids.

Though all these do's and don'ts may seem overwhelming, remember, if you want to stay healthy, when it comes to food safety, the old
saying rules are made to be broken does not apply.

Food Safety Musts

- Get perishable foods into the refrigerator as quickly as possible
  after buying them.

- Wash raw fruits and vegetables thoroughly.

- Keep your kitchen or food preparation areas clean.

- Wash your hands before preparing food and after handling raw
  foods.

- Keep hot foods hot and cold foods cold after they are prepared.

Chapter 57

Parasites and Foodborne Illness

Parasites may be present in food or in water and can cause disease. Ranging in size from tiny, single-celled organisms to worms visible to the naked eye, parasites are more and more frequently being identified as causes of foodborne illness in the United States. The illnesses they can cause range from mild discomfort to debilitating illness and possibly death.

Parasites are organisms that derive nourishment and protection from other living organisms known as hosts. They may be transmitted from animals to humans, from humans to humans, or from humans to animals. Several parasites have emerged as significant causes of foodborne and waterborne disease. These organisms live and reproduce within the tissues and organs of infected human and animal hosts, and are often excreted in feces.

They may be transmitted from host to host through consumption of contaminated food and water, or by putting anything into your mouth that has touched the stool (feces) of an infected person or animal.

Parasites are of different types and range in size from tiny, single-celled, microscopic organisms (protozoa) to larger, multi-cellular worms (helminths) that may be seen without a microscope.

Some common parasites are *Giardia duodenalis, Cryptosporidium parvum, Cyclospora cayetanensis, Toxoplasma gondii, Trichinella*

"Parasites and Foodborne Illness," a fact sheet produced by the Food Safety and Inspection Service (FSIS), U.S. Department of Agriculture (USDA), 2001. Available online at http://www.fsis.usda.gov/OA/pubs/parasite.htm.

spiralis, *Taenia saginata* (beef tapeworm), and *Taenia solium* (pork tapeworm).

Giardia Duodenalis *(Formerly Called* G. lamblia*)*

Giardia duodenalis, cause of giardiasis (GEE-are-DYE-uh-sis), is a one-celled, microscopic parasite that can live in the intestines of animals and people. It is found in every region throughout the world and has become recognized as one of the most common causes of water-borne (and occasionally foodborne) illness.

How do people get giardiasis?

People get giardiasis the following ways:

- By consuming food or water contaminated with *G. duodenalis* cysts (the infective stage of the organism).
- By putting anything into your mouth that has touched the stool of a person or animal with giardiasis.

Symptoms of Giardiasis

Diarrhea, abdominal cramps, and nausea are the most common symptoms. Some cases may be without symptoms.

When will symptoms appear? What is the duration?

Symptoms will usually appear 1 to 2 weeks after ingestion of a *G. duodenalis* cyst. They may last 4 to 6 weeks in otherwise healthy persons, but there are cases of chronic illnesses lasting months or even years.

Who is at risk for contracting giardiasis?

Those at risk include:

- persons working in child daycare centers and children attending daycare centers;
- international travelers (traveler's diarrhea);
- hikers, campers, or any other persons who may drink from untreated water supplies; and
- persons with weakened immune systems including those with HIV/AIDS infection, organ transplant recipients, or those individuals undergoing chemotherapy.

How to Prevent Giardiasis

- Wash hands with hot, soapy water before handling foods and eating, and after using the toilet, diapering young children, and handling animals.
- Make sure infected individuals wash their hands frequently to reduce the spread of infection.
- Drink water only from treated municipal water supplies.
- When hiking, camping, or traveling to countries where the water supply may be unsafe to drink, either avoid drinking the water or boil it for 1 minute to kill the parasite. Drinking bottled beverages or hot coffee and tea are safe alternatives.
- Do not swallow water while swimming.
- Do not swim in community pools if you or your child has giardiasis.
- Drink only pasteurized milk, juices, or cider.
- Wash, peel, or cook raw fruits and vegetables before eating.
- Do not use untreated manure to fertilize fruits and vegetables.

Cryptosporidium Parvum

Cryptosporidium parvum, cause of the disease cryptosporidiosis (KRIP-toe-spo-RID-e-O-sis), is a one-celled, microscopic parasite, and a significant cause of waterborne illness worldwide. It is found in the intestines of many herd animals including cows, sheep, goats, deer, and elk.

How do people get cryptosporidiosis?

People get cryptosporidiosis the following ways:

- By consuming food or water contaminated with *C. parvum* oocysts (infective stage of the parasite). The oocysts are the environmentally resistant stage of the organism and are shed in the feces of a host (human or animal).
- By putting anything into your mouth that has touched the stool of a person or animal with cryptosporidiosis.

Symptoms of Cryptosporidiosis

Symptoms include watery diarrhea, stomach cramps, upset stomach, and slight fever. Some cases may be without symptoms.

When will symptoms appear? What is the duration?

Symptoms appear 2 to 10 days after ingestion of *C. parvum* oocysts. The illness usually goes away without medical intervention in 3 to 4 days, but in some outbreaks in daycare centers, diarrhea has lasted 1 to 4 weeks. In people with AIDS and other individuals with weakened immune systems, cryptosporidiosis can be serious, long-lasting, and sometimes fatal.

Who is at risk for contracting cryptosporidiosis?

Those at risk include:

- persons working in child daycare centers and children attending daycare centers;
- persons with weakened immune systems including those with HIV/AIDS infection, organ transplant recipients, or those individuals undergoing chemotherapy;
- international travelers (traveler's diarrhea); and
- hikers, campers, or any other persons who may drink from untreated water supplies.

How to Prevent Cryptosporidiosis

- Wash hands with hot, soapy water before handling foods and eating, and after using the toilet, diapering young children, and handling animals.
- Make sure infected individuals wash their hands frequently to reduce the spread of infection.
- Drink water only from treated municipal water supplies.
- When hiking, camping, or traveling to countries where the water supply may be unsafe to drink, either avoid drinking the water or boil it for 1 minute to kill the parasite. Drinking bottled beverages or hot coffee and tea are safe alternatives.
- Do not swallow water while swimming.
- Do not swim in community swimming pools if you or your child has cryptosporidiosis.
- Drink only pasteurized milk, juices, or cider.
- Wash, peel, or cook raw fruits and vegetables before eating.

- Do not use untreated manure to fertilize fruits and vegetables.

Cyclospora Cayetanensis

Cyclospora cayetanensis (SIGH-clo-SPOR-uh KYE-uh-tuh-NEN-sis), cause of cyclosporiasis, is a one-celled, microscopic parasite. Currently little is known about this organism, although cases of cyclosporiasis are being reported from various countries with increasing frequency.

How do people get cyclosporiasis?

People get cyclosporiasis the following ways:

- By consuming food or water contaminated with *C. cayetanensis* oocysts (the infective stage of the organism).

- By putting anything into your mouth that has touched the stool of a person or animal with cyclosporiasis.

Symptoms of Cyclosporiasis

Symptoms include watery diarrhea (sometimes explosive), stomach cramps, nausea, vomiting, muscle aches, low-grade fever, and fatigue. Some cases are without symptoms. Symptoms are more severe in persons with weakened immune systems.

When will symptoms appear? What is the duration?

Symptoms typically appear about 1 week after ingestion of *C. cayetanensis* oocysts. If untreated, the symptoms may last a week to more than a month. Symptoms may return.

Who is at risk for contracting cyclosporiasis?

Persons of all ages are at risk for infection. Persons with weakened immune systems including those with HIV/AIDS infection, organ transplant recipients, or those individuals undergoing chemotherapy may be at greater risk for infection.

How to Prevent Cyclosporiasis

- Wash hands with hot, soapy water before handling foods and eating, and after using the toilet, diapering young children, and handling animals.

- Make sure infected individuals wash their hands frequently to reduce the spread of infection.

- Drink water only from treated municipal water supplies.

- When hiking, camping, or traveling to countries where the water supply may be unsafe to drink, either avoid drinking the water or boil the water for 1 minute to kill the parasite. Drinking bottled beverages or hot coffee and tea are safe alternatives.

- Do not swallow water while swimming.

- Do not swim in community swimming pools if you or your child has cyclosporiasis.

- Wash, peel, or cook raw fruits and vegetables before eating.

- Do not use untreated manure to fertilize fruits and vegetables.

Toxoplasma Gondii

Toxoplasma gondii, cause of the disease, toxoplasmosis (TOX-o-plaz-MO-sis), is a single-celled, microscopic parasite found throughout the world. It is interesting to note that these organisms can only carry out their reproductive cycle within members of the cat family. In this parasite-host relationship, the cat is the definitive host. The infective stage (oocyst) develops in the gut of the cat. The oocysts are then shed into the environment with cat feces.

How do people get toxoplasmosis?

People get toxoplasmosis the following ways:

- By consuming foods (such as raw or undercooked meats, especially pork, lamb, or wild game) or drinking untreated water (from rivers or ponds) that may contain the parasite.

- Fecal-oral: Touching your hands to your mouth after gardening, handling cats, cleaning a cat's litter box, or anything that has come into contact with cat feces.

- Mother-to-fetus (if mother is pregnant when first infected with *T. gondii*).

- Through organ transplants or blood transfusions, although these modes are rare.

Symptoms of Toxoplasmosis and Severe Toxoplasmosis

Toxoplasmosis is relatively harmless to most people, although some may develop flu-like symptoms such as swollen lymph glands and/or muscle aches and pains. In otherwise healthy individuals, the disease is usually mild and goes away without medical treatment. However, dormant tissue stages can remain in the infected individual for life.

However, persons with weakened immune systems such as those with HIV/AIDS infection, organ transplant recipients, individuals undergoing chemotherapy, and infants may develop severe toxoplasmosis. Severe toxoplasmosis may result in damage to the eyes or brain. Infants becoming infected before birth can be born retarded or with other mental or physical problems.

When will symptoms appear? What is the duration?

The time that symptoms appear varies, but generally symptoms will appear 1 week to 1 month after consuming the parasite.

The duration of the illness depends on the health and immune status of the host. Persons with weakened immune systems may experience illnesses of long duration, possibly resulting in death.

Who is at risk for contracting severe toxoplasmosis?

Those at risk include:

- Persons with weakened immune systems including those with HIV/AIDS infection, organ transplant recipients, or those individuals undergoing chemotherapy.

- Infants born to mothers who become infected with *T. gondii* shortly before becoming pregnant or during pregnancy. Those mothers exposed to *T. gondii* longer than 6 months before becoming pregnant rarely transmit toxoplasmosis to their infants.

How to Prevent Toxoplasmosis

- If you are pregnant or if you have a weakened immune system, you should discuss your risk of contracting toxoplasmosis with your health care provider.

- Wear clean latex gloves when handling raw meats, or have someone who is healthy, and not pregnant, handle the meats for you.

- Cook all meats thoroughly to 160° F.

- Wash hands, cutting boards, and other utensils thoroughly with hot, soapy water after handling raw meats.

- Clean cat litter boxes daily because cat feces more than a day old can contain mature parasites.

- Wash hands thoroughly with hot, soapy water after handling cats, cleaning and cat litter boxes, especially before you handle or eat food.

- Wear gloves when you handle garden soil or sandboxes. Cats may use gardens or sandboxes as litter boxes.

- Cover sandboxes to prevent cats from using them as litter boxes.

- Help prevent cats from becoming infected with *T. gondii* by discouraging them from hunting and scavenging.

- Feed cats commercially made cat foods or cook their food.

Trichinella Spiralis

Trichinella spiralis, cause of trichinosis (TRICK-a-NO-sis) is an intestinal roundworm whose larvae may migrate from the digestive tract and form cysts in various muscles of the body. Infections occur worldwide, but are most prevalent in regions where pork or wild game is consumed raw or undercooked. The incidence of trichinosis has declined in the United States due to changes in hog feeding practices. Presently, most cases in this country are caused by consumption of raw or undercooked wild game.

How do people get trichinosis?

People get trichinosis by consuming raw or undercooked meats such as pork, wild boar, bear, bobcat, cougar, fox, wolf, dog, horse, seal, or walrus containing Trichinella larvae.

The illness is not spread directly from person to person.

Symptoms of Trichinosis

The first symptoms are nausea, diarrhea, vomiting, fever, and abdominal pain, followed by headaches, eye swelling, aching joints and muscles, weakness, and itchy skin. In severe infections, persons may experience difficulty with coordination and have heart and breathing problems. Death may occur in severe cases.

When will symptoms appear? What is the duration?

Abdominal symptoms may appear within 1 to 2 days after eating contaminated meat. Further symptoms (eye swelling and aching muscles and joints) may begin 2 to 8 weeks after infection. Mild cases may assumed to be flu.

Who is at risk for contracting trichinosis?

• Persons consuming raw or under cooked pork or wild game.

• Persons with weakened immune systems including those with HIV/AIDS infection, organ transplant recipients, or those individuals undergoing chemotherapy may be at a greater risk for infection.

How to Prevent Trichinosis

• Cook pork and wild game to 160° F to kill any *Trichinella* larvae that may be present.

Taenia Saginata/Taenia Solium *(Tapeworms)*

Taenia saginata (beef tapeworm) and *Taenia solium* (pork tapeworm) are parasitic worms (helminths). Taeniasis is the name of the intestinal infection caused by adult-stage tapeworms (beef or pork tapeworms). Cysticercosis is the name of the tissue (other than intestinal) infection caused by the larval-stage of the pork tapeworm only.

It is interesting to note that humans are the definitive hosts of both organisms. This means that the reproductive cycle, and thus egg production by the organisms, occurs only within humans. Eggs are passed in human feces and they may be shed into the environment for as long as the worms remain in the intestines (for as long as 30 years). In addition, the eggs may remain viable in the environment for many months.

These diseases are more prevalent in underdeveloped countries where sanitation practices may be substandard and in areas where pork and beef are consumed raw or undercooked. They are relatively uncommon in the U.S., although travelers and immigrants are occasionally infected.

How do people get taeniasis?

People get taeniasis by consuming infected beef or pork (raw or undercooked).

How do people get cysticercosis?

People get cysticercosis the following ways:

- By consuming food or water contaminated with the eggs of *T. solium* (pork tapeworm). Worm eggs hatch and the larvae then migrate to various parts of the body and form cysts called cysticerci. This can be a serious or fatal disease if it involves organs such as the central nervous system, heart, or eyes.

- By putting anything into your mouth that has touched the stool of a person infected with *T. solium*.

- Some persons with intestinal tapeworms may infect themselves with eggs from their own feces as a result of poor personal hygiene.

Symptoms of Taeniasis

Most cases of infection with adult worms are without symptoms. Some persons may experience abdominal pain, weight loss, digestive disturbances, and possible intestinal obstruction.

Irritation of the perianal area can occur, caused by worms or worm segments exiting the anus.

When will symptoms appear? What is the duration?

T. saginata (beef tapeworm) infections appear within 10 to 14 weeks. *T. solium* (pork tapeworm) infections appear within 8 to 12 weeks.

Taeniasis may last many years without medical treatment.

Who is at risk for contracting taeniasis?

- Anyone consuming infected beef or pork (raw or undercooked).

- Persons with weakened immune systems including those with HIV/AIDS infection, organ transplant recipients, or those individuals undergoing chemotherapy may be at a greater risk for infection.

Symptoms of Cysticercosis

Symptoms may vary depending on the organ or organ system involved. For example, an individual with cysticercosis involving the central nervous system (neurocysticercosis) may exhibit neurological symptoms such as psychiatric problems or epileptic seizures. Death is common.

When will symptoms appear? What is the duration?

Symptoms usually appear from several weeks to several years after becoming infected with the eggs of the pork tapeworm (*T. solium*). Symptoms may last for many years if medical treatment is not received.

Who is at risk for contracting cysticercosis?

- Persons traveling to countries where sanitation may be substandard and the water supply may be unsafe.

- Persons with weakened immune systems including those with HIV/AIDS infection, organ transplant recipients, or those individuals undergoing chemotherapy may be at a greater risk for infection.

How to Prevent Taeniasis

- Cook beef and pork to 160° F to kill encysted tapeworm larvae that may be present.

How to Prevent Cysticercosis

- Drink water only from treated municipal water supplies.

- When traveling to countries where the water supply may be unsafe, either avoid the water or boil it for 1 minute to kill parasite eggs. Drinking bottled beverages or hot coffee and tea are safe alternatives.

- Do not swallow water while swimming.

- Do not swim in community swimming pools if you or your child are infected with tapeworms.

- Wash, peel, or cook raw fruits and vegetables before eating.

- Make sure that infected individuals wash their hands frequently to reduce the spread of infection.

Chapter 58

Escherichia Coli

Escherichia coli O157:H7 is an emerging cause of foodborne illness. An estimated 73,000 cases of infection and 61 deaths occur in the United States each year. Infection often leads to bloody diarrhea, and occasionally to kidney failure. Most illness has been associated with eating undercooked, contaminated ground beef. Person-to-person contact in families and child care centers is also an important mode of transmission. Infection can also occur after drinking raw milk and after swimming in or drinking sewage-contaminated water.

Consumers can prevent *E. coli* O157:H7 infection by thoroughly cooking ground beef, avoiding unpasteurized milk, and washing hands carefully. Because the organism lives in the intestines of healthy cattle, preventive measures on cattle farms and during meat processing are being investigated.

E. coli O157:H7 is one of hundreds of strains of the bacterium *Escherichia coli*. Although most strains are harmless and live in the intestines of healthy humans and animals, this strain produces a powerful toxin and can cause severe illness.

E. coli O157:H7 was first recognized as a cause of illness in 1982 during an outbreak of severe bloody diarrhea; the outbreak was traced to contaminated hamburgers. Since then, most infections have come from eating undercooked ground beef.

"*Escherichia Coli* O157:H7," a fact sheet produced by the Centers for Disease Control and Prevention (CDC), 2001. Available online at http://www.cdc.gov/ncidod/dbmd/diseaseinfo/escherichiacoli_g.htm.

The combination of letters and numbers in the name of the bacterium refers to the specific markers found on its surface and distinguishes it from other types of *E. coli*.

How E. Coli *O157:H7 Is Spread*

The organism can be found on a small number of cattle farms and can live in the intestines of healthy cattle. Meat can become contaminated during slaughter, and organisms can be thoroughly mixed into beef when it is ground. Bacteria present on the cow's udders or on equipment may get into raw milk.

Eating meat, especially ground beef, that has not been cooked sufficiently to kill *E. coli* O157:H7 can cause infection. Contaminated meat looks and smells normal. Although the number of organisms required to cause disease is not known, it is suspected to be very small.

Among other known sources of infection are consumption of sprouts, lettuce, salami, unpasteurized milk and juice, and swimming in or drinking sewage-contaminated water. Bacteria in diarrheal stools of infected persons can be passed from one person to another if hygiene or handwashing habits are inadequate. This is particularly likely among toddlers who are not toilet trained. Family members and playmates of these children are at high risk of becoming infected.

Young children typically shed the organism in their feces for a week or two after their illness resolves. Older children rarely carry the organism without symptoms.

Illnesses Caused by E. Coli *O157:H7*

E. coli O157:H7 infection often causes severe bloody diarrhea and abdominal cramps; sometimes the infection causes nonbloody diarrhea or no symptoms. Usually little or no fever is present, and the illness resolves in 5 to 10 days.

In some persons, particularly children under 5 years of age and the elderly, the infection can also cause a complication called hemolytic uremic syndrome, in which the red blood cells are destroyed and the kidneys fail. About 2%-7% of infections lead to this complication. In the United States, hemolytic uremic syndrome is the principal cause of acute kidney failure in children, and most cases of hemolytic uremic syndrome are caused by *E. coli* O157:H7.

480

Diagnosis of E. Coli *O157:H7 Infection*

Infection with *E. coli* O157:H7 is diagnosed by detecting the bacterium in the stool. Most laboratories that culture stool do not test for *E. coli* O157:H7, so it is important to request that the stool specimen be tested on sorbitol-MacConkey (SMAC) agar for this organism. All persons who suddenly have diarrhea with blood should get their stool tested for *E. coli* O157:H7.

Treatment

Most persons recover without antibiotics or other specific treatment in 5-10 days. There is no evidence that antibiotics improve the course of disease, and it is thought that treatment with some antibiotics may precipitate kidney complications. Antidiarrheal agents, such as loperamide (Imodium), should also be avoided.

Hemolytic uremic syndrome is a life-threatening condition usually treated in an intensive care unit. Blood transfusions and kidney dialysis are often required. With intensive care, the death rate for hemolytic uremic syndrome is 3%-5%.

Long-Term Consequences of Infection

Persons who only have diarrhea usually recover completely.

About one-third of persons with hemolytic uremic syndrome have abnormal kidney function many years later, and a few require long-term dialysis. Another 8% of persons with hemolytic uremic syndrome have other lifelong complications, such as high blood pressure, seizures, blindness, paralysis, and the effects of having part of their bowel removed.

Prevention

E. coli O157:H7 will continue to be an important public health concern as long as it contaminates meat. Preventive measures may reduce the number of cattle that carry it and the contamination of meat during slaughter and grinding. Research into such prevention measures is just beginning.

Cook all ground beef and hamburger thoroughly. Because ground beef can turn brown before disease-causing bacteria are killed, use a digital instant-read meat thermometer to ensure thorough cooking.

Ground beef should be cooked until a thermometer inserted into several parts of the patty, including the thickest part, reads at least 160° F. Persons who cook ground beef without using a thermometer can decrease their risk of illness by not eating ground beef patties that are still pink in the middle.

If you are served an undercooked hamburger or other ground beef product in a restaurant, send it back for further cooking. You may want to ask for a new bun and a clean plate, too.

Avoid spreading harmful bacteria in your kitchen. Keep raw meat separate from ready-to-eat foods. Wash hands, counters, and utensils with hot soapy water after they touch raw meat. Never place cooked hamburgers or ground beef on the unwashed plate that held raw patties. Wash meat thermometers in between tests of patties that require further cooking.

Drink only pasteurized milk, juice, or cider. Commercial juice with an extended shelf life that is sold at room temperature (e.g. juice in cardboard boxes, vacuum sealed juice in glass containers) has been pasteurized, although this is generally not indicated on the label. Juice concentrates are also heated sufficiently to kill pathogens.

Wash fruits and vegetables thoroughly, especially those that will not be cooked. Children under 5 years of age, immunocompromised persons, and the elderly should avoid eating alfalfa sprouts until their safety can be assured. Methods to decontaminate alfalfa seeds and sprouts are being investigated.

Drink municipal water that has been treated with chlorine or other effective disinfectants. Avoid swallowing lake or pool water while swimming. Make sure that persons with diarrhea, especially children, wash their hands carefully with soap after bowel movements to reduce the risk of spreading infection, and that persons wash hands after changing soiled diapers. Anyone with a diarrheal illness should avoid swimming in public pools or lakes, sharing baths with others, and preparing food for others.

Chapter 59

Salmonellosis

What is salmonellosis?

Salmonellosis is an infection with a bacteria called *Salmonella*. Most persons infected with *Salmonella* develop diarrhea, fever, and abdominal cramps 12 to 72 hours after infection. The illness usually lasts 4 to 7 days, and most persons recover without treatment. However, in some persons the diarrhea may be so severe that the patient needs to be hospitalized. In these patients, the *Salmonella* infection may spread from the intestines to the blood stream, and then to other body sites and can cause death unless the person is treated promptly with antibiotics. The elderly, infants, and those with impaired immune systems are more likely to have a severe illness.

What sort of germ is **Salmonella***?*

The *Salmonella* germ is actually a group of bacteria that can cause diarrheal illness in humans. They are microscopic living creatures that pass from the feces of people or animals, to other people or other animals. There are many different kinds of *Salmonella* bacteria. *Salmonella* serotype *typhimurium* and *Salmonella* serotype *enteritidis*, are the most common in the United States. *Salmonella* has been known to cause illness for over 100 years. They were discovered by an American scientist named Salmon, for whom they are named.

"Salmonellosis," a fact sheet produced by the Centers for Disease Control and Prevention (CDC), 2001. Available online at http://www.cdc.gov/ncidod/dbmd/diseaseinfo/salmonellosis_g.htm.

483

How can Salmonella *infections be diagnosed?*

Many different kinds of illnesses can cause diarrhea, fever, or abdominal cramps. Determining that *Salmonella* is the cause of the illness depends on laboratory tests that identify *Salmonella* in the stools of an infected person. These tests are sometimes not performed unless the laboratory is instructed specifically to look for the organism. Once *Salmonella* has been identified, further testing can determine its specific type, and which antibiotics could be used to treat it.

How can Salmonella *infections be treated?*

Salmonella infections usually resolve in 5-7 days and often do not require treatment unless the patient becomes severely dehydrated or the infection spreads from the intestines. Persons with severe diarrhea may require rehydration, often with intravenous fluids. Antibiotics are not usually necessary unless the infection spreads from the intestines, then it can be treated with ampicillin, gentamicin, trimethoprim/sulfamethoxazole, or ciprofloxacin. Unfortunately, some *Salmonella* bacteria have become resistant to antibiotics, largely as a result of the use of antibiotics to promote the growth of feed animals.

Are there long term consequences to a Salmonella *infection?*

Persons with diarrhea usually recover completely, although it may be several months before their bowel habits are entirely normal. A small number of persons who are infected with *Salmonella*, will go on to develop pains in their joints, irritation of the eyes, and painful urination. This is called Reiter's syndrome. It can last for months or years, and can lead to chronic arthritis which is difficult to treat. Antibiotic treatment does not make a difference in whether or not the person later develops arthritis.

How do people catch Salmonella*?*

Salmonella live in the intestinal tracts of humans and other animals, including birds. *Salmonella* are usually transmitted to humans by eating foods contaminated with animal feces. Contaminated foods usually look and smell normal. Contaminated foods are often of animal origin, such as beef, poultry, milk, or eggs, but all foods, including vegetables may become contaminated. Many raw foods of animal origin are frequently contaminated, but fortunately, thorough cooking kills *Salmonella*. Food may also become contaminated by the unwashed hands of an infected food handler, who forgot to wash his or her hands with soap after using the bathroom.

Salmonella may also be found in the feces of some pets, especially those with diarrhea, and people can become infected if they do not wash their hands after contact with these feces. Reptiles are particularly likely to harbor *Salmonella* and people should always wash their hands immediately after handling a reptile, even if the reptile is healthy. Adults should also be careful that children wash their hands after handling a reptile.

What can a person do to prevent this illness?

There is no vaccine to prevent salmonellosis. Since foods of animal origin may be contaminated with *Salmonella*, people should not eat raw or undercooked eggs, poultry, or meat. Raw eggs may be unrecognized in some foods such as homemade hollandaise sauce, caesar and other salad dressings, tiramisu, homemade ice cream, homemade mayonnaise, cookie dough, and frostings. Poultry and meat, including hamburgers, should be well-cooked, not pink in the middle. Persons also should not consume raw or unpasteurized milk or other dairy products. Produce should be thoroughly washed before consuming.

Cross-contamination of foods should be avoided. Uncooked meats should be kept separate from produce, cooked foods, and ready-to-eat foods. Hands, cutting boards, counters, knives, and other utensils should be washed thoroughly after handling uncooked foods. Hand should be washed before handling any food, and between handling different food items.

People who have salmonellosis should not prepare food or pour water for others until they have been shown to no longer be carrying the *Salmonella* bacterium.

People should wash their hands after contact with animal feces. Since reptiles are particularly likely to have *Salmonella*, everyone should immediately wash their hands after handling reptiles. Reptiles (including turtles) are not appropriate pets for small children and should not be in the same house as an infant.

How common is salmonellosis?

Every year, approximately 40,000 cases of salmonellosis are reported in the United States. Because many milder cases are not diagnosed or reported, the actual number of infections may be twenty or more times greater. Salmonellosis is more common in the summer than winter.

Children are the most likely to get salmonellosis. Young children, the elderly, and the immunocompromised are the most likely to have severe infections. It is estimated that approximately 1,000 persons die each year with acute salmonellosis.

What else can be done to prevent salmonellosis?

It is important for the public health department to know about cases of salmonellosis. It is important for clinical laboratories to send isolates of *Salmonella* to the City, County, or State Public Health Laboratories so the specific type can be determined and compared with other *Salmonella* in the community. If many cases occur at the same time, it may mean that a restaurant, food or water supply has a problem which needs correction by the public health department.

Some prevention steps occur everyday without you thinking about it. Pasteurization of milk and treating municipal water supplies are highly effective prevention measures that have been in place for many years. In the 1970s, small pet turtles were a common source of salmonellosis in the United States, and in 1975, the sale of small turtles was halted in this country. Improvements in farm animal hygiene, in slaughter plant practices, and in vegetable and fruit harvesting and packing operations may help prevent salmonellosis caused by contaminated foods. Better education of food industry workers in basic food safety and restaurant inspection procedures, may prevent cross-contamination and other food handling errors that can lead to outbreaks. Wider use of pasteurized egg in restaurants, hospitals, and nursing homes is an important prevention measure. In the future, irradiation or other treatments may greatly reduce contamination of raw meat.

What is the government doing about salmonellosis?

The Centers for Disease Control and Prevention (CDC) monitors the frequency of *Salmonella* infections in the country and assists the local and State Health Departments to investigate outbreaks and devise control measures. CDC also conducts research to better identify specific types of *Salmonella*. The Food and Drug Administration inspects imported foods, milk pasteurization plants, promotes better food preparation techniques in restaurants and food processing plants, and regulates the sale of turtles. The FDA also regulates the use of specific antibiotics as growth promotants in food animals. The U.S. Department of Agriculture monitors the health of food animals, inspects egg pasteurization plants, and is responsible for the quality of slaughtered and processed meat. The U.S. Environmental Protection Agency regulates and monitors the safety of our drinking water supplies.

What can I do to prevent salmonellosis?

- Cook poultry, ground beef, and eggs thoroughly before eating. Do not eat or drink foods containing raw eggs, or raw unpasteurized milk.

- If you are served undercooked meat, poultry or eggs in a restaurant, don't hesitate to send it back to the kitchen for further cooking.

- Wash hands, kitchen work surfaces, and utensils with soap and water immediately after they have been in contact with raw meat or poultry.

- Be particularly careful with foods prepared for infants, the elderly, and the immunocompromised.

- Wash hands with soap after handling reptiles or birds, or after contact with pet feces.

- Avoid direct or even indirect contact between reptiles (turtles, iguanas, other lizards, snakes) and infants or immunocompromised persons.

- Don't work with raw poultry or meat, and an infant (e.g., feed, change diaper) at the same time.

- Mother's milk is the safest food for young infants. Breast-feeding prevents salmonellosis and many other health problems.

Chapter 60

Shigellosis

What is shigellosis?

Shigellosis is an infectious disease caused by a group of bacteria called *Shigella*. Most who are infected with *Shigella* develop diarrhea, fever, and stomach cramps starting a day or two after they are exposed to the bacterium. The diarrhea is often bloody. Shigellosis usually resolves in 5 to 7 days. In some persons, especially young children and the elderly, the diarrhea can be so severe that the patient needs to be hospitalized. A severe infection with high fever may also be associated with seizures in children less than 2 years old. Some persons who are infected may have no symptoms at all, but may still pass the *Shigella* bacteria to others.

What sort of germ is Shigella*?*

The *Shigella* germ is actually a family of bacteria that can cause diarrhea in humans. They are microscopic living creatures that pass from person to person. *Shigella* were discovered over 100 years ago by a Japanese scientist named Shiga, for whom they are named. There are several different kinds of *Shigella* bacteria: *Shigella sonnei*, also known as group D *Shigella*, accounts for over two-thirds of the shigellosis in the United States. A second type, *Shigella flexneri*, or group B *Shigella*, accounts for almost all of the rest. Other types of

"Shigellosis," a fact sheet produced by the Centers for Disease Control and Prevention (CDC), 2001. Available online at http://www.cdc.gov/ncidod/dbmd/ diseaseinfo/shigellosis_g.htm.

Shigella are rare in this country, though they continue to be important causes of disease in the developing world. One type found in the developing world, *Shigella dysenteriae* type 1, causes deadly epidemics there.

How can Shigella *infections be diagnosed?*

Many different kinds of diseases can cause diarrhea and bloody diarrhea, and the treatment depends on which germ is causing the diarrhea. Determining that *Shigella* is the cause of the illness depends on laboratory tests that identify *Shigella* in the stools of an infected person. These tests are sometimes not performed unless the laboratory is instructed specifically to look for the organism. The laboratory can also do special tests to tell which type of *Shigella* the person has and which antibiotics, if any, would be best to treat it.

How can Shigella *infections be treated?*

Shigellosis can usually be treated with antibiotics. The antibiotics commonly used for treatment are ampicillin, trimethoprim/sulfamethoxazole (also known as Bactrim or Septra), nalidixic acid, or ciprofloxacin. Appropriate treatment kills the *Shigella* bacteria that might be present in the patient's stools, and shortens the illness. Unfortunately, some *Shigella* bacteria have become resistant to antibiotics and using antibiotics to treat shigellosis can actually make the germs more resistant in the future. Persons with mild infections will usually recover quickly without antibiotic treatment. Therefore, when many persons in a community are affected by shigellosis, antibiotics are sometimes used selectively to treat only the more severe cases. Antidiarrheal agents such as loperamide (Imodium) or diphenoxylate with atropine (Lomotil) are likely to make the illness worse and should be avoided.

Are there long term consequences to a Shigella *infection?*

Persons with diarrhea usually recover completely, although it may be several months before their bowel habits are entirely normal. About 3% of persons who are infected with one type of *Shigella*, *Shigella flexneri*, will later develop pains in their joints, irritation of the eyes, and painful urination. This is called Reiter's syndrome. It can last for months or years, and can lead to chronic arthritis which is difficult to treat. Reiter's syndrome is caused by a reaction to *Shigella* infection that happens only in people who are genetically predisposed to it.

Once someone has had shigellosis, they are not likely to get infected with that specific type again for at least several years. However, they can still get infected with other types of *Shigella*.

How do people catch Shigella?

The *Shigella* bacteria pass from one infected person to the next. *Shigella* are present in the diarrheal stools of infected persons while they are sick and for a week or two afterwards. Most *Shigella* infections are the result of the bacterium passing from stools or soiled fingers of one person to the mouth of another person. This happens when basic hygiene and handwashing habits are inadequate. It is particularly likely to occur among toddlers who are not fully toilet-trained. Family members and playmates of such children are at high risk of becoming infected.

Shigella infections may be acquired from eating contaminated food. Contaminated food may look and smell normal. Food may become contaminated by infected food handlers who forget to wash their hands with soap after using the bathroom. Vegetables can become contaminated if they are harvested from a field with sewage in it. Flies can breed in infected feces and then contaminate food. *Shigella* infections can also be acquired by drinking or swimming in contaminated water. Water may become contaminated if sewage runs into it, or if someone with shigellosis swims in it.

What can a person do to prevent this illness?

There is no vaccine to prevent shigellosis. However, the spread of *Shigella* from an infected person to other persons can be stopped by frequent and careful handwashing with soap. Frequent and careful handwashing is important among all age groups. Frequent, supervised handwashing of all children should be followed in day care centers and in homes with children who are not completely toilet-trained (including children in diapers). When possible, young children with a *Shigella* infection who are still in diapers should not be in contact with uninfected children.

People who have shigellosis should not prepare food or pour water for others until they have been shown to no longer be carrying the *Shigella* bacterium.

If a child in diapers has shigellosis, everyone who changes the child's diapers should be sure the diapers are disposed of properly in a closed-lid garbage can, and should wash his or her hands carefully with soap and warm water immediately after changing the diapers.

After use, the diaper changing area should be wiped down with a disinfectant such as household bleach, Lysol or bactericidal wipes.

Basic food safety precautions and regular drinking water treatment prevents shigellosis. At swimming beaches, having enough bathrooms near the swimming area helps keep the water from becoming contaminated.

Simple precautions taken while traveling to the developing world can prevent getting shigellosis. Drink only treated or boiled water, and eat only cooked hot foods or fruits you peel yourself. The same precautions prevent traveler's diarrhea in general.

How common is shigellosis?

Every year, about 18,000 cases of shigellosis are reported in the United States. Because many milder cases are not diagnosed or reported, the actual number of infections may be twenty times greater. Shigellosis is particularly common and causes recurrent problems in settings where hygiene is poor and can sometimes sweep through entire communities. Shigellosis is more common in summer than winter. Children, especially toddlers aged 2 to 4, are the most likely to get shigellosis. Many cases are related to the spread of illness in childcare settings, and many more are the result of the spread of the illness in families with small children.

In the developing world, shigellosis is far more common and is present in most communities most of the time.

What else can be done to prevent shigellosis?

It is important for the public health department to know about cases of shigellosis. It is important for clinical laboratories to send isolates of *Shigella* to the City, County or State Public Health Laboratory so the specific type can be determined and compared to other *Shigella*. If many cases occur at the same time, it may mean that a restaurant, food or water supply has a problem which needs correction by the public health department. If a number of cases occur in a day-care center, the public health department may need to coordinate efforts to improve handwashing among the staff, children, and their families. When a community-wide outbreak occurs, a community-wide approach to promote handwashing and basic hygiene among children can stop the outbreak. Improvements in hygiene for vegetables and fruit picking and packing may prevent shigellosis caused by contaminated produce.

Some prevention steps occur everyday, without you thinking about it. Making municipal water supplies safe and treating sewage are highly effective prevention measures that have been in place for many years.

What is the government doing about shigellosis?

The Centers for Disease Control and Prevention (CDC) monitors the frequency of *Shigella* infections in the country, and assists local and State health departments to investigate outbreaks, determine means of transmission and devise control measures. CDC also conducts research to better understand how to identify and treat shigellosis. The Food and Drug Administration inspects imported foods, and promotes better food preparation techniques in restaurants and food processing plants. The Environmental Protection Agency regulates and monitors the safety of our drinking water supplies. The government has also maintained active research into the development of a *Shigella* vaccine.

How can I learn more about this and other public health problems?

You can discuss any medical concerns you may have with your doctor or other heath care provider. Your local city or county health department can provide more information about this and other public health problems that are occurring in your area. General information about the public health of the nation is published every week in the *Morbidity and Mortality Weekly Report*, by the CDC in Atlanta, GA. Epidemiologists in your local and State Health Departments are tracking a number of important public health problems, investigating special problems that arise, and helping to prevent them form occurring in the first place, or from spreading if they do occur.

Some tips for preventing the spread of shigellosis:

- wash hands with soap carefully and frequently, especially after going to the bathroom, after changing diapers, and before preparing foods or beverages
- dispose of soiled diapers properly
- disinfect diaper changing areas after using them
- keep children with diarrhea out of child care settings
- supervise handwashing of toddlers and small children after they use the toilet
- persons with diarrheal illness should not prepare food for others

- if you are traveling to the developing world, "boil it, cook it, peel it, or forget it"

- avoid drinking pool water

Chapter 61

Shellfish-Associated Toxins

Shellfish poisoning is caused by a group of toxins elaborated by planktonic algae (dinoflagellates, in most cases) upon which the shellfish feed. The toxins are accumulated and sometimes metabolized by the shellfish. The 20 toxins responsible for paralytic shellfish poisonings (PSP) are all derivatives of saxitoxin. Diarrheic shellfish poisoning (DSP) is presumably caused by a group of high molecular weight polyethers, including okadaic acid, the dinophysis toxins, the pectenotoxins, and yessotoxin. Neurotoxic shellfish poisoning (NSP) is the result of exposure to a group of polyethers called brevetoxins. Amnesic shellfish poisoning (ASP) is caused by the unusual amino acid, domoic acid, as the contaminant of shellfish.

The types of shellfish poisoning are:

- Paralytic Shellfish Poisoning (PSP)

- Diarrheic Shellfish Poisoning (DSP)

- Neurotoxic Shellfish Poisoning (NSP)

- Amnesic Shellfish Poisoning (ASP)

"Various Shellfish-Associated Toxins," from *Foodborne Pathogenic Microorganisms and Natural Toxins Handbook: The Bad Bug Book,* produced by the U.S. Food and Drug Administration (FDA), Center for Food Safety and Applied Nutrition (CFSAN), 1992, deemed current by the FDA as of February 2003. Available online at http://www.cfsan.fda.gov/~mow/chap37.html.

Nature of Disease

Ingestion of contaminated shellfish results in a wide variety of symptoms, depending upon the toxins(s) present, their concentrations in the shellfish and the amount of contaminated shellfish consumed. In the case of PSP, the effects are predominantly neurological and include tingling, burning, numbness, drowsiness, incoherent speech, and respiratory paralysis. Less well characterized are the symptoms associated with DSP, NSP, and ASP. DSP is primarily observed as a generally mild gastrointestinal disorder, i.e., nausea, vomiting, diarrhea, and abdominal pain accompanied by chills, headache, and fever. Both gastrointestinal and neurological symptoms characterize NSP, including tingling and numbness of lips, tongue, and throat, muscular aches, dizziness, reversal of the sensations of hot and cold, diarrhea, and vomiting. ASP is characterized by gastrointestinal disorders (vomiting, diarrhea, abdominal pain) and neurological problems (confusion, memory loss, disorientation, seizure, coma).

Diagnosis of Human Illness

Diagnosis of shellfish poisoning is based entirely on observed symptomatology and recent dietary history.

Associated Foods

All shellfish (filter-feeding mollusks) are potentially toxic. However, PSP is generally associated with mussels, clams, cockles, and scallops; NSP with shellfish harvested along the Florida coast and the Gulf of Mexico; DSP with mussels, oysters, and scallops, and ASP with mussels.

Relative Frequency of Disease

Good statistical data on the occurrence and severity of shellfish poisoning are largely unavailable, which undoubtedly reflects the inability to measure the true incidence of the disease. Cases are frequently misdiagnosed and, in general, infrequently reported. Of these toxicoses, the most serious from a public health perspective appears to be PSP. The extreme potency of the PSP toxins has, in the past, resulted in an unusually high mortality rate.

Course of Disease and Complications

PSP: Symptoms of the disease develop fairly rapidly, within 0.5 to 2 hours after ingestion of the shellfish, depending on the amount of toxin consumed. In severe cases respiratory paralysis is common, and death may occur if respiratory support is not provided. When such support is applied within 12 hours of exposure, recovery usually is complete, with no lasting side effects. In unusual cases, because of the weak hypotensive action of the toxin, death may occur from cardiovascular collapse despite respiratory support.

NSP: Onset of this disease occurs within a few minutes to a few hours; duration is fairly short, from a few hours to several days. Recovery is complete with few after effects; no fatalities have been reported.

DSP: Onset of the disease, depending on the dose of toxin ingested, may be as little as 30 minutes to 2 to 3 hours, with symptoms of the illness lasting as long as 2 to 3 days. Recovery is complete with no after effects; the disease is generally not life threatening.

ASP: The toxicosis is characterized by the onset of gastrointestinal symptoms within 24 hours; neurological symptoms occur within 48 hours. The toxicosis is particularly serious in elderly patients, and includes symptoms reminiscent of Alzheimer's disease. All fatalities to date have involved elderly patients.

Target Populations

All humans are susceptible to shellfish poisoning. Elderly people are apparently predisposed to the severe neurological effects of the ASP toxin. A disproportionate number of PSP cases occur among tourists or others who are not native to the location where the toxic shellfish are harvested. This may be due to disregard for either official quarantines or traditions of safe consumption, both of which tend to protect the local population.

Chapter 62

Hepatitis A Virus

Hepatitis A is usually a mild illness characterized by sudden onset of fever, malaise, nausea, anorexia, and abdominal discomfort, followed in several days by jaundice.

The term hepatitis A (HA) or type A viral hepatitis has replaced all previous designations: infectious hepatitis, epidemic hepatitis, epidemic jaundice, catarrhal jaundice, infectious icterus, Botkins disease, and MS-1 hepatitis.

Diagnosis of Human Illness

Hepatitis A is diagnosed by finding IgM-class anti-HAV in serum collected during the acute or early convalescent phase of disease. Commercial kits are available.

Associated Foods

HAV is excreted in feces of infected people and can produce clinical disease when susceptible individuals consume contaminated water or foods. Cold cuts and sandwiches, fruits and fruit juices, milk and milk products, vegetables, salads, shellfish, and iced drinks are

---

"Hepatitis A Virus," from *Foodborne Pathogenic Microorganisms and Natural Toxins Handbook: The Bad Bug Book,* produced by the U.S. Food and Drug Administration (FDA), Center for Food Safety and Applied Nutrition (CFSAN), 1992, deemed current by the FDA as of February 2003. Available online at http://www.cfsan.fda.gov/~mow/chap31/html.

commonly implicated in outbreaks. Water, shellfish, and salads are the most frequent sources. Contamination of foods by infected workers in food processing plants and restaurants is common.

Relative Frequency of Disease

Hepatitis A has a worldwide distribution occurring in both epidemic and sporadic fashions. About 22,700 cases of hepatitis A representing 38% of all hepatitis cases (5-year average from all routes of transmission) are reported annually in the U.S. In 1988 an estimated 7.3% cases were foodborne or waterborne. HAV is primarily transmitted by person-to-person contact through fecal contamination, but common-source epidemics from contaminated food and water also occur. Poor sanitation and crowding facilitate transmission. Outbreaks of HA are common in institutions, crowded house projects, and prisons and in military forces in adverse situations. In developing countries, the incidence of disease in adults is relatively low because of exposure to the virus in childhood. Most individuals 18 and older demonstrate an immunity that provides lifelong protection against reinfection. In the U.S., the percentage of adults with immunity increases with age (10% for those 18-19 years of age to 65% for those over 50). The increased number of susceptible individuals allows common source epidemics to evolve rapidly.

Course of Disease and Complications

The incubation period for hepatitis A, which varies from 10 to 50 days (mean 30 days), is dependent upon the number of infectious particles consumed. Infection with very few particles results in longer incubation periods. The period of communicability extends from early in the incubation period to about a week after the development of jaundice. The greatest danger of spreading the disease to others occurs during the middle of the incubation period, well before the first presentation of symptoms. Many infections with HAV do not result in clinical disease, especially in children. When disease does occur, it is usually mild and recovery is complete in 1-2 weeks. Occasionally, the symptoms are severe and convalescence can take several months. Patients suffer from feeling chronically tired during convalescence, and their inability to work can cause financial loss. Less than 0.4% of the reported cases in the U.S. are fatal. These rare deaths usually occur in the elderly.

Target Populations

All people who ingest the virus and are immunologically unprotected are susceptible to infection. Disease however, is more common in adults than in children.

Hepatitis A is endemic throughout much of the world. Major national epidemics occurred in 1954, 1961 and 1971. Although no major epidemic occurred in the 1980s, the incidence of hepatitis A in the U.S. increased 58% from 1983 to 1989. Foods have been implicated in over 30 outbreaks since 1983. The most recent ones and the suspected contaminated foods include:

- 1987—Louisville, Kentucky. Suspected source: imported lettuce.

- 1990—North Georgia. Frozen strawberries; Montana. Frozen strawberries; Baltimore. Shellfish.

Food Analysis

The virus has not been isolated from any food associated with an outbreak. Because of the long incubation period, the suspected food is often no longer available for analysis. No satisfactory method is presently available for routine analysis of food, but sensitive molecular methods used to detect HAV in water and clinical specimens, should prove useful to detect virus in foods. Among those, the polymerase chain reaction (PCR) amplification method seems particularly promising.

Chapter 63

Color Additives

Color additives have long been a part of human culture. Archae-ologists date cosmetic colors as far back as 5000 B.C.

The U.S. Food and Drug Administration (FDA) separates color additives into two categories. These are colors that the agency certi-fies (derived primarily from petroleum and known as coal-tar dyes) and colors that are exempted from certification (obtained largely from mineral, plant, or animal sources). Only approved substances may be used to color foods, drugs, cosmetics, and medical devices.

FDA requires domestic and foreign manufacturers of certain col-ors to submit samples from each batch of color produced. FDA scien-tists test each sample of these colors to confirm that each batch of the color is within established specifications. These certified colors are listed on labels as FD&C, D&C or external D&C. Using the uncertified versions of color additives that require certification is illegal in foods, drugs, cosmetics, and medical devices.

The color certification program is self-supporting because the law requires manufacturers to pay FDA a user fee for each pound of color the agency certifies. In Fiscal Year 2000 FDA certified more than 13 million pounds of color additives.

The 1993 *FDA Consumer* magazine article reprinted below pro-vides additional information on the regulation of color additives.

"Color Additives Fact Sheet," produced by the U. S. Food and Drug Admin-istration (FDA), Center for Food Safety and Applied Nutrition (CFSAN), 2001. Available online at http://www.cfsan.fda.gov/~dms/cos-221.html.

From Shampoo to Cereal: Seeing to the Safety of Color Additives

It starts when you get up in the morning. You snatch a bar of soap and scrub your face. That's likely your first dab into the palette of added tints and hues that will color much of your day. Most of us hardly notice them, but color additives surround us. They're in shampoos. In shaving cream. Toothpaste. Deodorant. Contact Lenses. Lipstick, eyeliner, and mascara. At breakfast, the colors keep coming. Juice, cereal, pastry, coffee creamer, vitamins—all are likely to have added colors.

Color additives make things attractive, appealing, appetizing. They also serve as a code of sorts, allowing us to identify products on sight, like medicine dosages and candy flavors. We might reason, for example, that a pale green candy is mint flavored, while a darker green one is lime. Based on our color analysis alone, there will probably be no surprises when we pop the candy into our mouths.

With this rainbow hodgepodge bombarding us daily, it's only natural that consumers might wonder: Just how safe are all these colors? "Very," says John E. Bailey, Ph.D., acting director of FDA's Office of Cosmetics and Colors.

He explains that FDA has, over nearly a century, refined its process of monitoring and controlling color additive use. By law, industry must prove the safety of colors it sells. FDA ensures that colors on the market are safe for their intended purposes and do not cover up product inferiority or otherwise deceive consumers. FDA watches domestic color use closely, seizing products found unsafe.

Still, Bailey says, some consumers believe color additives can cause health problems or even be hazardous. This notion stems, he says, from persistent public attitudes about colors banned in the past. He says consumer confidence in the safety of all colors can be shaken when FDA removes a color from the market. But he emphasizes: "I think we can say with assurance that today's colors are safe if used properly and that consumers need not be worried."

Yellow Means Caution

Two categories make up FDA's list of permitted colors: those the agency certifies by batch (derived primarily from petroleum and coal sources) and ones exempt from batch certification (obtained largely from plant, animal, or mineral sources—fruit juice, carmine, and titanium dioxide, for example). Colors found to be potentially hazardous have been purged from the list of permissible additives. What remains is a wide color spectrum approved for use in foods, over-the-counter and prescription drugs, cosmetics, or in medical devices such as surgical sutures and contact lenses.

Though these colors have a good safety record, one commonly used additive reportedly has prompted minor adverse reactions in some people. It is FD&C Yellow No. 5, listed as tartrazine on medicine labels, a color found widely in beverages, desserts, processed vegetables, drugs, makeup, and many other products. FDA certifies more than 2 million pounds of it yearly.

In 1986, an FDA advisory committee concluded that Yellow No. 5 may cause itching or hives in a small population sub-group. This kind of skin reaction usually is not a serious one, says Linda Tollefson, D.V.M., an FDA epidemiologist "Reactions are classified as hypersensitive and are not true allergic reactions, which would be more severe."

Nonetheless, since 1980 (for drugs) and 1981 (for foods), FDA has required all products containing Yellow No. 5 to list the color on their labels so consumers sensitive to the dye can avoid it. (As of May 8, 1993, labels must list all certified colors as part of the requirements of the Nutrition Labeling and Education Act of 1990.)

A Certified Success

FDA requires domestic and foreign certifiable color manufacturers to submit samples taken from every batch of color produced. The agency has listed each certifiable color based on a specific chemical formula shown to produce no harmful effects in laboratory animals.

Each color has chemical specifications that place restrictions on the levels of impurities allowed in the additive. In some cases, these limitations are designed to ensure that the color contains no cancer-causing substances. Using chromatography and other sophisticated analytical techniques, FDA scientists probe sample compositions to confirm that each batch is within these limitations.

"We analyze every batch because every batch is a little different from the one before it," says Bailey. He explains that complex organic chemical reactions occurring during manufacturing can throw off a sample's composition. It's like baking a cake: Even though you follow a recipe closely, the cake turns out just a little different each time.

With certifiable colors, a shift in composition can mean rejection of an entire batch. In fiscal year 1992, of 3,943 batches tested, the agency rejected 40. FDA also regularly inspects color manufacturers and end users such as candy makers.

FDA is especially vigilant in monitoring products from foreign countries, which may contain color additives that are illegal domestically. The agency regularly seizes entire product shipments that contain prohibited colors. Often, this detective work comes easily. FDA, through its import alerts, flags certain products. "You look for a pattern," says Bailey.

The batch certification program supports itself because the law requires manufacturers to pay FDA a user fee for every pound of color the agency certifies. "We like to think of batch certification as a government success story," Bailey says.

The Red Scare

In 1960, amendments to the Food, Drug, and Cosmetic Act of 1938 added the so-called Delaney anti-cancer clause to FDA's legal mandate. Among other things, the clause prohibits marketing any color additive the agency has found to cause cancer in animals or humans, regardless of amount.

In recent years, regulators have faced a dilemma in light of technological advances that enable scientists to identify smaller and smaller concentrations of a substance and conduct more sensitive toxicological tests. Are such tiny amounts a health threat? Scientists have yet to answer this question. Congress has held hearings to examine the pros and cons of liberalizing the Delaney clause. At press time, debates on the issue were in progress.

FDA applied the Delaney clause in 1990 when it outlawed several uses of the strawberry-toned FD&C Red No. 3. The banned uses include cosmetics and externally applied drugs, as well as uses of the color's non-water-soluble "lake." FDA previously had allowed these provisional uses while studies were in progress to evaluate the color's safety. Research later showed large amounts of the color causes thyroid tumors in male rats.

Though FDA viewed Red No. 3 cancer risks as small—about 1 in 100,000 over a 70-year lifetime—the agency banned provisional listings because of Delaney directives. At the same time, Red No. 3 has permanent listings for food and drug uses that are still allowed although the agency has announced plans to propose revoking these uses as well. For now, Red No. 3 can be used in foods and oral medications. Products such as maraschino cherries, bubble gum, baked goods, and all sorts of snack foods and candy may contain Red No. 3.

According to the International Association of Color Manufacturers, Red No. 3 is widely used in industry and hard to replace. It makes a very close match for primary red, which is important in creating color blends. It doesn't bleed, so drug companies use it to color pills with discernible shades for identification.

If Red No. 3 joins the ranks of colors forbidden for all uses, it won't be the first FD&C Red in recent years to be pulled from the market. FDA banned FD&C Red No. 2, a tint that continues to be an enigma, in 1976.

In the early 1970s, data from Russian studies raised questions about Red No. 2's safety. Several subsequent studies showed no hazards. FDA conducted its own tests, which were inconclusive. The consumer-oriented Health Research Group petitioned FDA to ban the color, while congressional and public interest mounted.

FDA turned the matter over to its Toxicology Advisory Committee, which evaluated numerous reports and decided there was no evidence of a hazard. The committee then asked FDA to conduct follow-up analyses. Agency scientists evaluated biological data and concluded that "it appears that feeding FD&C Red No. 2 at a high dosage results in a statistically significant increase" in malignant tumors in female rats.

There still was no positive proof of either potential danger or safety. FDA ultimately decided to ban the color because it had not been shown to be safe. The agency based its decision in part on the presumption that the color might cause cancer.

The judgment had a profound effect on consumer attitudes toward certifiable colors, says FDA's John E. Bailey. "The Red No. 2 decision will always be with us, he says. For example, some candy manufacturers reacted by removing red-colored pieces from their products, even if there was no Red No. 2 present. They were afraid sales would plummet because of public perception that red candies were dangerous.

Though long gone from U.S. shelves, products tinted with Red No. 2 still can be found in Canada and Europe. Whether the color is gone forever in the United States remains to be seen. FDA and industry officials say it could stage a comeback. Industry could petition FDA to list Red No. 2 as a certifiable color if animal study data adequately show safety. If FDA then agrees, consumers could once again be munching on candies and using other products tinted with the deep-red dye.

Animal-Less Studies

Because of the cost, it is unlikely that industry will commission new animal studies to measure Red No. 2's safety. But advances in toxicological trial methods could enable scientists to assess potential hazards without using animals. Technology is moving toward a time when chemical substances could be evaluated accurately with a battery of short-term tests conducted in the test tube. Such analyses would greatly shorten the time and expense of evaluating not only colors but other food additives and environmental chemicals.

These test tube trials are not here yet. But if and when they arrive, they may have government and industry taking another look at certain color additives, including Red No. 2.

As for the colors that remain in use, consumers can rest assured that color additives are among the most scrutinized of all food ingredients. Next time you quaff a glass of red fruit punch or pop a blue pill, consider that those colors have been studied, studied, and restudied, sometimes dozens of times. And remember that FDA inspects every batch of certifiable colors used in consumer products.

You may, however, want to avoid consuming huge quantities of any one color additive. As Bailey says: "Good sense is the best policy. As with many other food ingredients, don't overuse any one product. Practice everything in moderation."

A Colorful History

Color additives have long been a part of human culture. Archaeologists date cosmetic colors as far back as 5000 B.C. Ancient Egyptian writings tell of drug colorants, and historians say food colors likely emerged around 1500 B.C.

Through the years, color additives typically came from substances found in nature, such as turmeric, paprika and saffron. But as the 20th century approached, new kinds of colors appeared that offered marketers wider coloring possibilities. These colors, many whipped up in the chemist's lab, also created a range of safety problems.

In the late 1800s, some manufacturers colored products with potentially poisonous mineral- and metal-based compounds. Toxic chemicals tinted certain candies and pickles, while other color additives contained arsenic or similar poisons. Historical records show that injuries, even deaths, resulted from tainted colorants. Food producers also deceived customers by employing color additives to mask poor product quality or spoiled stock.

By the turn of the century, unmonitored color additives had spread through the marketplace in all sorts of popular foods, including ketchup, mustard, jellies, and wine. Sellers at the time offered more than 80 artificial coloring agents, some intended for dyeing textiles, not foods. Many color additives had never been tested for toxicity or other adverse effects.

As the 1900s began, the bulk of chemically synthesized colors were derived from aniline, a petroleum product that in pure form is toxic. Originally, these were dubbed coal-tar colors because the starting materials were obtained from bituminous coal. (These formulations still are used today—albeit safely—for most certifiable color additives.)

Though colors from plant, animal and mineral sources—at one time the only coloring agents available—remained in use early in this century, manufacturers had strong economic incentives to phase them out. Chemically synthesized colors simply were easier to produce, less expensive, and superior in coloring properties. Only tiny amounts were needed. They blended nicely and didn't impart unwanted flavors to foods. But as their use grew, so did safety concerns.

In 1906, Congress passed the Pure Food and Drugs Act. This marked the first of several laws allowing the federal government to scrutinize and control additives use. The act covered only food coloring. It was not until passage of the Federal Food, Drug, and Cosmetic Act of 1938 that FDA's mandate included the full range of color designations consumers still can read on product packages: "FD&C" (permitted in food, drugs and cosmetic); "D&C" (for use in drugs and cosmetics) and "Ext. D&C" (colors for external-use drug and cosmetics).

Public hearings and regulations following the 1938 law gave colors the numbers that separate their hues. These letter and number combinations—FD&C Blue No. 1 or D&C Red No. 17, for example—make it easy to distinguish colors used in food, drugs or cosmetics from dyes made for textiles and other uses. Only FDA certified color additives can carry these special designations. The law also created a listing of color lakes. These water-insoluble forms of certain approved colors are used in coated tablets, cookie fillings, candies, and other products in which color bleeding could make a mess or otherwise cause problems.

Though the 1938 law did much to bring color use under strict control, nagging questions lingered about tolerance levels for color additives. One incident in the 1950s, in which scores of children contracted diarrhea from Halloween candy and popcorn colored with large amounts of FD&C Orange No. 1, led FDA to retest food colors. As a result, in 1960, the 1938 law was amended to broaden FDA's scope and allow the agency to set limits on how much color could be safely added to products.

FDA also instituted a pre-marketing approval process, which requires color producers to ensure, before marketing, that products are safe and properly labeled. Should safety questions arise later, colors can be reexamined. The 1960 measures put color additives already on the market into a provisional listing. This allowed continued use of the colors pending FDA's conclusions on safety.

From the original 1960 catalog of about 200 provisionally listed colors, which included straight colors and lakes, only lakes of some colors remain on the provisional list. Industry withdrew or FDA banned many, while the rest became permanently listed and are still used. Some of these colors, derived from coal or petroleum sources, are subject to certification and carry the F, D, or C prefix. Others, exempt from certification, are pigments and colors derived from plant, animal and mineral sources. They are found in a myriad of products—from the caramel that tints cola drinks to the orange annatto that gives color to cheese.

FDA certified over 11.5 million pounds of color additives last fiscal year. Of all those colors straight dye FD&C Red No. 40 is by far the most popular. Manufacturers use this orange-red color in all sorts of gelatins, beverages, dairy products and condiments. FDA certified more than 3 million pounds of the dye in fiscal year 1992—almost a million pounds more than the runner-up, FD&C Yellow No. 5.

Color Additive Terms

Allura Red (AC): The common name for uncertified FD&C Red No. 40.

Certifiable Color Additives: Colors manufactured from petroleum and coal sources listed in the Code of Federal Regulations for use in foods, drugs, cosmetics, and medical devices.

Coal-Tar Dyes: Coloring agents originally derived from coal sources.

D&C: A prefix designating that a certifiable color has been approved for use in drugs and cosmetics.

Erythrosine: The common name of FD&C Red No. 3.

Exempt Color Additives: Colors derived primarily from plant, animal and mineral (other than coal and petroleum) sources that are exempt from FDA certification.

Ext. D&C: A prefix designating that a certifiable color may be used only in externally applied drugs and cosmetics.

FD&C: A prefix designating that a certified color can be used in foods, drugs or cosmetics.

Indigotine: The common name for uncertified FD&C Blue No. 2.

Lakes: Water-insoluble forms of certifiable colors that are more stable than straight dyes and ideal for product in which leaching of the color is undesirable (coated tablets and hard candies, for example).

Permanent Listing: A list of allowable colors determined by tests to be safe for human consumption under regulatory provisions.

Provisional Listing: A list of colors, originally numbering about 200, that FDA allows to continue to be used pending acceptable safety data.

Straight Dye: certifiable colors that dissolve in water and are manufactured as powders, granules, liquids, or other special forms (used in beverages, baked goods, and confections, for example).

Tartrazine: A common name for uncertified FD&C Yellow No. 5.

—by John Henkel, staff writer for FDA Consumer

Chapter 64

Are Bioengineered Foods Safe?

Since 1994, a growing number of foods developed using the tools of the science of biotechnology have come onto both the domestic and international markets. With these products has come controversy, primarily in Europe where some question whether these foods are as safe as foods that have been developed using the more conventional approach of hybridization.

Ever since the latter part of the 19th century, when Gregor Mendel discovered that characteristics in pea plants could be inherited, scientists have been improving plants by changing their genetic makeup. Typically, this was done through hybridization in which two related plants were cross-fertilized and the resulting offspring had characteristics of both parent plants. Breeders then selected and reproduced the offspring that had the desired traits.

Today, to change a plant's traits, scientists are able to use the tools of modern biotechnology to insert a single gene—or, often, two or three genes—into the crop to give it new, advantageous characteristics. Most genetic modifications make it easier to grow the crop. About half of the American soybean crop planted in 1999, for example, carries a gene that makes it resistant to an herbicide used to control weeds. About a quarter of U.S. corn planted in 1999 contains a gene that produces a

"Are Bioengineered Foods Safe?" by Larry Thompson, *FDA Consumer* magazine, January-February 2000, produced by the U.S. Food and Drug Administration (FDA). Available online at http://www.fda.gov/fdac/features/2000/100_bio.html.

protein toxic to certain caterpillars, eliminating the need for certain conventional pesticides.

In 1992, the Food and Drug Administration published a policy explaining how existing legal requirements for food safety apply to products developed using the tools of biotechnology. It is the agency's responsibility to ensure the safety of all foods on the market that come from crops, including bioengineered plants, through a science-based decision-making process. This process often includes public comment from consumers, outside experts and industry. FDA established, in 1994, a consultation process that helps ensure that foods developed using biotechnology methods meet the applicable safety standards. Over the last five years, companies have used the consultation process more than 40 times as they moved to introduce genetically altered plants into the U.S. market.

Although the agency has no evidence that the policy and procedure do not adequately protect the public health, there have been concerns voiced regarding FDA's policy on these foods. To understand the agency's role in ensuring the safety of these products, *FDA Consumer* sat down with Commissioner Jane E. Henney, M.D., to discuss the issues raised by bioengineered foods:

FDA Consumer: Dr. Henney, what does it mean to say that a food crop is bioengineered?

Dr. Henney: When most people talk about bioengineered foods, they are referring to crops produced by utilizing the modern techniques of biotechnology. But really, if you think about it, all crops have been genetically modified through traditional plant breeding for more than a hundred years.

Since Mendel, plant breeders have modified the genetic material of crops by selecting plants that arise through natural or, sometimes, induced changes. Gardeners and farmers and, at times, industrial plant breeders have crossbred plants with the intention of creating a prettier flower, a hardier or more productive crop. These conventional techniques are often imprecise because they shuffle thousands of genes in the offspring, causing them to have some of the characteristics of each parent plant. Gardeners or breeders then look for the plants with the most desirable new trait.

With the tools developed from biotechnology, a gene can be inserted into a plant to give it a specific new characteristic instead of mixing all of the genes from two plants and seeing what comes out. Once in the plant, the new gene does what all genes do: It directs the production of a specific protein that makes the plant uniquely different.

This technology provides much more control over, and precision to, what characteristic breeders give to a new plant. It also allows the changes to be made much faster than ever before. No matter how a new crop is created—using traditional methods or biotechnology tools—breeders are required by our colleagues at the U.S. Department of Agriculture to conduct field testing for several seasons to make sure only desirable changes have been made. They must check to make sure the plant looks right, grows right, and produces food that tastes right. They also must perform analytical tests to see whether the levels of nutrients have changed and whether the food is still safe to eat.

As we have evaluated the results of the seeds or crops created using biotechnology techniques, we have seen no evidence that the bioengineered foods now on the market pose any human health concerns or that they are in any way less safe than crops produced through traditional breeding.

FDA Consumer: What kinds of genes do plant breeders try to put in crop plants?

Dr. Henney: Plant researchers look for genes that will benefit the farmer, the food processor, or the consumer. So far, most of the changes have helped the farmer. For example, scientists have inserted into corn a gene from the bacterium *Bacillus thuringiensis*, usually referred to as BT. The gene makes a protein lethal to certain caterpillars that destroy corn plants. This form of insect control has two advantages: It reduces the need for chemical pesticides, and the BT protein, which is present in the plant in very low concentrations, has no effect on humans.

Another common strategy is inserting a gene that makes the plant resistant to a particular herbicide. The herbicide normally poisons an enzyme essential for plant survival. Other forms of this normal plant enzyme have been identified that are unaffected by the herbicide. Putting the gene for this resistant form of the enzyme into the plant protects it from the herbicide. That allows farmers to treat a field with the herbicide to kill the weeds without harming the crop.

The new form of the enzyme poses no food safety issues because it is virtually identical to nontoxic enzymes naturally present in the plant. In addition, the resistant enzyme is present at very low levels and it is as easily digested as the normal plant enzyme.

Modifications have also been made to canola and soybean plants to produce oils with a different fatty acid composition so they can be used in new food processing systems. Researchers are working diligently to develop crops with enhanced nutritional properties.

FDA Consumer: Do the new genes, or the proteins they make, have any effect on the people eating them?

Dr. Henney: No, it doesn't appear so. All of the proteins that have been placed into foods through the tools of biotechnology that are on the market are nontoxic, rapidly digestible, and do not have the characteristics of proteins known to cause allergies.

As for the genes, the chemical that encodes genetic information is called DNA. DNA is present in all foods and its ingestion is not associated with human illness. Some have noted that sticking a new piece of DNA into the plant's chromosome can disrupt the function of other genes, crippling the plant's growth or altering the level of nutrients or toxins. These kinds of effects can happen with any type of plant breeding—traditional or biotech. That's why breeders do extensive field-testing. If the plant looks normal and grows normally, if the food tastes right and has the expected levels of nutrients and toxins, and if the new protein put into food has been shown to be safe, then there are no safety issues.

FDA Consumer: You mentioned allergies. Certain proteins can cause allergies, and the genes being put in these plants may carry the code for new proteins not normally consumed in the diet. Can these foods cause allergic reactions because of the genetic modifications?

Dr. Henney: I understand why people are concerned about food allergies. If one is allergic to a food, it needs to be rigorously avoided. Further, we don't want to create new allergy problems with food developed from either traditional or biotech means. It is important to know that bioengineering does not make a food inherently different from conventionally produced food. And the technology doesn't make the food more likely to cause allergies.

Fortunately, we know a lot about the foods that do trigger allergic reactions. About 90 percent of all food allergies in the United States are caused by cow's milk, eggs, fish and shellfish, tree nuts, wheat, and legumes, especially peanuts and soybeans.

To be cautious, FDA has specifically focused on allergy issues. Under the law and FDA's biotech food policy, companies must tell consumers on the food label when a product includes a gene from one of the common allergy-causing foods unless it can show that the protein produced by the added gene does not make the food cause allergies.

We recommend that companies analyze the proteins they introduce to see if these proteins possess properties indicating that the proteins might be allergens. So far, none of the new proteins in foods evaluated through the FDA consultation process have caused allergies. Because proteins resulting from biotechnology and now on the market are sensitive to heat, acid and enzymatic digestion, are present in very low levels in the food, and do not have structural similarities to known allergens, we have no scientific evidence to indicate that any of the new proteins introduced into food by biotechnology will cause allergies.

FDA Consumer: Let me ask you one more scientific question. I understand that it is common for scientists to use antibiotic resistance marker genes in the process of bioengineering. Are you concerned that their use in food crops will lead to an increase in antibiotic resistance in germs that infect people?

Dr. Henney: Antibiotic resistance is a serious public health issue, but that problem is currently and primarily caused by the overuse or misuse of antibiotics. We have carefully considered whether the use of antibiotic resistance marker genes in crops could pose a public health concern and have found no evidence that it does.

I'm confident of this for several reasons. First, there is little if any transfer of genes from plants to bacteria. Bacteria pick up resistance genes from other bacteria, and they do it easily and often. The potential risk of transfer from plants to bacteria is substantially less than the risk of normal transfer between bacteria. Nevertheless, to be on the safe side, FDA has advised food developers to avoid using marker genes that encode resistance to clinically important antibiotics.

FDA Consumer: You've mentioned FDA's consultative process a couple of times. Could you explain how genetically engineered foods are regulated in the United States?

Dr. Henney: Bioengineered foods actually are regulated by three federal agencies: FDA, the Environmental Protection Agency, and the U.S. Department of Agriculture. FDA is responsible for the safety and labeling of all foods and animal feeds derived from crops, including biotech plants. EPA regulates pesticides, so the BT used to keep caterpillars from eating the corn would fall under its jurisdiction. USDA's Animal and Plant Health Inspection Service oversees the agricultural environmental safety of planting and field-testing genetically engineered plants.

Let me talk about FDA's role. Under the federal Food, Drug, and Cosmetic Act, companies have a legal obligation to ensure that any food they sell meets the safety standards of the law. This applies equally to conventional food and bioengineered food. If a food does not meet the safety standard, FDA has the authority to take it off the market.

In the specific case of foods developed utilizing the tools of biotechnology, FDA set up a consultation process to help companies meet the requirements. While consultation is voluntary, the legal requirements that the foods have to meet are not. To the best of our knowledge, all bioengineered foods on the market have gone through FDA's process before they have been marketed.

Here's how it works. Companies send us documents summarizing the information and data they have generated to demonstrate that a bioengineered food is as safe as the conventional food. The documents describe the genes they use: whether they are from a commonly allergenic plant, the characteristics of the proteins made by the genes, their biological function, and how much of them will be found in the food. They tell us whether the new food contains the expected levels of nutrients or toxins and any other information about the safety and use of the product.

FDA scientists review the information and generally raise questions. It takes several months to complete the consultation, which is why companies usually start a dialog with the agency scientists nearly a year or more before they submit the data. At the conclusion of the consultation, if we are satisfied with what we have learned about the food, we provide the company with a letter stating that they have completed the consultation process and we have no further questions at that time.

FDA Consumer: Since genes are being added to the plant, why doesn't FDA review biotech products under the same food additive regulations that it reviews food colors and preservatives?

Dr. Henney: The food additive provision of the law ensures that a substance with an unknown safety profile is not added to food without the manufacturer proving to the government that the additive is safe. This intense review, however, is not required under the law when a substance is generally recognized as safe (GRAS) by qualified experts. A substance's safety can be established by long history of use in food or when the nature of the substance and the information generally available to scientists about it is such that it doesn't raise significant safety issues.

In the case of bioengineered foods, we are talking about adding some DNA to the plant that directs the production of a specific protein. DNA already is present in all foods and is presumed to be GRAS. As I described before, adding an extra bit of DNA does not raise any food safety issues.

As for the resulting proteins, they too are generally digested and metabolized and don't raise the kinds of food safety questions as are raised by novel chemicals in the diet. The proteins introduced into plants so far either have been pesticides or enzymes. The pesticide proteins, such as BT, would actually be regulated by EPA and go through its approval process before going on the market. The enzymes have been considered to be GRAS, so they have not gone through the food additive petition process. FDA's consultation process aids companies in determining whether the protein they want to add to a food is generally recognized as safe. If FDA has concerns about the safety of the food, the product would have to go through the full food additive premarket approval process.

FDA Consumer: Why doesn't FDA require companies to tell consumers on the label that a food is bioengineered?

Dr. Henney: Traditional and bioengineered foods are all subject to the same labeling requirements. All labeling for a food product must be truthful and not misleading. If a bioengineered food is significantly different from its conventional counterpart—if the nutritional value changes or it causes allergies—it must be labeled to indicate that difference. For example, genetic modifications in varieties of soybeans and canola changed the fatty acid composition in the oils of those plants. Foods using those oils must be labeled, including using a new standard name that indicates the bioengineered oil's difference from conventional soy and canola oils. If a food had a new allergy-causing protein introduced into it, the label would have to state that it contained the allergen.

We are not aware of any information that foods developed through genetic engineering differ as a class in quality, safety, or any other attribute from foods developed through conventional means. That's why there has been no requirement to add a special label saying that they are bioengineered. Companies are free to include in the labeling of a bioengineered product any statement as long as the labeling is truthful and not misleading. Obviously, a label that implies that a food is better than another because it was, or was not, bioengineered, would be misleading.

FDA Consumer: Overall, are you satisfied that FDA's current system for regulating bioengineered foods is protecting the public health?

Dr. Henney: Yes, I am convinced that the health of the American public is well protected by the current laws and procedures. I also recognize that this is a rapidly changing field, so FDA must stay on top of the science as biotechnology evolves and is used to make new kinds of modifications to foods. In addition, the agency is seeking public input about our policies and will continue to reach out to the public to help consumers understand the scientific issues and the agency's policies.

Not only must the food that Americans eat be safe, but consumers must have confidence in its safety, and confidence in the government's role in ensuring that safety. Policies that are grounded in science, that are developed through open and transparent processes, and that are implemented rigorously and communicated effectively are what have assured the consumers' confidence in an agency that has served this nation for nearly 100 years.

Part Eight

Environmental Hazards to Specific Populations

Chapter 65

Children's Environmental Health

This chapter discusses children's exposures to environmental chemicals and other agents, such as radiation, sunlight, and infectious organisms. It focuses on how patterns of exposure differ between children and adults and the implications of these differences for children's environmental health.

What Is Exposure?

Exposure is defined as any combination of circumstances that brings a "receptor," for example, a child, in contact with an environmental agent. The magnitude of exposure may be measured in terms of the concentration or level of an agent in the environmental medium that the receptor encounters, such as parts per million (ppm) sulfur dioxide in air. Exposure also involves the concept of duration. Acute exposure means any exposure that occurs over a very short period, such as a minute or 24 hours. Longer exposures may be referred to as subchronic (up to a few months) or chronic (years, or over the whole life-span). Some exposures include measures of both concentration and duration, such as 100 ppm for six months. The severity and nature of

Text in this chapter is excerpted from "Children's Environmental Exposures," from the *Critical Periods in Development*, Office of Children's Health Protection (OCHP) Paper Series on Children's Health and the Environment, Paper 2003-3, OCHP, U.S. Environmental Protection Agency (EPA), March 2003. Full text of this document, including bibliographic citations, is available online at http://www.yosemite.epa.gov/ochp/ochpweb.nsf/content/2003_33.htm/$File/2003_3.pdf.

adverse impacts from environmental agents usually depend strongly on both exposure level and duration.

Human exposure to environmental agents may occur via several pathways. Pathways are the avenues through which the agent comes in contact with the body. The most commonly considered pathways in environmental health are inhalation (through the respiratory system), ingestion (through the digestive system), and dermal absorption (through contact with the skin). For radiation and sunlight, exposure may be measured as the amount of energy that impinges on the skin or that is emitted by ingested or inhaled substances. As discussed in the following sections, there are many reasons why the nature of children's exposure through these pathways may be different that that of adults.

Developing infants also may be exposed in the womb (*in utero*) to environmental chemicals and other agents encountered by the mother during pregnancy, a pathway that is unique to this developmental stage. This exposure occurs when agents in the mother's bloodstream pass through the placenta and enter the fetal circulation.

Why Are We Concerned about Children's Environmental Exposures?

The first reason for studying children's environmental exposures is that the patterns of exposure to environmental agents are likely to differ between children and adults. These differences arise, as the following sections discuss, because of differences in child and adult behavior patterns and physiological characteristics. Children and adults divide their time very differently across locations (e.g., the amount of time spent indoors versus outdoors, or the amount of time spent on the floor versus sitting in a chair), and across activities (e.g., playing, crawling, and mouthing objects). In many instances, children's behavior patterns result in exposures over time that are greater than those of adults, or result in exposures that adults do not experience at all. Much of this chapter discusses how children's exposure patterns differ per se from those of adults.

Second, children are physiologically different from adults. Children tend to have higher basal (resting) metabolic rates. Combined with the fact that children are growing rapidly and generally are more active than adults, their higher metabolic rate means that they eat more, drink more, and breathe more air than adults do in proportion to their body size. Thus children may receive a higher dose (the amount of an agent absorbed into the body over time) of an environmental contaminant than would adults living in the same house. Since the nature and severity of adverse effects of environmental exposures are closely related to the size of the dose, higher doses translate into increased concern for adverse effects.

Finally, children and adults may process environmental agents differently once they enter the body. This chapter describes how environmental agents are absorbed, distributed, and excreted differently by children than by adults. In addition, children's metabolic capacity (i.e., their ability to chemically process environmental agents) may be less well-developed than that of adults. Both of these factors contribute to differences in the persistence of environmental agents in children's and adult's bodies and the concentration of the agents in specific organs. Concern over children's environmental exposures arises when agents persist for longer periods and at higher concentrations in children's bodies than in adults. Evidence of exposure comes from the levels of contaminants measured in children's blood, urine, or body tissues. Other such biomarkers of exposure include metabolites of environmental chemicals and measurements of physiological responses to exposures that occur before obvious toxic effects. An example of the latter is the altered metabolism of iron-carrying blood components caused by low-level exposure to lead.

Environmental Factors Affecting Children's Exposure

Numerous environmental (or external) factors affect the quantity of an agent or contaminant that can enter the developing human body. These factors include the composition of the child's diet, contaminants in other exposure media (e.g., air, soil), and the location and activities of the child in relation to the environmental agent. This section discusses these and other factors and how they work in concert with physiological (or internal) factors. This section is organized by the following topics:

- The limited diet of children;
- Behaviors unique to children;
- How and where children spend their time; and
- The impact of short stature.

The Limited Diet of Children

The patterns of exposure to ingested toxicants differ between children and adults in several ways. For example, young children eat three to four times more food in proportion to their body size than adults do, and therefore children ingest larger amounts of chemical and infectious agents per unit of body mass (CEC, 2000; Plunkett, 1992). Children also eat fewer types of foods. For example, human milk or cow milk-based products are the predominant source of energy and nutrients throughout the first year of life. When averaged over the first year, cow milk products comprise 36 percent and 58 percent of the diets of nursing and non-nursing infants, respectively (NRC, 1993), while in adults these products amount to only about 29 percent. Milk has a high fat content (about 3 percent in breast milk) (Rogan, 1986). Fat-soluble chemicals can be stored in fat and released during lactation. Both cow milk and breast milk have been shown to contain environmental pollutants such as lead, PCBs, and dioxins, although generally at low levels (Ong, 1985; Pluim, 1994; Rogan, 1986). The infant is potentially exposed to the same chemicals in milk. Unfortunately, although many chemicals may not be harmful to an adult in concentrations typically encountered on a daily basis, those chemicals can be detrimental to a young child (Kacew, 1992).

Young children typically consume large quantities of specific foods compared with adults, in proportion to body weight. The average infant (a child younger than 1 year old) consumes 15 to 17 times more apple juice and 14 to 15 times more pears than the national average consumption rate for these foods (NRC, 1993). Therefore, if these foods are contaminated with toxicants, children may be disproportionately exposed (Goldman, 1998).

Young children drink more water relative to their body mass than adults do. For example, infants less than 6 months of age, on average, consume 88 mL/kg/day (millimeters of water per kilogram body weight) of tap water through direct sources and indirect sources, such as water added in the preparation of formula or fruit juice (U.S. EPA, 2000c). (Infants who consume formula instead of breast milk drink a higher than average amount of tap water.) Infants from 6 months to one year of age ingest 56 mL/kg/day of tap water, on average. Adults 20 years of age and older, in contrast, ingest 15 mL/kg/day. Children younger than 7 years old drink more tap water in proportion to their body mass than older individuals do.

Teenagers generally drink the least tap water relative to body mass than do any age group. Bottled water consumption follows a similar pattern (US EPA, 2000c). As a result of this greater consumption of water, children may be disproportionately exposed to chemicals and infectious agents found in drinking water, including the water used to make infant formula (Bearer, 1995; Chance, 1998; U.S. EPA, 1997).

Food and fluid intake patterns and trends among adolescents also differ from those of adults. Between 1965 and 1996, 11 to 18 year olds in the United States reduced their consumption of dietary fat from 39 to 32 percent of dietary calories and saturated fat from 15 to 12 percent (Cavadini, 2000; Harnack, 1999). During the same period, total milk consumption decreased by 36 percent, while consumption of soft drinks, non-citrus juices, and high fat potato products increased. These changes in adolescent food and fluid consumption patterns were far larger than the corresponding changes among U.S. adults. If chemical contaminants are present in the ingredients used in highly consumed food and drink products, adolescents may be disproportionately exposed to contaminants.

One recent example is the finding of high levels of acrylamide, a potentially toxic chemical, in French fries and other fried foods (Becalski, 2003; Tareke, 2002). A study of mercury exposure from contaminated fish in the Madeira Basin of the Amazon provides another example of dietary exposure to environmental contaminant that was disproportionately higher for young children than for adults (Boischio, 1996). In the Madiera Basin, gold mining caused widespread environmental releases of mercury. The mercury exposure study, which used hair samples from mothers and their children to assess mean daily intake of mercury, showed that children were at the highest risk of exposure within the fish-eating population. Almost all infants (95 percent) were exposed to mercury above recommended maximum levels. The exposures came from breast milk or fish consumption, and the infants' mean daily intake was 4.5 micrograms/kg. Among children younger than five years old, the mean daily intake was 6.4 micrograms/kg and 60 percent ingested mercury above recommended levels. In contrast, only 45 percent of the mothers ingested mercury above recommended levels.

Behaviors Unique to Children

Three behaviors that influence a child's exposure to environmental agents include mouthing behavior, pica behavior, and participation in certain athletics and/or risky activities. Infants and toddlers pass through a developmental stage, characterized by intense oral exploratory behavior, when they indiscriminately place objects in their mouths. This behavior results in oral exposures in addition to those that occur from food intake, inhalation, or dermal exposure (Weaver, 1998 as cited in U.S. EPA, 2000b).

Basis for Vulnerability: Children often explore their environment by oral contact. This behavior can increase exposure to a variety of environmental agents; either by direct ingestion of soil, coatings such as paint, or other objects, or by mouthing hands that have contacted contaminated objects. Children also are disproportionately exposed to disinfection byproducts, such as chloroform, found in swimming pools because, among other reasons, they swim more often and have a great surface area relative to body weight to absorb contaminants that do adults. Exposure to disinfection byproducts from ingesting swimming pool water, however, may be negligible compared with exposure to contaminants form drinking tap water. Further, risk taking or other behaviors may disproportionately expose children to excessive sun or to environmental contaminants at locations such as industrial sites.

Ingestion of environmental toxicants from non-dietary sources is relatively high in young children because they often touch or place objects on potentially contaminated surfaces, then place the contaminated fingers or the contaminated objects in their mouths. A larger quantity of toxicant may adhere to wet fingers than dry fingers (Gurunathan, 1998, as cited in U.S. EPA, 2000b).

Recent date, however suggest that children aged 2 to 6 typically touch their hands to their mouths about nine times every hour and thereby are exposed to any toxicants in dust or soil that may be on their hands (Landrigan, 1998; Reed, 1999). Reed (1999) employed a videotape to quantify the types and frequencies of hand and mouthing activities of 20 children, ages 2 to 5 years, in their own homes. The range and average frequency of various behaviors are shown in Table 65.1.

Consumption of soil is a common behavior among young children. Soil may be ingested wither inadvertently or, in some instances, through deliberate or compulsive behavior (pica). An estimated 95 percent of children ingest 0.2 grams of soil per day or less, but studies have shown that children with pica behavior ingest up to 60 grams of soil per day (Calabrese, 1997). Soil consumption may be of longer duration and greater concern in mentally retarded children (Calabrese, 1997). Factors affecting exposure from pica behavior include the frequency and magnitude of pica events, access to contaminated soil, and the quality of adult supervision. Some data suggest that soil contaminant concentrations considered safe for short-term exposure in children who ingest less than 0.2 grams mg per day may be too high for the small portion of children who regularly exhibit pica behavior (Calabrese, 1997).

Soil ingestion estimates are important in the risk assessment of contaminated sites, and therefore the methods for obtaining these estimates are of special interest. Current estimates of soil ingestion are trace-element specific and vary widely among elements. Although estimates typically are expressed as amounts ingested daily, the values are generated by averaging soil ingestion over a study period of several days. The wide variability in the results has created uncertainty as to which method is most reliable for estimating soil ingestion (Stanek, 1995).

Many studies have documented examples of children being exposed to hazardous compounds in residential neighborhoods constructed on

Table 65.1. Frequency of Hand and Mouthing Behaviors (contacts/hour)

Behavior	Minimum	Maximum	Mean
Hand-to-Clothing	22.8	129.2	66.6
Hand-to-Dirt	0.0	146.3	11.4
Hand-to-Hand	6.3	116.4	21.1
Hand-to-Mouth	0.4	25.7	9.5
Hand-to-Object	56.2	312.0	122.9
Object-to-Mouth	0.0	86.2	16.3
Hand-to-Other Item*	8.3	243.6	82.9
Hand-to-Smooth Surface	13.6	190.4	83.7
Hand-to-Textured Surface	0.2	68.7	22.1

* Including paper, grass, and pets.

Young children have busy hands. On average, for example, the 2 to 6 year olds studied touched their hands to some object twice a minute, put their hands in their mouths every six minutes, and placed an object in their mouths every four minutes. These and other hand and mouthing behaviors provide numerous opportunities for children to ingest environmental toxicants.

Source: Reed, 1999.

contaminated soils or near pollution sources. When residential neighborhoods were built on soil contaminated with coalmine tailings, children were at risk of exposure to soil contaminated with heavy metals (such as led), aromatic hydrocarbons, and other compounds (Cook, 1993; van Wijnen, 1996). For example, children living in Leadville, Colorado, and historic mining and smelting community, were found to be at increased risk for elevated blood levels if they took food or a bottle outdoors when going to play (Cook, 1993).

Young swimmers may receive excessive exposure to chlorination byproducts, such as chloroform, created in the treatment of the water in swimming pools. Exposure may occur through inhalation of volatilized chemicals, ingestion of pool water, or dermal exposure (Levesque, 1994). Children may be at increased risk for this exposure because they may spend more time swimming, swim more vigorously, and have greater surface area per unit of body mass than adults do.

Children frequently engage in risky behavior. As children become more independent and free from parental authority and supervision, they may place themselves in risky situations because they are still developing their abstract reasoning skills and ability to assess danger. Because growing children tend to explore, they could be unknowingly at increased risk from exposure to toxicants in gardens and fields and from pollutants at industrial sites (Chance, 1998).

One example of adolescent risk-taking behavior or the lack of parental supervision is staying out in the sun without proper protection. Excessive sun exposure that occurs in the first 15 years of life is a risk factor for melanoma (Autier, 1998). In childhood and adolescence, cells in the skin that produce melanin may be more sensitive to sunlight than those same cells in adults. This increased sensitivity can cause damage to skin cells that may increase skin cancer risks later in life (AAP, 1999). Adolescents appear to have increased sun exposure compared with younger children, according to a study on sunbathing habits among 150 children (Grob, 1993). In a group of 3 year olds, 33 percent were highly overexposed to sunlight, compared with 62 percent of a group of 13 to 14 year olds. Because of parental supervision, most of the young children (63 percent) used good sun protection measures, but only 38 percent of the adolescents did so.

Risk-taking behavior is associated not only with injuries, but also with other serious health problems, especially in adolescence. Two prominent examples are initiation of smoking and unprotected sexual activity. Studies involving different age groups of smokers found an increased risk of lung cancer for individuals who began smoking between the ages of 7 and 15 years compared with individuals who began smoking later

(Engeland, 1996; Wiencke, 1999). One adverse effect of unprotected sex is contraction of the human immunodeficiency virus (HIV). HIV infection represented the third, fifth, and sixth most common cause of death for 15 to 34 year old African-Americans, Hispanics, and Whites, respectively (U.S. CDC, 2001c). For 35 to 44 year olds, HIV represented the third, second, and fifth most common cause of death for African-Americans, Hispanics, and Whites, respectively. According to the natural history of the disease, many of these HIV infections were transmitted during adolescence or young adulthood (Jenkins, 2000).

How and Where Children Spend Their Time

A necessary step in measuring the extent of children's exposure is documenting how and where they spend their time in order to estimate the likelihood of contact with various contaminant sources. Several studies that address activity patterns demonstrate that both adults and children spend most of their time indoors (Silvers, 1994; U.S. EPA, 2000b). Thus exposure is more likely to occur to toxicants that are applied or released indoors. Indoor air pollutants can originate indoors, or may be applied outdoors and then enter the home through open airways, such as windows or cracks in basement walls. Some pollutants may be encountered outside and then tracked into homes, schools, offices, or other indoor environments.

Most potential exposures of children to pesticides in the United States occur within the home; further, while in the home, children can be more highly exposed than adults are. Home pesticide use can include professionally applied pesticides for structural pest control, and the application of pesticides by family members inside the home or applied outdoors and carried inside. About 90 percent of U.S. households use pesticides. Since individuals spend most of their time indoors, they have the opportunity for significant contact with this category of indoor contaminants (Gurunathan, 1998). Data from an investigation of inappropriate residential use of methyl parathion found an association between surface contamination and elevated levels of pesticide metabolites in the urine of children under 3 years of age (Faustman, 2000).

Studies have found higher levels of pesticides in farm worker households in agricultural areas compared with those in non-farm-worker households in the same area (Bradman, 1997; Simcox, 1995). Pesticides applied outdoors may enter the household, where degradation is slower than outdoors, causing greater likelihood of exposure (Simcox, 1995). For example, residue levels of pesticides adhering to

Table 65.2. Pesticide Levels in Soil and House Dust

Compound	Population	Exposure Concentration	References
Diazinon	Families in California's Central Valley (an agricultural area)	0.7-169 ppm (farm worker homes) 0.2-2.5 ppm (non-farm worker homes)	Bradman, 1997
	Hands of children in families in California's Central Valley	52-220 ng/hand[a]	Bradman, 1997
Chlorpynifos[b]	Families in California's Central Valley	0.2-33 ppm (farm worker homes) <1 ppm (non-farm worker homes)	Bradman, 1997
	Hands of children in families in California's Central Valley	20-100 ng/hand[a]	Bradman, 1997
	Three occupied single-family homes after professional application in cracks and crevices	0.07-0.44 µg/kg/day	Byrne, 1998
	Two apartments after spraying entire floor	208 µg/kg/day[c]	Gurunathan, 1998
Four organo-phosphorus insecticides[d]	Agricultural family in Washington State	nondetect-0.93 ppm (soil) nondetect-17 ppm (dust)	Simcon, 1995
	Farm families in Washington State	62% of people (66% with at least one insecticide at 1000 ≥ ng/g)	Gurunathan, 1998

[a] Exposure likely exceeded oral reference dose (Bradman, 1997).

[b] Recommended maximum exposure dose for chlorpyrifos is 10 µg/kg/day for acute exposure and 4 µg/kg/day for chronic exposure (Gurunathan, 1998).

[c] Oral and dermal exposure assuming a 3 to 6 year old child living in the home 1 week after application; estimated exposure of 356 µg/kg/day for children with high frequency mouthing behavior.

[d] Azinphos-methyl, chlorpyrifos, parathion, and phosmet.

These studies demonstrate potential concern about exposure to pesticides in agricultural areas. For example, children in California's Central Valley had levels of diazinon and chlorpyrifos on their hands at levels likely exceeding the oral reference dose (Bradman, 1997).

dust particles were at least 3 to 5 times higher in the homes of farm worker families. Parathion levels from household dust samples were 13 times higher among agricultural families than non-agricultural families (Simcox, 1995). Table 65.2 summarizes some of the data addressing this issue.

Increased outdoor activity also may cause children to be exposed to higher concentrations of outdoor pollutants than adults are, including pollutants in the air or settled on the ground. The total estimated time that children spend outdoors is 2.8 hours per day at ages 3 to 5 years, 2.2 hours per day at ages 6 to 8 years, and 1.8 hours per day at ages 9 to 14 years (Timmer, 1985, as cited in U.S. EPA 2000b). Based on a review of the available studies, children are estimated to spend on average about one hour per day playing on grass. This activity could be important if insecticides or herbicides are applied to lawns or if grass is contaminated with other toxicants.

The Impact of Stature

During infancy and the toddler years, play patterns, crawling, and short stature cause disproportionate exposure to any contaminants that may be on or near the floor. The breathing zone for adults is 4 to 6 feet above the floor or ground, while the breathing zone for children is much lower. Particularly in indoor environments, dense vapors, large respirable particulates, and infectious agents settle out of the air and concentrate near the floor. House dust may become enriched in heavy metals and other pollutants tracked in from outdoors or entering through ventilation systems. Radon, a heavy gaseous pollutant released from soils, can infiltrate houses through foundations and collect in basements and crawl spaces. These factors increase the likelihood of intake of these agents by young children (Bearer, 1995), and therefore children are at greater risk for health effects due to these agents (Blot, 1990). Children also are at particular risk through dermal absorption because they have a much higher surface-area-to-body mass ratio than adults do. Other chemicals that accumulate near the floor after indoor release include formaldehyde, volatile organic chemicals, and pesticide residues (Chance, 1998).

Physiological Factors Affecting Absorption Intake of Environmental Pollutants

Physiological (internal) factors affect the concentration and persistence of chemical or other agent after it enters the body. In children, these factors include enhanced absorption of a compound from the environment and increased distribution of the compound to susceptible tissues. Children have higher metabolic rates and are more active than adults are, which lead to increased consumption of food, water, and air relative to their body weights. The limited ability to biotransform and eliminate toxic substances during certain periods in development also contributes to developmental vulnerability.

Physiological factors related to differences between adults and children are discussed in this section. These physiological factors do not represent a comprehensive list of differences between adults and children. Other factors include differences in repair mechanisms or capacity for repair to cellular damage and differences in both the amount of fat its distribution within the body. These differences are beyond the scope of this chapter and will not be discussed.

Enhanced Absorption of Contaminants

For a toxicant to cause health problems, it must first be absorbed into the body and pass through cell membranes to produce an internal dose. The duration of exposure affects the internal dose because with increasing duration of contact, more time is available for the toxicant to be absorbed. The duration of skin contact can be particularly important because children do not wash their hands as often as adults do. The dose of environmental chemicals entering children's bodies also may differ from that of adults because of unique aspects of transplacental, dermal, gastrointestinal, and respiratory absorption and absorption through the blood-brain barrier.

Transplacental Absorption

As noted previously, a fetus may be exposed to toxicants through the placenta from maternal circulation. Toxicants present in amniotic fluid also can be absorbed through fetal skin, alveoli (lungs), and gastrointestinal tract. Most compounds readily cross the placenta, including compounds of low molecular weight such as carbon monoxide, lipophilic compounds such as polycyclic aromatic hydrocarbons and ethanol, and PCBs (Rogan, 1986). The drugs chloramphenicol (Leeder, 1997; Levin, 1996), theophylline (Leeder, 1997), morphine (Leeder, 1997), aspirin (Briggs, 1994; Levin, 1996), and acetaminophen (Levin, 1996; Briggs, 1994) all readily cross the placental barrier. Their concentration in fetal tissues may be higher and elevated levels may persist for longer than in the mother, because of the fetus's limited capacity to metabolize the agent.

Dermal Absorption

Dermal absorption occurs mostly through unbroken skin, although some toxicants can be absorbed to a small extent by hair follicles, sweat glands, and sebaceous glands, or through open cuts or abrasions. Children's skin contact with surfaces while crawling or playing contributes to exposure to environmental compounds. Because children have higher ratios of skin surface area to body weight than adults do and experience more intensive contact with home surroundings, increased dermal absorption may occur.

Some compounds are easily absorbed through the skin when dermal contact occurs. Because the skin of children is generally more permeable than that of adults, dermal exposure to significant quantities of some compounds during development is more likely to result in a significant internal dose. The skin of a newborn in particular is highly vulnerable to absorption of toxic chemicals because keratinization (thickening and toughening of the skin) does not occur until 3 to 5 days after birth at term, and is even more delayed in pre-term infants (Bearer, 1995). Few date, however, are available to quantify the differential absorption through the skin by age (Gurunathan, 1998; Weaver, 1998). Nevertheless, many studies have demonstrated enhanced absorption of toxicants through the skin of newborns (Eichenfield, 1999). Evidence that chemicals can be absorbed significantly through an infant's skin comes from findings of systemic adverse effects, that is, effects occurring in organs distant from the point of application. Examples of systemic adverse affects associated with dermal exposures to chemicals include the following:

- Aniline dyes in diapers: methemoglobinemia (impaired oxygen uptake) in infants (Corradini, 1965).

- Ethanol applied with gauze pads: intoxication (Dalt, 1991).

- Phenolic disinfectant compounds applied to the skin: poisoning, hyperbilirubinemia (liver disease), and possibly hemolytic anemia (Robson, 1969; Vitkun, 1983; Wysowski, 1978).

- Hexachlorophene in disinfectant soaps and creams: neurotoxicity and death (Shuman, 1975; Tyrala, 1977).

- Iodine-containing disinfectants on the skin: hypothyroidism and goiter (Chabrolle, 1978: l'Alemand, 1987).

- Warfarin-containing skin powders: hemorrhagic disease among infants (Martin-Bouyer, 1983).

- Hydrocortisone, a steroid, which is absorbed more readily through the skin of infants: immune suppression following prolonged exposure (Turpeinen, 1988).

Gastrointestinal Absorption

Absorption takes place along the entire gastrointestinal (GI) tract; however, most absorption occurs in the stomach and small intestines (Lu, 1991; Rozman, 1996). The large surface area of the intestines and the prolonged time that ingested substances are confined to the intestines increases absorption from this site. In children younger than 6 to 8 months old, characteristics of the immature GI tract such as a prolonged gastric emptying time, up to 6 to 8 hours, and a prolonged intestinal transit time (Morselli, 1980) increase the potential for absorption through the GI tract. Since children need more calcium than adults for continued bone growth, their gastrointestinal absorption of calcium is increased compared with adults. Lead is absorbed by way of the calcium transport mechanism, which may explain why children absorb a larger fraction of ingested lead than adults. Children absorb an estimated 50 percent of ingested lead, while adults absorb only about 10 percent (Bearer, 1995).

Developmental age affects gastrointestinal absorption in other ways. In laboratory animals, newborn rats absorb 12 percent of administered cadmium (a toxic metal, compared with adults rats, which absorb 0.5 percent of the same dose. In humans, newborns do not achieve adult levels of stomach acidity until several months of age. This reduced acidity affects the form of some chemicals in a way that may either increase or decrease their absorption (Bearer, 1995). In addition, during infancy, bacterial overgrowth may occur in the more alkaline environment of the GI tract. These bacteria can form toxic nitrites when the infant consumes well water contaminated with nitrates or ingests nitrate from other sources (Bearer, 1995; Freeman, 1996).

Respiratory Absorption

Young children breathe about twice as much air in proportion to their body mass as adults do and therefore inhale proportionately more airborne chemicals and infectious agents (Bearer, 1995). The lungs of young children may absorb gases, vapors of volatile liquids, aerosols, or particulates. Inhaled gases and vapors diffuse through the alveoli and dissolve in the blood. How fast a toxicant is absorbed from the lungs depends on how soluble it is in blood (Rozman, 1996).

Absorption through the Blood-Brain Barrier

Exposure of the brain to toxicants depends on the permeability of the blood-brain barrier for the specific agent. This barrier impedes, but does not absolutely block chemicals from entering the central nervous system (Lu, 1991; Rozman, 1996). The more lipid-soluble a compound is, the more readily it is absorbed by the central nervous system. The effectiveness of the blood-brain barrier against absorption of toxicants varies by region of the brain (Rozman, 1996). The lipid content of the brain is high, potentially increasing the likelihood that lipophilic (oily) compounds will be absorbed.

The effectiveness of the blood-brain barrier is age-dependent. The blood-brain barrier is a term used to describe the limited ability of most chemicals to penetrate into the brain from general blood circulation. The blood-brain barrier develops gradually during fetal growth and infancy, and matures during childhood. Higher permeability to chemicals may result in higher exposures in the infants' central nervous system, which plays an important role in causing the greater toxicity of compounds such as morphine and lead in newborns (Rozman, 1996).

Blood Volume and Organ Size

In proportion to body mass, a child has a greater blood flow to the brain and other organs than a mature adult has, which means that exposures of these organs to blood-borne contaminants may be greater in children (Roberts, 1984). Also, the size of some organs relative to body mass is greater in children than in adults. For example, the infant brain represents 13 percent of the total body mass, while an adult's brain constitutes only 2 percent of the total mass (Dekaban, 1978). In addition, cerebral blood flow is greater per unit mass of brain weight in children compared to adults. Cerebral blood flow in a 10 year old child is approximately 50 L/kg brain weight per hour, compared with a typical flow in a 65 year old adult of 40 L/kg brain weight per hour. The greater relative brain mass and cerebral blood flow may result in a greater distribution and storage of certain environmental chemicals in children than in adults (Behrman, 1987; Snodgrass, 1990). The apparent increase in storage can extend the duration of exposure to a chemical as it is slowly re-released over time.

Distribution of Contaminants in Blood and Body Fluids

Certain components in the blood help prevent toxic chemicals from reaching body organs where the chemicals might cause damage. In other words, these components decrease the biologically available dose. Protein binding can effectively sequester a chemical and prevent its access to target sites in the body organs. The free or unbound fractions of chemicals are more likely to cause adverse effects inside the body. Most binding is to serum albumin. Chemical binding to serum albumin is lower in infants than in older children and adults, but it reaches adult levels by about 10 to 12 months of age (Roberts, 1984). Thus, the toxic chemicals stay in the blood longer, potentially causing adverse effects (Snodgrass, 1990).

Body composition also influences the distribution of chemicals. Infants have a greater percentage of water in their bodies and a greater volume of extracellular fluid than adults. Total body water can vary from as much as 75 percent of body weight at birth for full-term infants to only 50 to 60 percent of body weight in an adult. Similarly, the amount of body fat can affect the distribution of lipophilic chemicals in the body.

Biotransformation Processes

Many important chemical processes are less developed or entirely absent in young children. These processes are important for environmental health because they can affect how environmental agents are processed in the body after exposures. Biotransformation may either increase or decrease the toxicity of a chemical agent, or make it easier or harder to eliminate it from the body. Thus, the immaturity of biotransformation processes during development can be a disadvantage to the fetus or child, in situations where biotransformation in an adult detoxifies hazardous substances. In children many important detoxifying pathways may not function effectively (Adam, 1999; de Wildt, 1999; Faustman, 2000; Graeter, 1996; Leeder, 1997; Parkinson, 1996; Perera, 1999; Raunio, 1995; Strolin-Benedetti, 1998). Immaturity could be an advantage however, in those instances when biotransformation serves to create an even more hazardous compound through activation. Given the evolutionary role of many metabolic pathways in protecting the body against adverse effects of foreign chemicals, the reduced metabolic capacity of infants and children probably predisposes them to the risk of more sever adverse effects than adults face from many environmental exposures.

Energy Metabolism

Because children have a relatively large skin surface area in proportion to their body mass compared with adults, they lose body heat more rapidly. Therefore, to maintain their body temperature, they may have a higher resting (basal) metabolic rate than adults do and, consequentially, require more oxygen relative to their body mass. In addition, children tend to be more active than adults, further increasing their respiration rate and energy metabolism. Consequently, exposure to any air pollutant for children is greater per nit of body mass than it is for adults. Food intake in proportion to body mass tends to decrease with age.

Excretion and Elimination

Following absorption and distribution, toxicants are eliminated by excretion, which may occur rapidly or slowly (Lu, 1991; Rozman, 1996). Chemicals may be excreted in the form of the parent chemicals, their biotransformation products, or conjugates (that is, linked to other compounds). The major routes of elimination are urinary excretion, fecal excretion, and exhalation, although urinary excretion generally predominates. Some chemicals have to be biotransformed to water-soluble products to allow excretion in the urine. The kidney removes toxicants by glomerular filtration, tubular diffusion, and tubular secretion. Glomerular filtration eliminates most toxicants, unless they are tightly bound to plasma proteins.

Since the liver and kidneys of newborns are not completely developed at birth, toxicants are eliminated more slowly and may accumulate in the system, leading to greater time-averaged internal doses (Rozman, 1996). Glomerular filtration rates and renal tubular secretion rates at birth are much lower than they are in adults (Bearer, 1995; Levin, 1996). Both systems only work at 30 percent capacity or less in premature newborns (Levin, 1996). Fifty percent of the adult capacity is reached in 3 to 4 week old infants, increasing to full capacity at 9 to 12 months postpartum.

Conclusions

Exposure monitoring and analyses of human blood and urine samples have shown that exposure to damaging environmental agents occurs during human development. Children, because of the combined effects of physiology and behaviors specific to their age-group, may experience exposure to higher levels of intoxicants than do adults living in the same environment. In addition, children may absorb environmental contaminants more efficiently, process them more slowly, and eliminate them from the body less efficiently than adults do. Thus, concern over children's environmental exposure and the disproportionate impacts they may have on children.

Specific areas of concern associated with children's environmental exposures include the following:

- Children's behavior may contribute to higher exposures. Children spend more time outdoors than adults do, where they may come in contact with environmental toxicants. They tend to have more contact with soils and house dust, and infants and toddlers engage in mouthing behaviors that may increase exposure to environmental agents.

- Children's metabolic rate and activity levels tend to be greater than those of adults. Children consume more water and food per unit of body weight than adults do, and consume larger amounts of a narrower range of specific foods. Children have higher respiratory rates and generally are more active than adults, and therefore may be exposed to relatively larger amounts of airborne contaminants.

- Because of their size and mode of locomotion, children, particularly toddlers, may experience more exposure to house dust and heavy vapor contaminants, especially indoors.

- Children tend to absorb environmental agents more efficiently. The skin of infants and children is more permeable to many environmental chemicals than the skin of adults is. Similarly, the blood-brain barrier is less well developed in children. Some substances, such as lead, for example, are absorbed more efficiently from the gastrointestinal tract in children than in adults.

- Children and adults exhibit differences in their metabolism and excretion of absorbed environmental contaminants. Metabolic pathways are generally less developed in infants and young children than in adults. Depending on the specific substances involved, impaired metabolism may either increase or decrease the toxicity of environmental agents. Metabolic and degradative processes may not be developed well enough in children to quickly inactivate or eliminate some toxic chemicals. The liver and kidneys of infants and young children also are less effective at removing environmental toxicants from the bloodstream than those of adults.

For all these reasons, children's exposures are of concern from the perspective of environmental health.

Because of the inherent differences between children and adults, it is important to continue to quantify the exposures of children to environmental contaminants and develop methods to reduce, where possible and appropriate, the environmental (external) factors contributing to these exposures.

Chapter 66

Ten Tips to Protect Children from Pesticide and Lead Poisonings around the Home

These simple steps can help you save children from environmental hazards around the home:

1. Always store pesticides and other household chemicals, including chlorine bleach, out of children's reach—preferably in a locked cabinet.

2. Always read directions carefully because pesticide products, household cleaning products, and pet products can be dangerous or ineffective if too much or too little is used.

3. Before applying pesticides or other household chemicals, remove children and their toys, as well as pets, from the area. Keep children and pets away until the pesticide has dried or as long as is recommended on the label.

4. If your use of a pesticide or other household chemical is interrupted (perhaps by a phone call), properly re-close the container and remove it from children's reach. Always use household products in child-resistant packaging.

"Ten Tips to Protect Children from Pesticide and Lead Poisonings around the Home," a fact sheet produced by the U.S. Environmental Protection Agency (EPA), EPA 735-F-97-001, 1997. Available online at http://www.epa.gov/oppfead1/cb/10_tips. Despite the older date of this document, the information is valuable in helping to avoid environmental hazards around the home.

5. Never transfer pesticides to other containers that children may associate with food or drink (like soda bottles), and never place rodent or insect baits where small children can get to them.

6. When applying insect repellents to children, read all directions first; do not apply over cuts, wounds or irritated skin; do not apply to eyes, mouth, hands or directly on the face; and use just enough to cover exposed skin or clothing, but do not use under clothing.

7. Wash children's hands, bottles, pacifiers and toys often, and regularly clean floors, window sills, and other surfaces to reduce potential exposure to lead dust.

8. Get your child tested for lead if you suspect he or she has been exposed to lead in either your home or neighborhood.

9. Inquire about lead hazards. When buying or renting a home or apartment built before 1978, the seller or landlord is now required to disclose known lead hazards.

10. If you suspect that lead-based paint has been used in your home or if you plan to remodel or renovate, get your home tested. Do not attempt to remove lead paint yourself. Call 1-800-424-LEAD (1-800-424-5323) for guidelines.

For more information about pesticides, call the National Pesticide Information Center (NPIC) at 1-800-858-7378.

For more information about lead, call the National Lead Information Center at 1-800-LEADFYI, (in the District of Columbia, call 202-833-4726). For information about how to get your home or child tested for lead poisoning, call your local/state health department.

Chapter 67

Women's Health and the Environment

Women have a particular stake in environmental health research. Not only do they share many of the same diseases as men and children—in which the environment, along with genetic susceptibility, has an important role—but women also have particular environmental diseases related to their gender. Some, such as osteoporosis, involve aging as well—and women on average live longer than men.

Other diseases involve women's role in reproduction and in the bearing and nursing of children. Women tend to carry more fat, in which substances introduced lower in the food chain may accumulate.

Women also greatly influence the health of their children. Studies indicate they can pass along substances—lead stored in their bone, for example—to their fetuses. Taking drugs, including prescription drugs and nonprescription drugs as common as aspirin, may affect a pregnancy. Smoking is linked to lower birth weight, douching to reduced fertility.

Following are some additional conditions in which an environmental factor is being studied as a possible cause, trigger or influence:

"Women's Health and the Environment," NIEHS Fact Sheet #10, produced by the National Institute of Environmental Health Sciences, (NIEHS), 1997. Available online at http://www.niehs.nih.gov/oc/factsheets/womens.htm. Despite the older date of this document, it contains a good overview of the issues involved in women's health and the environment; And "Finding Causes of Breast Cancer," by Keri Brenner, *Marin Independent Journal*, October 8, 2002. Reprinted with permission from the *Marin Independent Journal*.

Breast Cancer—National Institute of Environmental Health Sciences (NIEHS) scientists co-discovered the first breast cancer gene, BRCA1, and played a role in the multi-national discovery of BRCA2. Together, these genes may account for much familial breast cancer, the kind that clusters in some families. The genes may be involved in 5 to 10 percent of all breast cancer—and a higher percentage of early breast cancers (affecting women under 45). A test has been devised to identify women carrying the defective BRCA1 gene.

In another attack on this multi-faceted disease, NIEHS is studying a growth factor called transforming growth factor alpha that responds to the female hormone estrogen and may play a role in normal breast development—and could lead to new ways to detect breast cancer.

Grantees are studying the possible role of pesticides that may mimic some of the activity of estrogen. Institute scientists also collaborated on a study that showed that late first pregnancy and late menopause were associated with a higher risk of breast cancer, while women with four or more pregnancies had a significantly lower risk.

Environmental estrogens are a variety of synthetic chemicals and natural plant compounds that are thought to mimic the female hormone estrogen. They may act like estrogens or may block the natural hormone.

The body's estrogen controls the growth of cells by attaching to proteins called estrogen receptors throughout the body. Many environmental estrogens can attach to these same proteins, fooling the body or tissues by giving them an inappropriate estrogen signal. These compounds are found all around us. We eat them, drink them, breathe them and use them at work, at home and in the garden. They include pesticides such as the now-banned DDT; kepone, polychlorinated biphenyls (PCBs), natural plant products in our diet, and the drug diethylstilbestrol (DES), which was widely used for more than 20 years beginning in the 1940s to prevent spontaneous abortions in women. In 1971, researchers showed that daughters of women who took DES had a high rate of a rare form of cervico-vaginal cancer. DES's common use as a growth promoter in cattle also was banned by the Food and Drug Administration in the 1970s.

NIEHS is supporting and conducting studies of environmental estrogen exposures, including a testing of the blood and urine of a representative group of Americans to determine how much of these chemicals are accumulating in the body. There is a possibility they might play a role in diseases such as cancers of the breast, uterus and ovaries; endometriosis and uterine fibroids. There is also a possibility that some of these estrogen-like substances, such as the ones occurring naturally in vegetables, may be beneficial.

Endometriosis is a condition which occurs when endometrial tissue, the tissue that lines the uterus and is shed during menstruation, grows outside the uterus. When this abnormal growth occurs, painful implants can develop, most commonly on the ovaries, the fallopian tubes and the ligaments that support the uterus. Other possible sites for endometrial growths are the bladder, bowel and vagina. Endometriosis affects an estimated 10%-15% of premenopausal women. The cause of it is unknown. Many of the risk factors for this disease are related to estrogen exposure. Thus, environmental estrogens may contribute to the development of endometriosis in susceptible individuals.

Uterine Fibroids—The most common tumors in women are benign (non-malignant) uterine fibroids, or leiomyomas. These tumors are present in 20%-30% of women over age 30; uterine fibroids are more common in African-American women.

Fibroids can cause significant pain and discomfort and are associated with reproductive problems. They are the leading reason for hysterectomies—major operations in which the uterus is surgically removed, either through the abdominal wall or the vagina.

NIEHS epidemiologists are conducting a study of uterine fibroids in black and white women in their late-reproductive years who are members of the George Washington University Health Plan in Washington, D.C.

Osteoporosis is a debilitating condition characterized by fragility of the bone. It sometimes occurs in men but is generally found in postmenopausal women. Cadmium, lead and possibly other heavy metals found in the environment may be significant factors in developing this disease. NIEHS-supported research has shown that cadmium exposure results in increased loss of bone mineral in mice whose ovaries have been removed. The bone loss appears to occur from a direct action of cadmium on bone, not through an indirect effect on kidney reabsorption of calcium. Thus, cadmium exposure may be a significant factor contributing to osteoporosis in older women. Continued efforts to study the basic physiology of bone metabolism as well as the mechanisms of heavy metal toxicity in bone tissue should provide insight into the disease mechanisms of osteoporosis.

Other NIEHS-supported studies are investigating the health consequences of lead released into the blood stream and soft tissue due to osteoporosis. One health effect that has been identified is an increased risk for hypertension. Some of these studies are using lead as a marker to develop hormonal therapies to prevent bone reabsorption.

Autoimmune Diseases—Women are disproportionately susceptible to autoimmune diseases such as multiple sclerosis, rheumatoid arthritis, scleroderma (a disease of the connective tissue), and systemic lupus erythematosus (SLE).

The body produces antibodies that fight foreign proteins known as antigens. In lupus, the antibodies mistake the body's own cells as foreign and attack them. The disease may range from mild to severe and is characterized by periods of flare-ups and remissions. Lupus may cause weight loss, fever, fatigue, aching, and weakness and may involve different organ systems such as the central nervous system, the heart, lungs, kidneys, muscles, and joints. A gene on chromosome 1 has been linked with susceptibility to lupus in Caucasians, Asians, and African Americans.

Exposures to various chemicals such as pharmaceuticals and solvents have been linked to autoimmune diseases. For example, exposure to hydrazine, an industrial chemical, or tartrazine, a food additive, is associated with lupus. And scleroderma has been associated with workplace exposure to vinyl chloride and silica dust.

Women have particular environmental diseases related to their gender, as well as sharing other environment-related diseases with men and children.

While some environmental estrogens may cause harm, there is a possibility some may reduce risks. Fibroids, the leading reason for hysterectomies, are being studied in black and white women in a Washington health plan.

Finding Causes of Breast Cancer

Researchers are on the verge of finding links between chemical toxins and the human gene changes that create breast cancer, the head of one of the nation's top environmental health agencies said yesterday in San Rafael.

"We now have the right tools to address diseases—such as breast cancer—that are occurring in epidemic proportions," said Kenneth Olden, director of the National Institute of Environmental Health Sciences. "I'm very excited that we can now do research on the interaction between the environment and genetics."

Olden, speaking before more than 100 people on the first of two days of a Marin County Town Meeting on "Breast Cancer and the Environment," said the NIEHS is seeking federal funds to create eight Centers of Excellence across the nation. At the centers, researchers would build a database of those chemical/environmental interactions in relation to breast cancer.

Such interactions can now be explored with the recent completion of the mapping of the human genome, Olden said. That technological advance is what researchers were waiting for to begin cataloging thousands of chemicals and determining whether they are carcinogenic—and, if so, at what levels of exposure.

"It's a new science, toxicogenomics," said Olden, referring to the blend of toxicology and genomics, or gene research. Rep. Lynn Woolsey, D-Petaluma, a strong proponent of breast cancer research, is sponsoring a bill that would allocate funds for the Centers of Excellence, said Anita Franzi, Woolsey's field representative. "She has a very personal stake in this," Franzi added. "Both her mother and her grandmother died of breast cancer."

If the bill, which is still in committee, is passed, the Bay Area is likely to be the site of one of those centers, said Janice Barlow, executive director of Marin Breast Cancer Watch, event co-sponsor. "Clearly it makes sense that there will be a center here," Barlow said. Olden said even if the bill is not forthcoming, the NIEHS will likely fund at least three centers using existing fiscal 2003 funding.

"I kind of share (Olden's) optimism" that the environmental cause of breast cancer will be found soon," Barlow said. "The next couple of years may be a major breakthrough. "We've been kind of stymied the last few years," Barlow added, referring to uncovering the cause of Marin's sky-high breast cancer rate.

"There's a saying that there are years of questions, followed by years of answers," she added. "We've already had the years of questions—hopefully now we'll have the years of answers."

"We look for the greatest contrast possible between rates and exposures," said Patricia Buffler, a professor of epidemiology at the University of California at Berkeley, School of Public Health. Buffler organized an international summit on breast cancer, including comparisons of the incidence of breast cancer in various populations around the world.

"The highest incidence is with white women in America, here in Marin, where it's 110 women per 100,000," Buffler said. "The lowest is in Southeast Asia, where it's five women per 100,000." Peggy Reynolds, a cancer epidemiologist at the California Department of

Health Services' Environmental Health Investigations Branch, said her studies have found a strong relationship between socioeconomic status and breast cancer rates—the rates were 40 percent higher in the top socioeconomic classes compared with the lowest levels. Also, the rates were 27 percent higher in the urban metro areas than in the rural sections.

Tina Clarke, research scientist with the surveillance research division of the Northern California Cancer Center, said the biggest increase in the rate of breast cancer was in women ages 45 to 64.

"There's something about women 45 to 64 that's driving a different trend in Marin," Clarke said. Clarke and her team, based in Union City, study data from the California Cancer Registry reported from nine counties, including Marin.

Dr. Chris Benz, of the Buck Institute for Age Research in Novato, said breast cancer in women whose tumors are positive for increased estrogen receptors and increased progesterone receptors is the fastest growing segment of the illness in Marin. Receptors for estrogen and progesterone—the two main female sex hormones—are the parts of human cells that allow a buildup of those hormones.

"There seems to be an unequal distribution of known risk factors (in Marin) leading to estrogen-receptor-positive and progesterone-receptor-positive tumors," Benz said. Such risk factors as longer exposure to estrogen over a woman's lifetime via early menarche (the start of menstruation) or late menopause (the end of menstruation).

"Drugs such as tamoxifen can act to prevent estrogen-receptor-positive tumors," he said. A series of studies are also under way by Marin County officials and various Bay Area agencies and universities, but results won't be available until later this year.

Chapter 68

Workers and Noise Hazards

Noise is one of the most common hazards encountered by U.S. workers. It is estimated that about 10 million U.S. workers are regularly
exposed to dangerous noise levels on the job. This noise can cause
damage to the sensitive cells lining the inner parts of the human ear.
When loud sounds damage your hearing, your ability to detect high
frequency sounds goes first. Initially you won't notice the effects of
this because the sound frequency affected first is 4,000 Hertz, that
is, 4,000 cycles per second. This is higher than the ordinary sound
frequencies of human speech (which go from about 200 to 3,000 Hertz),
so your ability to hear other people's speech and communicate with
them won't be affected.

But if these loud sounds continue, your hearing will continue to
deteriorate. Within a few years your hearing will be damaged at the
frequencies below (and above) 4,000 Hertz. Eventually your ability
to hear sounds below 3,000 Hertz will be affected. Then you will begin having a hard time hearing what other people are saying to you.

For example, you might not be able to understand a waitress in a
noisy restaurant, or hear what someone is saying to you at a noisy
party. Perhaps you will have difficulty hearing the doorbell or the
phone ringing—since these are usually designed to ring at high frequencies. Also, many consonants such as F, X and S, which have high

Reprinted with permission from "Noise Hazards," by David Kotelchuck, *UE
News,* June 1998. © United Electrical, Radio and Machine Workers of America
(UE). Despite the older date of this document the information about occupa-
tional noise hazards will be helpful to the reader.

frequency sounds in them, become hard to distinguish. So you may not be able to tell the difference between the words "fifteen" and "sixteen."

Get a Checkup

How can you find out about the earliest (4,000 Hertz) hearing losses, the ones that happen before you begin to notice problems hearing others speak? The answer is to have your ears checked by an audiologist. This is a person trained to measure the ability of human ears to hear sounds over a wide range of sound frequencies. When this person gives you an audiological exam, he or she will be able to pick up any hearing loss at 4,000 Hertz long before you notice any loss. (The results of such a test are called an audiogram.)

The next step is to work with your union to get management to quiet down the noise in your shop. You can try to get a provision in your contract guaranteeing free earplugs and earmuffs for those who want to wear them.

Audiograms are costly, but remember if noise levels on your job average 85 decibels or more (on the A scale of a sound level meter) then your employer is required by law to give you an annual audiogram free of cost to you and during working hours. You must also be given a full, confidential report of what the audiogram shows. Also, if the average sound level you are exposed to exceeds 85 decibels, your employer must by law provide (at no cost to you) earplugs or earmuffs, which you have the option of wearing. (Above 90 decibels, the earplugs or earmuffs not only must be provided, they must be worn.) When earplugs or earmuffs are provided by your employer, at any decibel level, they must be fit-tested on you individually by a qualified person.

Legal Exposure

How do you know if the sound you are exposed to is 85 decibels or more? You need a meter to tell you exactly. And remember the sound must average above 85 decibels or more over an eight-hour workshift. You are legally allowed to be exposed above 85 decibels for a few minutes to a few hours, but over the whole workshift the average must be 85 decibels or below. (As a rule of thumb, if you are in a room where you have to shout at a person two feet away from you in order to be heard, then the sound in the room is about 85 decibels.)

If the sound level averages more than 90 decibels during an 8-hour shift, then your employer is in violation of the federal safety and health law. (Rule of thumb: At 90 decibels you have to shout at a person whose ear is one foot away from you in order to be heard.) Exposures between 85 and 90 decibels are legal, but you are entitled to a free annual audiogram once the levels are 85 or more.

If a sound level meter is needed to measure noise levels, the union health and safety committee or your local officers should ask management to provide one. Sometimes a local COSH (Committee on Occupational Safety and Health) group can lend their meter to you, or a local clinic might have one to lend. Remember, though, check the battery on the meter before you begin and check that the meter has been calibrated before the measurement with a sound source of known frequency and loudness. (Also, many people now use so-called sound dosimeters instead of sound level meters. You wear these dosimeters on your lapel, usually, and they give you your personal average daily dose of sound at the end of the workshift. A dose of 1.0 over an 8-hour shift corresponds to an average daily sound exposure of 90 decibels, and a dose of 0.5 to a daily average of 85 decibels.)

Workers' Compensation

Finally, if you have been exposed to loud noises on the job for many years, say 10 years or more, you may be eligible to receive workers' compensation payments for partial permanent hearing loss. If you are showing unusual signs of hearing loss as you age (we all lose some hearing with age, but exposed workers lose more and at younger ages), ask your union officers for a referral to a workers' comp lawyer. Only 10 percent of workers who have suffered a compensable hearing loss on the job ever apply for compensation.

While loss of hearing won't kill you, it can make communication with family and friends very difficult, if not impossible. For many victims of hearing loss due to noise on the job, this medical condition can lead to withdrawal, depression and even to suicide in some cases. Hearing loss due to noise on the job is irreversible. Once the loss has occurred, you can never recover your old hearing. So take noise on the job seriously, and don't let job-related hearing loss creep up on you. Almost all work situations can be quieted when the employer is persuaded to do something about noise on the job.

Chapter 69

Prioritizing Environmental Health Threats to Older Persons

On October 29, 2002 the Environmental Protection Agency (EPA) Administrator Christie Whitman met with the heads of the nation's leading aging organizations to announce that the agency is developing a new Aging Initiative that will result in a national agenda designed to examine and prioritize environmental health threats to older persons.

The Initiative will examine the impact that a rapidly growing aging population will have on ecosystems as well as encourage older persons to volunteer in their own communities to reduce hazards and protect the environment for future generations. This will be the first coordinated approach by the agency to address environmental hazards that affect the health of the elderly.

"Protecting the health of older Americans must be one of EPA's priorities," said Whitman. "There is much we can do together to make older persons and their families aware of—and safe from—environmental hazards that may impact their health and quality of life."

Speaking on behalf of the 50-member Leadership Council of Aging Organizations (LCAO), President and CEO of the National Council on the Aging James Firman said, "We commend the EPA for focusing on the health and safety of older Americans. We know many LCAO members will want to work with the EPA to educate seniors about

"EPA Announces New Aging Initiative to Protect Older Persons from Environmental Health Threats," U.S. Environmental Protection Agency (EPA), 2002. Available online at http://www.epa.gov/epahome/headline_103002.htm.

such threats and promote civic engagement of seniors nationwide in combating these problems."

Currently there are 35 million people in the United States 65 years of age and older, and that number is expected to double over the next 30 years. In 2011, the first of the baby boomers will begin to turn 65. Among older Americans there is an increasing number who are at risk of chronic diseases and disabling conditions that may be caused or exacerbated by environmental conditions. Hazards that may adversely impact the health of older Americans are lead, indoor and outdoor air pollution, microorganisms in water and pesticides. As part of the Initiative, the agency will build on ongoing projects.

The National Academy of Sciences will hold a workshop in Washington, D.C., to examine the susceptibility of older persons to environmental health hazard, and what interventions can be undertaken to reduce the exposure to environmental hazards.

The Aging Initiative will draw on the expertise of professionals and researchers at the federal, state and local levels in the fields of environment and health. EPA will also work with the public and service provider organizations dealing with the aging population. Whitman announced that public meetings to get input for the Initiative would be held in the spring in California, Florida, Iowa, Pennsylvania, Texas and Washington, D.C.

Chapter 70

Environmental Health: Are Minority Populations at Greater Risk?

The affluent citizens of this Nation enjoy better health than do its minority and poorer citizens. The most striking health disparities involve shorter life expectancy among the poor, as well as higher rates of cancer, birth defects, infant mortality, asthma, diabetes, and cardiovascular disease. Although health care access might account for some of this disparity, the differences in environmental and occupational exposures are also thought to play a role. Minority and poorer communities are more likely to live in polluted environments and to work in hazardous occupations. There may also be a disproportionate placement of pollution-intensive industries and hazardous waste sites in low-income and minority communities. Clearly research into the influence of poverty and environmental pollution on human health needs to be encouraged, and the training and support of researchers in this field needs to be increased.

The National Institute of Environmental Health Sciences (NIEHS) has been a leader in the area of understanding how poverty, environmental pollution, and health interrelate. The NIEHS has developed a number of projects and grant programs designed to define the health disparities issue and to arm policy makers with the necessary information to reduce these disparities. Additionally the NIEHS has developed innovative grants programs aimed at empowering local

"Health Disparities Research," a fact sheet produced by the National Institute of Environmental Health Science (NIEHS), National Institutes of Health (NIH), updated 2001. Available online at http://www.niehs.nih.gov/oc/factsheets/disparity/phome.htm.

communities to deal with the environmental health problems in their regions. Many of these efforts are outlined in this chapter.

Agricultural Chemicals and Minority Health Issues

Agricultural Health Study

The NIEHS, in partnership with the National Cancer Institute (NCI), has a long-term Agricultural Health Study of farmers and pesticide applicators, as well as their spouses and children, to determine the health consequences of exposures typical in rural environments. The NIEHS was particularly instrumental in ensuring that a large part of this cohort included African-American families. The NIEHS component of this study will focus on non-cancer endpoints, which include reproductive outcomes, childhood development, asthma and other respiratory diseases, immunological effects, neurological symptoms, degenerative retinal disease, and neurological diseases.

Pesticide Exposure and Neurologic Function in Farmworkers

Pesticide use in the United States has increased greatly in the last 50 years, but the health effects of pesticide exposure are still unclear. NIEHS-funded researchers are planning a cross-sectional study of the neurologic effects of chronic, low-level exposure on exposed farmworkers. The study will be conducted in central Florida, in collaboration with a local grassroots organization. A large number of the participants are Hispanic and the cohort includes both men and women. The results of this study will elucidate the effects of pesticide exposure on neurologic function and also address the health problems of an underserved minority group. The Office of Research on Minority Health (ORMH) of the National Institutes of Health (NIH) might also join NIEHS in support of this project.

Migrant Farmworkers

California is a major agricultural state whose success relies heavily on the use of pesticides and the labor of farmworkers. To monitor potential adverse effects of pesticides in farmworkers, the State of California requires routine assays of blood levels of acetylcholinesterase, an enzyme that serves as a biomarker of exposure to the major pesticides used in California agriculture. As part of its outreach responsibilities, the NIEHS Center in Davis, California examined this monitoring program and discovered some surprising results. The commercial bioassays being used were inaccurate, often underestimating enzyme levels (and thus exposure effects) by as much as 40 percent. The result was an extensive monitoring system that could not provide accurate or useful information. As a result of the NIEHS Community Outreach and Education Program (COEP) study, this Center is now working with State regulatory agencies in an effort to develop more accurate testing methods.

Minority Farmers Highly Exposed to Agricultural Chemicals

The NIEHS Environmental Health Science Centers are academic institutions throughout the country that bring together many scientific disciplines to focus on particular environmental health problems. Three of these centers—the University of Iowa, the University of California at Davis, and Oregon State University—focus on health concerns of agricultural workers, many of whom are migrant workers or disadvantaged minorities. Results of this research will help define the risks to this occupational group so that better prevention/intervention strategies can be developed to protect their health.

Community-Based Prevention/Intervention Research (CBPIR)

The NIEHS is funding three grants as a part of the Community-Based Prevention and Intervention Research project related to pesticides: (1) A multiphase research project that will assess pesticide contamination in agricultural communities with an emphasis on pesticide exposure among children of agricultural workers. (2) A study focusing on disadvantaged and medically underserved populations will conduct formative research among farmworkers, growers, and service providers to help develop interventions to reduce exposure to agricultural chemicals. (3) A collaborative effort between a university-based research team and a community-based farmworker organization to test the effectiveness of an intervention that is proposed to help reduce exposure to agrichemicals.

Asthma

Five-Cities Study

Inner-city disadvantaged and minority children appear to be at greater risk of respiratory illness, especially asthma. Previous NIEHS-supported studies (the Six- and Twenty-Four Cities Studies) have demonstrated increased respiratory illness and lower lung function associated with air pollution among white children in suburban and rural communities. An ongoing study (Five-Cities Study) is assessing the degree to which minority and/or economically disadvantaged children are at increased risk for adverse respiratory health effects of ozone, acid aerosols, and particulate air pollution.

Inner-City Asthma Study

The NIEHS and the NIAID collaborate on the Inner-City Asthma Study (ICAS). This cooperative, multi-center study seeks to reduce the disproportionate burden of asthma morbidity among underserved, inner-city children and adolescents from 4 to 12 years of age. The goal of this study is to design and evaluate an asthma intervention aimed at reducing asthma morbidity in a cost-effective manner based in health care delivery settings. This study evaluates a culturally appropriate, comprehensive, and cost-effective intervention program aimed at reducing asthma morbidity by modifying potentially reversible factors shown to contribute to asthma morbidity, such as allergens and environmental tobacco smoke.

Developing a Geographic Framework for Studying Respiratory Health in Harlem

This study geographically characterizes the Harlem and Washington Heights communities with respect to potential environmental exposures such as diesel exhaust particles and manufacturing facilities, while also linking available respiratory health outcome data and sociodemographic characteristics with environmental exposure data. Other objectives are to target monitoring sites for collecting ambient air pollution exposure data (e.g., particulate matter), to perform preliminary monitoring at indicated sites, and to develop Geographic Information System (GIS) research capabilities and expertise at the Harlem Center for Health Promotion and Disease Prevention and the Center for Environmental Health in Harlem.

This study was designed to investigate variations in diesel bus and truck traffic in the communities of West Harlem and Central Harlem, and to assess whether the amount of soot in the air that people breathe correlates with diesel pollution sources. This project will not only serve as the underpinnings of a program to assess air quality, but will provide a framework for geographic analyses of other diseases and exposures in northern Manhattan.

Asthma-Related Projects of the Community-Based Prevention/Intervention Research (CBPIR) Program

The NIEHS CBPIR program funds a number of asthma studies in urban, socioeconomically disadvantaged populations. One study will evaluate whether nurse management and peer counseling help to reduce severe episodes of asthma. Another study focuses on methods to help control and prevent asthma with interventions such as case management and environmental control of asthma and community-based asthma interventions in pregnant women. A third community-based intervention project will evaluate the relationship between cockroach and dust allergens on asthma. These studies will develop and implement culturally appropriate methods and materials for communicating the study findings to the community involved.

National Allergen Survey

The NIEHS has partnered with the Department of Housing and Urban Development (HUD) to conduct a national survey of the levels of major allergens found in homes throughout the United States. Results of this survey will be instrumental in defining the demographics of allergen exposure and in better formulating public policy to address health effects from these exposures.

Other NIEHS Efforts

The NIEHS is funding a number of studies related to the effects of environmental exposures on lung function. For example, NIEHS-funded research is exploring the role of toxic effects of particulates and oxidants on lung function as well as the effects of acid aerosols and ozone on asthma in underserved urban populations.

The Environmental Intervention in the Primary Prevention of Asthma in Children Study

The Environmental Intervention In The Primary Prevention Of Asthma In Children Study (The EIPPAC Study) is a proposed NIEHS clinical trial aimed at the primary prevention of asthma in children by environmental intervention in their homes. This study will target individuals from low-income residences with the goal of developing primary prevention strategies that could be effective against asthma. It is anticipated that the EIPPAC study will provide important insights

561

on the role of environmental interventions in the primary prevention of asthma in children. An expected benefit of this study will be a reduced prevalence of asthma in children, thereby decreasing the economic burden of health care to the children's families and to the Nation. The Office of Research on Minority Health (ORMH) of the National Institutes of Health (NIH) might also join NIEHS in support of this project.

Lead

The Treatment of Lead-Exposed Children (TLC) Clinical Trial

NIEHS-supported studies have shown that even moderate-to-low blood lead levels in children can cause neurobehavioral problems later in life. The Institute is now investigating ways to reverse these effects. The NIEHS and the ORMH have joined to support a clinical trial designed to test if the chelating drug, succimer, can reverse the neurobehavioral consequences of moderate blood lead levels. In this study, treated and untreated children will be measured for cognitive and behavioral development three years after treatment. All children receive home lead abatement and vitamin and mineral supplementation. The study's principal aim is to determine whether succimer is both safe and effective and to track any behavior and developmental changes among these children.

Low Birth Weight in Babies

Low birth weight is associated with a number of adverse health outcomes, including reduced growth, lower cognitive performance, and greater morbidity. Low birth weight is more prevalent among infants in low-income families; thus, reducing the incidence of low birth weight is a necessary step in addressing this Nation's health disparities. A new NIEHS-supported study reveals an environmental component to low birth weight—a mother's lead burden. Lead, a common contaminant of inner-city environments, is stored in bone where, during pregnancy, it can be mobilized and cross the placenta to expose the fetus. This study measured pregnant women's bone lead levels and found that the higher the level, the greater the possibility her child was born with a low birth weight. This finding identifies a controllable environmental component to this intractable health disparity problem and reveals another possible benefit from the national remediation efforts to reduce environmental lead and from NIEHS-sponsored studies to identify effective therapeutic interventions for existing body burdens of lead.

The NIEHS has also joined with the National Institute of Nursing Research, the National Institute of Dental and Craniofacial Research, and the National Institute of Child Health and Human Development to support a Program Announcement on "Low Birth Weight in Minority Populations." This Program Announcement seeks to encourage research to develop innovative strategies to prevent low birth weight in minority populations and to expand our understanding of how psychosocial and environmental factors affect or interact with the biologic mechanisms that influence pregnancy outcomes.

Hypertension

African-Americans have a high incidence of hypertension, a leading risk factor for heart disease. A NIEHS-supported study in a group of middle-aged and older men has now shown that high lead levels, as measured in bone, is significantly associated with risk for hypertension.

Kidney Disease

Kidney, or renal, damage is a serious health problem that can translate into kidney failure, dependence on dialysis machines, and death itself. NIEHS-supported researchers have now shown that even low blood lead levels correlated with significant reductions in kidney function as measured by serum creatine concentration. These findings show that lead abatement and treatment programs might serve as new preventive strategies for kidney damage, as well as a number of other diseases prevalent in urban and inner-city environments where lead exposures are frequently high.

Lead-Related Community-Based Prevention/Intervention Research (CBPIR) Projects

The NIEHS funded Community-Based Prevention and Intervention Research project has two initiatives to help reduce lead exposures in children. In both studies, minority and disadvantaged children will be monitored for the prevalence of high blood lead levels. Behavioral and exposure interventions will be assessed for effectiveness in both individuals and communities.

Other Diseases That Adversely Affect Minority Health

Biomarkers of Lung Cancer Susceptibility in Minorities

While African-Americans share a disproportionate burden of lung cancer incidence and mortality, Mexican-Americans exhibit substantially lower rates. These racial differences may represent interactions of environmental and genetic influences. The NIEHS is merging and extending two existing ecogenetic studies. In the enhanced study design, researchers will integrate molecular and cytogenetic markers of lung cancer susceptibility into a case control study of 100 black African-American and 100 Mexican-American patients with previously untreated lung cancer. The molecular component will focus on estimating the prevalence of genetic polymorphisms in two cytochrome P450 genes (CYP 2D6, CYP lAl) and alleles of glutathione Stransferase type mu. Since lung cancer is the leading cause of cancer mortality, the identification of genetic markers of risk has great potential for cancer control. The use of multiple genetic markers of risk within the same population provides a highly efficient means to simultaneously test several hypotheses concerning genetic contributions to cancer risk in minority populations.

Environmental Genome Project (EGP)

The NIEHS is expanding its research program on genetic susceptibility to environmentally associated diseases through a new Environmental Genome Project. This project is aimed at the identification of allelic variants (polymorphisms) of environmental disease susceptibility genes in the U.S. population, developing a central database of polymorphisms for these genes, and fostering population-based studies of gene-environment interaction in disease etiology. By identifying those genes and allelic variants that affect individual response to environmental agents, scientists can better predict health risks and assist regulatory agencies in the development of environmental protection policies. One EGP research project will explore the increasing evidence that people of color are exposed to numerous environmental hazards, including hazardous air pollutants, such as polyaromatic hydrocarbons (PAHs) and environmental tobacco smoke (ETS). A molecular epidemiologic cohort study of African-American and Hispanic mothers and newborns is proposed to investigate the role of PAH and ETS in procarcinogenic and developmental damage. A combination of personal monitoring, questionnaires and biomarkers in peripheral blood will be used to quantify individual exposure to the toxicants of concern.

Other NIEHS Efforts

Understanding genetic changes as a result of environmental exposures helps researchers develop therapies and intervention strategies for environmental threats. The objective of one NIEHS-funded project is to refine and validate molecular biomarkers of human exposures to environmental pollutants such as aromatic and heterocyclic amines. Using these biomarkers in studies will help define the roles heterocyclic amines in the risk of colon cancer and aromatic amines in the risk of bladder cancer in smokers and nonsmokers in different racial and ethnic groups. Another NIEHS-supported project uses the CYP1A1 gene, which codes for a critical detoxifying enzyme, to monitor human exposure to aromatic hydrocarbons, and to explore the ways in which genetic variation of CYP1A1 related to cancer susceptibility in African-Americans.

Children's Health Disparities

PCBs Effects on the Health of Native American Children

An NIEHS-funded study seeks to identify the consequences of exposure to polychlorinated biphenyls (PCBs), mercury, lead, and fluoride on the health of children as measured by their physical, cognitive, and behavioral development. This population of Native American children is exposed to these environmental toxins through their diet, which is composed primarily of fish that may be contaminated with PCBs. Results of this study will help determine childhood health effects from exposure to PCBs and other environmental toxins, along with intervention efforts to prevent such exposures in the future.

Chronic Low-Level Methylmercury in Children

Two studies supported by NIEHS are examining the effects on children exposed to chronic low-level methylmercury (MeHg) as a result of their high intake of saltwater fish. The project is a longitudinal study in which the MeHg exposure of a cohort of children has been followed prenatally to the current age of 66 months. The study established that the amount of MeHg found in mother's hair during pregnancy correlates well with the MeHg level in prenatal brain as determined by the autopsy of the brains of 22 stillborns. Thus, these measures can be used to establish initial MeHg exposure in children recruited into this study.

Prenatal Exposure to PCBs

Many rural low-income communities rely on fishing as a major source of their diet. Unfortunately many of the waters in this country are polluted with PCBs and other contaminants. An NIEHS grantee has been following a population of children born to mothers who consumed large amounts of potentially PCB-contaminated fish. Because PCBs can cross the placenta, this maternal exposure could result in exposure to the fetus (i.e., in utero exposure). NIEHS-funded studies have already shown that in utero exposure to PCBs was associated with poorer short-term memory during infancy and childhood, and deficits in intellectual ability (6.2 deficits in IQ), short and long-term memory and focused and sustained attention in school age children up to 11 years of age. This study will measure PCB levels in umbilical cord blood and maternal blood and milk samples and correlate these values with the children's behavior, achievement and performance on reading mastery tests.

Children's Environmental Health and Prevention Centers

The NIEHS, the Environmental Protection Agency (EPA), and the Centers for Disease Control and Prevention (CDC) have teamed to create the first Federal research centers devoted exclusively to children's environmental health and disease prevention. This joint effort uses the expertise and resources of non-profit institutions across the Nation. These centers also incorporate the concept that research is made more meaningful when the public has input and access to scientists. Public outreach is a cornerstone of the program, with community involvement and information exchange between researchers and local citizens a requirement of each center. The first eight programs have the following research emphases:

1. University of Southern California, children's respiratory diseases;

2. University of California, Berkeley, the impact of pesticides on growth and development;

3. University of Washington, children's susceptibilities to pesticides;

4. University of Iowa, causes of airway disease in rural children;

5. University of Michigan, childhood asthma;

6. Johns Hopkins University, environmental pollutants, allergens and asthma in inner-city children;

7. Mount Sinai Medical Center, potential risks to inner-city children from pesticides, lead and PCBs; and

8. Columbia University, environmental risks to African-American and Hispanic infants and children.

Future plans call for recruiting more centers devoted to studying the neurodevelopmental and neurobehavioral effects of environmental exposures in children.

Women's Health Disparities

Systemic Lupus Erythematosus (SLE): The Carolina Lupus Study

Systemic lupus erythematosus (SLE) is an autoimmune disease that can cause severe damage to the kidneys, joints, and other tissues. Ninety percent of SLE patients are women, and compared to whites, African-Americans are 3 to 4 times more likely to develop the disease. Mortality is also higher among blacks, compared to white, SLE patients. Reasons for the African-American excess risk are not known. The NIEHS and the ORMH have joined to create The Carolina Lupus Study, a population-based, case-control study in eastern North Carolina and South Carolina designed to examine hormonal and environmental influences on the etiology of SLE. The Carolina Lupus Study offers the opportunity to examine occupational and environmental risk factors in a previously understudied population. These efforts may help illuminate etiologic pathways and develop prevention strategies for susceptible populations. Environmental exposures under study include silica dust, ultraviolet light, solvents, heavy metals, and pesticides. The study participants are 90 percent women and 55 percent African-American.

Uterine Leiomyomas or Fibroids

Uterine fibroids are the leading indication for hysterectomy among pre-menopausal women in the United States. Based on hysterectomy

567

statistics, African-American women appear to be at 3- to 9-fold higher risk than white women, although it is not done if this disparity reflects a true difference in incidence or prevalence of uterine fibroids or, instead, is due to differences in diagnosis and treatment. To better define the cause of this health disparity, the NIEHS and the ORMH have initiated a study of uterine fibroids among 35 to 49 year-old members of a large pre-paid health plan in Washington, D.C. After one year of data collection, 285 black and 123 white women have been enrolled. Data from ultrasound examinations have been completed for 226 black women and 167 white women. In this group, 73% of black women had uterine fibroids, compared to 48 percent of white women. These data indicate that the differences in hysterectomy rates are not just a result of diagnostic/treatment bias. There are real differences in uterine fibroid risk between blacks and whites and the NIEHS hopes to help define some of the environmental triggers for uterine fibroid development.

A conference co-sponsored by NIEHS was held in October, 1999 called Women's Health and the Environment—The Next Century: Advances in Uterine Leiomyoma Research. The goal of this conference was to bring together researchers working in the fields of medicine, epidemiology, basic research and therapeutics to foster an exchange of scientific information among members of the uterine leiomyoma research community. Participants were drawn from academia, medicine, government and industry. The outcomes from this conference are helping the NIEHS to evaluate the current state of knowledge and to develop a research agenda to fill any data gaps in the area of uterine fibroids.

Breast Cancer

African-American women appear to be at greater risk of developing more aggressive forms of breast cancer and are more likely to die from this disease than are white breast cancer victims. The reasons will most likely prove to be multifactorial, but environmental exposures might play a role. A recently published study supported by the NIEHS showed that women with higher blood levels of the organochlorine pesticide, dieldrin, had twice the risk of later breast cancer development than did women with low levels of this pesticide. Since many people of color engage in farm work, they and their families would be expected to have higher exposures to endocrine-disrupting compounds such as dieldrin and, consequently, would be at higher risk for breast cancer development. The NIEHS, in partnership with the

National Cancer Institute (NCI), has a long-term Agricultural Health Study of farmers and pesticide applicators, as well as their spouses and children, to determine the health consequences of exposures typical in rural environments. The NIEHS was particularly instrumental in ensuring that a large part of this cohort included African-American families.

The NIEHS has other epidemiologic studies into environmental causes of breast cancer, as well as a portfolio of research examining the basic mechanisms by which environmental toxicants could cause breast cancer. Work is ongoing in the areas of gene regulation of mammary tumorigenesis, signal transduction in breast cancer cells, and expression of the P450 genes and other genes in breast cells. The effects of electromagnetic field radiation, polycyclic biphenyls, and polycyclic aromatic hydrocarbons on mammary gland development after exposures in utero and at various times in the life cycle are also being explored. Some of this work has shown differences in cell cycle control and apoptosis in mammary cells in women who are young/nulliparous compared to those who are older/parous. This is the same aggregation that relates to major reproductive risk factors for breast cancer.

The NIEHS supports a number of other studies examining the relationship of organochlorine exposures to breast cancer risk. In collaboration with the NCI, the NIEHS is co-funding the Long Island Breast Cancer Study Project. This includes a case-control study to see if women with breast cancer have higher exposures to organochlorine pesticides and air pollutants. Special attention is being paid to risk in African-American women. All African-American breast cancer cases in this study will have complete environmental biological sampling done. Analysis of these data may provide clues about unique risks for these women.

Other NIEHS-supported research include an ongoing study in rural areas of North Carolina. This study is measuring blood levels of organochlorine pesticides, as well as exposure histories of study participants for all past pesticide use. This study will compare pesticide exposure levels and their importance as causal factors in breast cancer risks between African-American and white women. Another study, conducted in Los Angeles, California, is measuring organochlorine pesticide levels in inner-city African-American women and relating it to their risk of breast cancer.

The NIEHS has also joined with the NCI on an initiative entitled "Regional Variation in Breast Cancer." This project uses geographic information systems to look at trends and differences in breast cancer risk factors in regions across the U.S. to investigate the role of exposures to toxicants and traditional breast cancer risk factors in explaining these differences. The project is being conducted through five grants. Three will be concerned with understanding the trends in breast cancer incidence, mortality and survival, and the environmental influences on these trends. A fourth, in California, will study the reasons for regional variation in breast cancer rates across the state, with particular emphasis on phytoestrogens as a source for these differences. A fifth study, in Connecticut, is looking at the role of variation in metabolizing enzymes in affecting breast cancer risk.

The NIEHS has other ongoing and planned studies addressing the environmental and genetic factors involved in breast cancer development. One proposed study is the Sisterhood Study. This study is designed to clarify the joint effects of environmental and genetic factors in the development of breast cancer by following a cohort of the unaffected sisters of women with breast cancer. This cohort would allow examination of breast cancer risks in relation to endogenous hormones, environmental hormone disruptors, growth factors, and environmental contaminants of public concern such as pesticides and solvents. Such exposures need to be studied jointly with genes involved in metabolic activation, receptor binding, or detoxification, to elucidate genetic modifiers of response. The NIEHS would ensure recruitment of minority women into this study. The initial cohort is expected to yield sufficient new cases for examination of gene-environment interactions at five years of follow-up, although the cohort could be studied longer. Although the effort would target breast cancer, less common hormonally related cancers such as ovarian and endometrial cancer could also be studied.

Environmental Estrogens and Other Endocrine Disruptors

Breast cancer, as well as other cancers (including ovarian and uterine cancers) and pathologies (including uterine fibroids, endometriosis, and subfertility/infertility), have been implicated as possible outcomes from exposure to endocrine disruptors. Endocrine disruptors are environmental compounds that have the ability to interfere with natural hormonal processes. Among the chemicals suspected to be endocrine disruptors are insecticides such as DDT and dieldrin, herbicides such as 2,4-D, plasticizers such as phthalates, and important industrial compounds such as cadmium, lead, styrene, dioxin, and PCBs, as well as many naturally occurring compounds such as phytoestrogens found in the normal human diet. The NIEHS has been

570

a pioneer in conducting research on the health effects of endocrine disruptors. Since many of the potential health endpoints and putative environmental exposures of endocrine disruption are higher in low-income communities, results of this research might shed light on the health disparities seen in this country.

For many years, NIEHS has supported research on how reproductive toxicants disrupt normal endocrine functions. More recent research, however, has started to focus on the hypothesis that adverse effects of endocrine disrupting chemicals can be caused by relatively small doses during a unique window of vulnerability for the fetus or newborn during development with subsequent adverse effects that may not be detectable until much later in life. Scientists at the NIEHS are examining the long-term effects of exposure to various endocrine disrupting compounds during development using reproductive and carcinogenic, as well as developmental, endpoints. In collaboration with researchers at the National Center for Toxicological Research, NIEHS scientists are investigating five compounds for adverse effects over multiple generations in animals. Such studies should begin to address the concern that potential adverse effects of chemicals with endocrine modulating activity are affecting human health, for example, by increasing human breast cancer risks.

Community Partnerships: Translational Research: Outreach Activities

Community-Based Prevention/Intervention Research (CBPIR) Project

This NIEHS initiative aims to implement culturally relevant prevention and intervention activities in economically disadvantaged and underserved populations adversely affected by environmental contaminants. This project, composed of nine grants, is intended both to foster refinement of scientifically valid intervention methods and to strengthen the participation of affected communities in this effort. The long-range goal of this program is to improve the knowledge and behavior of disadvantaged or underserved community members regarding prevention, detection, and treatment of environmentally related diseases and health conditions, and to reduce the incidence and mortality rates of such diseases and conditions. Currently, the NIEHS supports eight CBPIR grants; the National Institute for Nursing Research, in coordination with the NIEHS, supports another CBPIR grant.

Community-based prevention/intervention research thus seeks to expand our knowledge and understanding of the potential causes and remedies of environmentally related disorders, while at the same time enhancing the capacity of communities to participate in the processes that shape research approaches and intervention strategies. Given the complexity and magnitude of environmental health problems, research endeavors aimed at improving our knowledge of and ability to resolve these issues can benefit from establishing collaborative relationships with communities experiencing these problems. Such community-research partnerships have benefits for both the researcher and the community. These partnerships can, for example, facilitate the definition of important environmental health issues and concerns, the development of measurement instruments that are culturally appropriate, and the establishment of trust that will enrich the value of data collected.

Research projects are conducted in a manner that reinforces collaboration between community members and research institutions. Relevant results are disseminated to the community in clear, useful terms. Moreover, these studies are designed to be culturally appropriate, i.e., due consideration is given to the social, economic, and cultural conditions that influence health status. Identifying and incorporating unique cultural factors into intervention strategies may result in increased acceptability, use, and adherence. This approach seeks to maximize the potential for change in knowledge, attitudes, and behavior.

CBPIR programs are located in Florida, North Carolina, St. Louis, Oklahoma, New York City, Seattle, Portland, Oregon, Chicago, and Philadelphia. Research programs in these sites address community based prevention/intervention strategies for agricultural pesticide exposure, asthma, and lead poisoning.

Developmental Centers

NIEHS initiated the Developmental Centers program to (1) encourage research programs that study environmentally associated health problems of economically disadvantaged and underserved populations, and (2) to develop promising programs that could later compete for the longer-funded Environmental Health Sciences Centers grants. As part of their program's research objectives, the NIEHS Developmental Centers disseminate their findings to surrounding communities in the form of disease prevention and intervention strategies. ORMH might also join NIEHS in support of this project.

The potential impact of this program is illustrated by the NIEHS-supported research at Columbia University's School of Public Health. These researchers have uncovered a possible source of respiratory distress in households in Northern Manhattan. In this area, there has been an alarming rise in asthma prevalence, morbidity, and mortality over the past 15 years. One factor that appears likely to play a role in the epidemic is exposure to indoor allergens. Of particular importance to the communities of Harlem and Washington Heights are exposures to allergens associated with cockroaches and rodents, two classes of pests that heavily infect these communities. This Developmental Center is currently investigating possible approaches to reduce exposures to indoor allergens, including roach and rodent antigens. These approaches may include education, behavior modification, and integrated pest management methods.

Community Outreach and Education Program (COEP)

NIEHS requires that all of its Centers develop and maintain community outreach and education programs (COEP). The objective of COEP is to translate research results into knowledge applied to public health. Appropriate activities may consist of continuing professional education, disease prevention programs, education (primary, secondary, and/or college), information dissemination, community issue programs, and public awareness seminars. As a part of this effort, each NIEHS Center defines the community and region that it serves and develops outreach efforts specifically designed to address environmental health issues and problems of greatest concern to that community. Particular importance is given to populations that may be more susceptible to environmental insults, e.g., children, the elderly, or socioeconomically disadvantaged communities. NIEHS Centers are encouraged to sponsor local efforts through community organizations and to collaborate with other existing outreach programs in their area, such as those supported by other Federal agencies and state or local agencies or health departments.

An excellent example of the potential of COEP to provide information relevant to their communities can be found in California, which has a large population of Hispanic farmworkers. The State of California requires routine assays in farmworkers of blood levels of acetylcholinesterase, an enzyme that serves as a biomarker of exposure to the major pesticides used in California agriculture. As part of its outreach responsibilities, the NIEHS Center at the University of California-Davis examined this monitoring program and discovered some levels (and thus exposure effects) by as much as 40 percent. Furthermore, the various assays available used completely different units of measurement, making meaningful comparisons difficult and cumbersome. The result was an extensive statewide monitoring program that could not provide accurate or useful information. As a result of these findings, the state's California Environmental Protection Agency rewrote its Public Worker Safety Regulations. It now requires standardized procedures for clinical laboratories for assessment of acetylcholinesterase activity in agricultural workers exposed to organophophate and carbamate insecticides. Thus the practice of the law is now in line with the public health intent of the law. Such would not have been possible, however, without the work done by the UC-Davis COEP, and their subsequent follow-up with state regulators.

Environmental Justice: Partnerships for Communication

The NIEHS initiated a special grant program, the "Environmental Justice: Partnerships for Communication" program, to create mechanisms that empower affected communities to have a demonstrable role in identifying and defining problems and risks related to environmental health and in shaping future research approaches to such problems.

The primary objective of this program is to establish methods for linking members of a community, who are directly affected by adverse environmental conditions, with researchers and health care providers. Development of community-based strategies to address environmental health problems requires approaches that are not typically familiar to the research and medical communities. The distinctive needs of individual communities and their inhabitants are only rarely considered in identifying environmental health problems and devising appropriate medical intervention tactics. This program is designed to develop new modes of communication and to ensure that the community actively participates with researchers and health care providers in developing responses and setting priorities for intervention strategies.

Twelve ongoing projects are committed to enhancing minority participation in research studies and to facilitating communication among environmental health researchers, community health care providers and community members. These projects address the development of partnerships among community members, research scientists and health care providers to design community-based and culturally based appropriate mechanisms for environmental health education and outreach. Some of the environmental health issues addressed in this program include asthma, elevated blood lead levels, radiation exposure, occupational exposures, pesticide exposures, and severe urban smog.

An example of the potential impact of this program can be found in Southeastern Los Angeles, an area in which heavy industry borders residential Hispanic neighborhoods. One such neighborhood was jolted by the discovery of a mountain of broken concrete and asphalt being created in its midst as part of clean-up efforts of earthquake-destroyed roads. The debris covered several acres and reached the height of a multi-storied building. Heavy dust was a constant reminder of the dump's presence. Concerned neighbors contacted a community group that was recently awarded an NIEHS Environmental Justice: Partnerships for Communication grant. This group was able to broker a partnership with a nearby NIEHS Environmental Health Sciences Center to collect monitoring data and to use this information to convince the local air pollution agency to demand remediation. The debris and dust will be removed in 12 months and residents will be consulted at all stages of development. The same grantee engineered a smaller clean-up, this time of ground glass deposited in an outside storage area next to a residential neighborhood. This group used contacts with NIEHS-supported scientists to collect dust samples in the homes adjacent to this site and to show a high proportion of glass-containing dust and higher-than-expected incidence of nose bleeds in children living in these homes. This information was instrumental in requiring the company to store its glass waste in a more responsible manner. These examples illustrate ways the NIEHS is using its resources to better serve the public, particularly the disadvantaged and minority populations which often bear the greatest burden of environmental hazards.

Mississippi Delta Project

The Mississippi Delta Project is a collaborative effort between government, academia, grass-roots communities, and local and state health agencies. It is the first effort of its kind to address environmental contamination in a key geographic area. This region is one of the poorest parts of the country and is greatly affected by environmental pollution. The NIEHS works cooperatively with other Federal agencies to identify key environmental hazards, promote environmental quality, and reduce and prevent these hazards, where appropriate, from affecting the health and environment of residents.

Other NIEHS Efforts

A number of NIEHS funded studies are exploring strategies to communicate and educate disadvantaged minority populations about the dangers and risks of some environmental exposures. Native Americans, Hispanics, African-Americans, and other minority populations should benefit from the results of studies researching health fertility and reproductive risk of pesticides and methods reducing pesticide exposure in minority families. Outreach efforts such as the Biennial Symposium on Minorities and Cancer will further strengthen the ties between scientists and communities.

Support of Colleges/Universities of Historically Underserved Populations

Colleges and universities that serve historically underserved populations can provide a rich resource for engaging in health disparities research. These institutions often have the credibility and access needed to recruit subjects from minority populations, they have the interest and commitment, and they have the student population that could serve as biomedical researchers in the future. What they often lack, however, are the resources and infrastructure necessary for the increasingly high technology field of environmental health sciences. The NIEHS has developed several programs that serve to use these institutions for such diverse purposes as: (1) conducting relevant outreach and empowerment projects to local disadvantaged communities, (2) partnering these institutions with major research universities to improve the access of minority students to the expertise and instrumentation necessary for environmental health research, and (3) enhancing the resources and infrastructure of these institutions so that they are better positioned to conduct competitive research.

Advanced Research Cooperation in Environmental Health (ARCH)

The Advanced Research Cooperation in Environmental Health (ARCH) Program is a pilot program developed to strengthen the capacity of Historically Black Colleges and Universities (HBCUs) and other minority-based institutions to engage in high quality competitive environmental health research. The ARCH Program, a multidisciplinary biomedical research effort, is based on a mutually beneficial collaborative partnership between an HBCU and another, more research intensive, academic institution. This program capitalizes on the unique positive features of each prototype institution and ensures the sharing of appropriate physical and human resources that will lead to the overall success of this program.

The first ARCH recipients are Xavier University of Louisiana, partnered with Tulane University, and Southern University at Baton Rouge, partnered with the University of Texas Medical Branch, in Galveston. Work at Xavier University will focus on the alteration of gene regulation by environmental compounds, including interaction with steroid receptors. Southern University at Baton Rouge will concentrate on the occupational compound, butadiene, and its effect on reproductive and neuroendocrine responses, on p53-mediated cellular responses, and on DNA damage and DNA repair.

Ponce University School of Medicine

In Puerto Rico, the NIEHS is supporting development of an environmental toxicology program at Ponce University School of Medicine. The goal is to strengthen four critical areas of research:

1. clinical toxicology, with special reference to asthma,

2. marine toxins,

3. oxygen-free radical toxicology, and

4. molecular toxicology.

Asthma is an emerging public health problem in Puerto Rico because of its high prevalence (17.5 percent) and severity, and there is a significant increase in emergency room visits due to asthma exacerbations in the last five years. Efforts are underway to identify and quantify known environmental irritants associated with a severe outcome for asthma. The effect of marine neurotoxins on subcellular transport and signal transduction pathways is also being investigated. Other studies examine the metabolic pathways determining the impact of environmental toxicants on humans. NIEHS support is designed not only to address environmental health issues of local concern in Puerto Rico but also to enhance the capacity of minority investigators at this institution to compete for NIH grant funding by connecting them with funded investigators at NIEHS Centers and supporting new facilities and resources.

Radiation Education Center at a Tribal College

An NIEHS-funded Environmental Justice grant called the Uranium Education Project has established a Radiation Education Center to implement an empowerment program for Navajo Native Americans. The focus will be health issues arising from the legacy of former uranium mining and milling operations on a Navajo reservation in New Mexico. Uranium mining and milling have left large areas of the Navajo reservation contaminated with mine and mill tailings and associated radiation. There are well-documented problems with lung cancer and silicosis in former Navajo uranium miners, and there is great concern among uranium millers and other Navajos who reside near contaminated areas about late effects of radiation exposure from these sources. A partnership between the local Navajo community, Dine College (a tribal community college), local primary care physicians, the Indian Health Service, local school districts, the University of New Mexico Center for Population Health, and scientists with expertise in radiation health issues has been created to provide information and skills for empowerment among this minority group.

University of Maryland at Baltimore County (UMBC)— Meyerhoff Scholars Program

The NIEHS has partnered with the University of Maryland and the National Science Foundation to support the Meyerhoff Scholars Program. This program, the Alliance for Minority Participation in Science Program, is designed to encourage African-American students at the UMBC to pursue undergraduate biological science degrees. The institutional support and encouragement made possible by this program positions these students to pursue postgraduate careers in biomedical research.

Morehouse College Public Health Science Institute

The NIEHS has partnered with Morehouse College in Atlanta to provide research opportunities for students in a cooperative summer program. The program is designed to train minorities in the areas of biostatistics, epidemiology, and environmental health sciences. These 3-month internships, to be conducted within the Office of the Director, NIEHS, will focus on engaging these students in the use of quantitative disciplines in areas of environmental justice and health.

578

Morehouse School of Medicine

NIEHS is helping support research efforts of a group of scientists at Morehouse School of Medicine investigating environmental effects on nervous tissue systems. Currently this group is focusing on the eye and is helping to define environmental influences that lead to near-sightedness, or myopia. The rhesus monkey is the model being used and NIEHS is also helping to support a colony of these animals for use by the researchers.

Durham Technical Community College

Higher education is expensive and many poorer students find the cost of community colleges and technical training to be more afford-able than Bachelor's Degree programs. The NIEHS is developing pro-grams that target these academic institutions. The first of these is at Durham Technical Community College in Durham, NC. This college has a large African-American student body and the NIEHS, in part-nership with the NC Biotechnology Center, supports the new Clini-cal Research Associates Program. This program awards an Associate's Degree in clinical trials research. In addition to courses in anatomy, pharmacology, and data analysis, this curriculum provides on-site training in working laboratories. Graduates of this program will have numerous job opportunities because of the high concentration of bio-medical and pharmaceutical research institutions in Durham and the nearby Research Triangle Park, NC. Thus this program will serve to increase the number of minorities engaged in biomedical research and, it is hoped, will provide a springboard for some of these graduates to pursue advanced training.

Training and Education

The Minority Worker Training Program (MWTP)

The Minority Worker Training Program is a national pilot program to recruit and train young people living near hazardous waste sites or in communities at risk of exposure to contaminated properties. Participants are trained for future employment in the fields of remediation and environmental health. This program promotes part-nerships or agreements with academic and other institutions, with a particular focus on historically black colleges and universities. This project is done in collaboration with the EPA and, in addition to train-ing minority inner-city youth for future jobs, it gives them the skill and knowledge to identify and address environmental problems within their own communities.

K-12 Environmental Health Science Education

In 1992, the NIEHS began development of an environmental health sciences education program at the K-12 grade levels. The objective of this program is to improve the understanding of environmental health issues by all students and to expand career awareness for those interested in pursuing research and service occupations in environmental health sciences. Initiatives within this grant program support development of instructional materials for use in grades K-12 and teacher enhancement and development activities to provide teachers with the disciplinary and pedagogical skills needed to teach environmental health science. An important element of these programs is that they are designed for the success of all students, regardless of background or ability, especially those from under represented populations, including women, people of color, persons with disabilities, and the economically disadvantaged. In addition, these projects promote parental and community involvement so that both students as well as their parents become more aware of environmental health concepts and issues.

The Myerhoff Program

A significant reason the NIEHS supports the Myerhoff program is to increase the number of minority students interested in pursuing careers in biomedical environmental health science research. The NIEHS is further enhancing opportunities for minority students by creating opportunities for research and mentoring through its Environmental Health Sciences Centers and intramural research programs.

Bridging Education, Science and Technology (BEST) Program

The Bridging Education, Science and Technology (BEST) program is a partnership between the NIEHS and the Durham Public Schools (DPS). It one of several NIEHS K-12 Programs. BEST is an effort to address science education concerns and needs particularly among disadvantaged and minority groups. The program is designed to heighten DPS students' science involvement, specifically in the area of molecular biology, and to engage them in related supplementary activities that will enhance their probability of success in the sciences.

Other NIEHS Efforts

In fiscal year 1992, a new program was initiated which provided a mechanism for supporting graduate studies leading to a Ph.D. degree. This program is called the Individual National Research Service Award for Predoctoral Fellowships for Minority Students. Currently, the NIEHS supports a total of 13 predoctoral fellows. The NIEHS will further increase the effect of this program on the development of environmental health scientists through our collaborative interactions with the National Institute of General Medical Sciences.

The Summers of Discovery Program established by the Institute's Division of Intramural Research is a science education outreach program designed to attract students, particularly women and minorities, to science careers. The program targets three separate populations—high school through graduate school students, pre-college science teachers, and science faculty members from women's colleges and minority universities. Participants spend between two and three months working on a research project where they are exposed to some of the latest techniques in environmental toxicology. This experience gives students and teachers a much better understanding of the field of environmental health sciences as it is practiced at NIEHS.

In addition, the NIEHS has a short-term training program, National Research Service Award institutional training grants, for undergraduate minorities to develop their interests and skills in research. The goal of this program is to attract talented students to Ph.D. programs in environmental health sciences.

The NIEHS also promotes the NIH Research Supplements for Underrepresented Minorities. The aim of these supplements is to attract and encourage minority individuals to enter and pursue biomedical and behavioral research careers in areas within the missions of all the awarding components of the NIH by providing supplemental funds to certain ongoing research grants. By providing research opportunities for underrepresented minorities at various career levels (high school through postdoctoral training), the number of minorities entering and remaining in biomedical research careers will increase.

Health Disparities Research Agenda

Regional Health Disparities Workshops

The NIEHS is sponsoring a series of regional workshops devoted to issues examining the relationships among poverty, pollution, and health status. The workshops are intended to generate ideas and stimulate discussion on research activities that will drive (1) the design of action plans to lessen the adverse health impact of hazardous environmental exposures on populations of low socioeconomic strata, and (2) the development of research directions to enhance our understanding of how socioeconomic status and hazardous environmental exposures interact to contribute to disparities in health.

NIEHS Leadership Retreat

The Director, NIEHS, holds an annual planning retreat for upper management and senior scientists of NIEHS. These retreats are attended by invited outside experts, as well as the NIEHS' Advisory Council. The 1999 retreat was devoted to the issue of health disparities and was designed to orient management and researchers to this issue and to help develop areas in which NIEHS research could make an impact.

Regional Town Meetings

The NIEHS holds four regional town meetings throughout the country each year. These meetings are designed to solicit community input into the NIEHS research agenda and to help ensure that the NIEHS portfolio of research is responsive to the needs of the American people. These meetings are usually hosted by NIEHS-supported Environmental Health Sciences Centers and special efforts are made to ensure that low-income communities and communities of color are able to come and to be heard.

Part Nine

Additional
Help and Information

Chapter 71

Glossary of Environmental Health Terms

This glossary is intended to help people become familiar with the terms they are likely to see in government reports, engineering studies and health literature. It is divided into two sections: Terms and Agencies.

Terms

Absorption: The process of taking in, as when a sponge takes up water. Chemicals can be absorbed into the bloodstream after breathing or swallowing. Chemicals can also be absorbed through the skin into the bloodstream and then transported to other organs. Not all of the chemical breathed, swallowed, or touched is always absorbed.

Acute: Occurring over a short time, usually a few minutes or hours. An acute exposure can result in short term or long term health effects. An acute effect happens within a short time after exposure.

Ambient: Surrounding. Ambient air usually means outdoor air (as opposed to indoor air).

Analyte: A chemical for which a sample (such as water, air, blood, urine or other substance) is tested. For example, if the analyte is mercury, the laboratory test will determine the amount of mercury in the sample.

Used with permission of the New York State Department of Health. © 2002. This glossary is posted under "Information for Consumers" on the Department's website at www.health.state.ny.us.

Aquifer: An underground source of water. This water may be contained in a layer of rock, sand or gravel.

Background level: A typical level of a chemical in the environment. Background often refers to naturally occurring or uncontaminated levels. Background levels in one region of the state may be different than those in other areas.

Bedrock: The solid rock underneath surface soils.

Biological monitoring: Analyzing chemicals, hormone levels or other substances in biological materials (blood, urine, breath, etc.) as a measure of chemical exposure, health status, etc. in humans or animals. A blood test for lead is an example of biological monitoring.

Body burden: The total amount of a chemical in the body. Some chemicals build up in the body because they are stored in body organs like fat or bone or are eliminated very slowly.

Case control study: A study in which people with a disease (cases) are compared to people without the disease (controls) to see if their past exposures to chemicals or other risk factors were different.

Central nervous system (CNS): The part of the nervous system that includes the brain and the spinal cord.

CERCLA: Comprehensive Environmental Response, Compensation and Liability Act. See "Superfund."

Chronic: Occurring over a long period of time, several weeks, months or years.

Cohort study: A study in which a group of people with a past exposure to chemicals or other risk factors are followed over time and their disease experience compared to that of a group of people without the exposure.

Composite sample: A sample which is made by combining samples from two or more locations. The sample can be of water, soil or another medium.

Concentration: The amount of one substance dissolved or contained in a given amount of another substance or medium. For example, sea water has a higher concentration of salt than fresh water does.

Contaminant: Any substance that enters a system (the environment, human body, food, etc.) where it is not normally found. Contaminants are usually referred to in a negative sense and include substances that spoil food, pollute the environment or cause other adverse effects.

Dermal: Referring to the skin. For example, dermal absorption means absorption through the skin.

Detection limit: The smallest amount of substance that a laboratory test can reliably measure in a sample of air, water, soil or other medium.

Dose: The amount of substance to which a person is exposed.

Epidemiology: The study of the occurrence and causes of health effects in human populations. An epidemiological study often compares two groups of people who are alike except for one factor such as exposure to a chemical or the presence of a health effect. The investigators try to determine if the factor is associated with the health effect.

Exposure: Contact with a chemical by swallowing, by breathing or by direct contact (such as through the skin or eyes). Exposure may be either short term (acute) or long term (chronic).

Exposure assessment: A process that estimates the amount of a chemical that enters or comes into contact with people or animals. An exposure assessment also describes how often and for how long an exposure occurred, and the nature and size of a population exposed to a chemical.

Feasibility Study (FS): A study that compares different ways to clean up a contaminated site. The feasibility study recommends one or more actions to remediate the site. See "Remedial investigation."

Gradient: The change in a property over a certain distance. For example, lead can accumulate in surface soil near a road due to automobile exhaust. As you move away from the road, the amount of lead in the surface soil decreases. This change in the lead concentration with distance from the road is called a gradient.

Health assessment for contaminated sites: Determination of actual or possible health effects due to environmental contamination or exposure. It includes a health-based interpretation of all the information known about the situation. The information may come from site investigations (environmental sampling and studies), exposure assessments, risk assessments, biological monitoring or health effects studies. The health assessment is used to advise people how to prevent or reduce their exposures, to determine remedial actions or the need for additional studies.

Health effects studies related to contaminants: Studies of the health of people who may have been exposed to contaminants. They include, but are not limited to, epidemiological studies, reviews of health status of people in exposure or disease registries, and doing medical tests.

Health registry: A record of people exposed to a specific substance (such as a heavy metal), or having a specific health condition (such as cancer or a communicable disease). New York State maintains several health registries.

Ingestion: Swallowing (such as eating or drinking). Chemicals in or on food, drink, utensils, cigarettes, hands, etc. can be ingested. After ingestion, chemicals may be absorbed into the blood and distributed throughout the body.

Inhalation: Breathing. People can take in chemicals by breathing contaminated air.

Interim Remedial Measure (IRM): An action taken at a contaminated site to reduce the chances of human or environmental exposure to site contaminants. Interim remedial measures are planned and carried out before comprehensive remedial studies. They can prevent additional damage during the study phase, but don't interfere in any way with the need to develop a complete remedial program. An example of an interim remedial measure is removing drums of chemicals to a storage facility from a site that has drums sitting in an empty field.

Latency period: The period of time between exposure to something that causes a disease and the onset of the health effect. Cancer caused by chemical exposure may have a latency period of 5 to 40 years.

Leaching: As water moves through soils or landfills, chemicals in the soil may dissolve in the water thereby contaminating the groundwater. This is called leaching.

Maximum Contaminant Level (MCL): The highest (maximum) level of a contaminant allowed to go uncorrected by a public water system under federal or state regulations. Depending on the contaminant, allowable levels might be calculated as an average over time, or might be based on individual test results. Corrective steps are implemented if the MCL is exceeded.

Media: Elements of a surrounding environment that can be sampled for contamination; usually soil, water, or air. Plants, as well as humans (when sampling blood, urine, etc.) and animals (such as sampling fish to update fish consumption advisories) can also be considered media. The singular of "media" is "medium."

Metabolism: All the chemical reactions that enable the body to work. For example, food is metabolized (chemically changed) to supply the body with energy. Chemicals can be metabolized by the body and made either more or less harmful.

Morbidity: Illness or disease. A morbidity rate for a certain illness is the number of people with that illness divided by the number of people in the population from which the illnesses were counted.

National Priority List (NPL): A list maintained by the U.S. Environmental Protection Agency (EPA) of certain inactive hazardous waste sites. The list is produced and updated periodically by the EPA. See "Superfund."

Odor threshold: The lowest concentration of a chemical that can be smelled. Different chemicals have different odor thresholds. Also, some people can smell a chemical at lower concentrations than others can.

Organic: Generally considered as originating from plants or animals, and made primarily of carbon and hydrogen. Scientists use the term organic to mean those chemical compounds which are based on carbon.

Permeability: The property of permitting liquids or gases to pass through. A highly permeable soil, such as sand, allows a liquid to pass through quickly. Clay has a low permeability.

Persistence: The quality of remaining for a long period of time (such as in the environment or the body). Persistent chemicals (such as DDT and PCBs) are not easily broken down.

Preliminary Site Assessment (PSA): A process followed by the New York State Department of Environmental Conservation (DEC) to determine if a site contains hazardous waste and its potential for harming the public health or environment. This process includes inspecting the site, sampling if needed, and taking physical or hydrological measurements as appropriate.

Plume: An area of chemicals moving away from its source in a long band or column. A plume, for example, can be a column of smoke from a chimney or chemicals moving with groundwater.

Protocol: The detailed plan for conducting a scientific procedure. A protocol for measuring a chemical in soil, water or air describes the way in which samples should be collected and analyzed.

Quality assurance and quality control (QA/QC): A system of procedures, checks and audits to judge and control the quality of measurements and reduce the uncertainty of data. Some quality control procedures include having more than one person review the findings and analyzing a sample at different times or laboratories to see if the findings are similar.

Remedial Investigation (RI): An in-depth study (including sampling of air, soil, water and waste) of a contaminated site needing remediation to determine the nature and extent of contamination. The remedial investigation (RI) is usually combined with a feasibility study (FS).

Remediation: Correction or improvement of a problem, such as work that is done to clean up or stop the release of chemicals from a contaminated site. After investigation of a site, remedial work may include removing soil and/or drums, capping the site or collecting and treating the contaminated fluids.

Risk: Risk is the possibility of injury, disease or death. For example, for a person who has measles, the risk of death is one in one million.

Risk assessment: A process which estimates the likelihood that exposed people may have health effects. The four steps of a risk assessment are: hazard identification (Can this substance damage health?); dose-response assessment (What dose causes what effect?); exposure assessment (How and how much do people contact it?); and risk characterization (combining the other three steps to characterize risk and describe the limitations and uncertainties).

Risk management: The process of deciding how and to what extent to reduce or eliminate risk factors by considering the risk assessment, engineering factors (Can procedures or equipment do the job, for how long and how well?), social, economic and political concerns.

Route of exposure: The way in which a person may contact a chemical substance. For example, drinking (ingestion) and bathing (skin contact) are two different routes of exposure to contaminants that may be found in water. See "Exposure."

Safe: Strictly, free from harm or risk. Exposure to a chemical usually has some risk associated with it, although the risk may be very small. However, many people use the word safe to mean something that has a very low risk or one that is acceptable to them.

Site inspection: A Department of Health visit to a site to evaluate the likelihood of human exposure to toxic chemicals, and to do an exposure assessment. See "Exposure assessment."

Solubility: The largest amount of a substance that can be dissolved in a given amount of a liquid, usually water. For a highly water-soluble compound, such as table salt, a lot can dissolve in water. Motor oil is only slightly soluble in water.

Superfund (federal and state): The federal and state programs to investigate and clean up inactive hazardous waste sites.

Target organ: An organ (such as the liver or kidney) that is specifically affected by a toxic chemical.

Volatile: Evaporating readily at normal temperatures and pressures. The air concentration of a highly volatile chemical can increase quickly in a closed room.

Volatile organic compound (VOC): An organic chemical that evaporates readily. Petroleum products such as kerosene, gasoline and mineral spirits contain VOCs. Chlorinated solvents such as those used by dry cleaners or contained in paint strippers are also VOCs. See "organic" and "volatile."

Agencies

American Conference of Governmental Industrial Hygienists (ACGIH): ACGIH is a professional society of government workers and educators who work to promote occupational safety and health. The organization publishes recommendations on ventilation, air sampling and air concentration guidelines (threshold limit values or TLVS) designed to control exposure of workers to chemicals, noise and radiation in the workplace.

Agency for Toxic Substances and Disease Registry (ATSDR): ATSDR is part of the U.S. Department of Health and Human Services. As mandated by the federal Superfund law, the agency assesses health risks from hazardous waste sites on the National Priority List. ATSDR determines if additional health studies are needed at these sites, provides health advisories and publishes toxicological profiles on chemicals found at hazardous waste sites. ATSDR also maintains exposure registries of people exposed to certain substances.

Centers for Disease Control and Prevention (CDC or CDCP): The CDC, part of the U.S. Department of Health and Human Services, provides federal leadership in the prevention and control of diseases. The CDC includes many programs that conduct research and provide information on public health issues such as occupational health, AIDS, cancer, infectious diseases and other diseases.

Consumer Product Safety Commission (CPSC): The CPSC, a federal commission, protects the public from injury caused by consumer products. The CPSC evaluates products, investigates the causes of product-related injuries and issues and enforces safety standards. For example, the CPSC has banned certain products containing asbestos. The CPSC also regulates the lead content of paints.

International Agency for Research on Cancer (IARC): IARC, part of the World Health Organization, is an international organization that evaluates the human cancer risk from chemical exposure. IARC evaluates scientific studies on chemicals and publishes critical reviews on the cancer risks of these substances. IARC also identifies further research that is needed to evaluate the cancer-causing ability of some chemicals.

National Academy of Sciences (NAS): NAS is a private, nonprofit corporation established by Congress to investigate and report on science and technology at the request of the federal government. The National Research Council (NRC) is a part of the NAS and has reported on public health problems such as chemical contamination of drinking water.

National Institute of Environmental Health Sciences (NIEHS): The NIEHS tries to reduce human illness from environmental causes by understanding environmental factors, individual susceptibility and age. The NIEHS conducts biomedical research programs, prevention and intervention efforts, and education.

National Institute for Occupational Safety and Health (NIOSH): NIOSH, part of the Centers for Disease Control, conducts research on worker safety and health and recommends standards for worker protection to OSHA. For example, NIOSH recommends guidelines for workplace exposure to hazardous substances and has published criteria documents on many chemicals.

National Institutes of Health (NIH): NIH, part of the U.S. Department of Health and Human Services, conducts scientific research into the causes, prevention and cure of diseases. For example, the National Cancer Institute (part of NIH) studies how some environmental chemicals cause cancer. Many other diseases, some related to chemical exposure, are also under study at NIH.

National Toxicology Program (NTP): NTP, part of the U.S. Department of Health and Human Services (DHHS), coordinates the toxicology research being conducted within DHHS. The NTP selects priority chemicals for study, develops necessary testing procedures and coordinates the research done by programs in three DHHS agencies: NIH, FDA and CDC.

NIEHS: *See:* National Institute of Environmental Health Sciences.

Occupational Safety and Health Administration (OSHA): OSHA, part of the U.S. Department of Labor, enforces federal laws that protect worker safety and health, such as maintaining standards for occupational exposure to chemicals, training employees and keeping records of chemical exposures.

U.S. Department of Energy (DOE): The DOE administers federal energy research, development, regulation and policy. DOE is in charge of federal research on the storage and disposal of radioactive waste and can provide information to the public on radioactive waste disposal and management.

U.S. Department of Health and Human Services (DHHS): DHHS carries out federal health and social programs such as social security, human development, family support, health care financing and public health. The Public Health Service, a part of DHHS, includes agencies such as the Centers for Disease Control, the Agency for Toxic

Substances and Disease Registry, the Food and Drug Administration and the National Institutes of Health.

U.S. Environmental Protection Agency (EPA): The EPA enforces federal environmental protection laws. It registers and regulates pesticides, enforces laws covering outdoor air and drinking water quality and regulates the disposal of hazardous and solid wastes. EPA's Integrated Risk Information System (IRIS) is an electronic database containing information on health effects that may result from exposure to chemicals. IRIS is intended for those without extensive training in toxicology, but with some knowledge of health sciences.

U.S. Food and Drug Administration (FDA): The FDA, part of the U.S. Department of Health and Human Services, carries out and enforces laws that protect the quality and safety of foods, food additives, cosmetics and medical drugs and devices. For example, the FDA monitors the quality of foods and drugs through product testing, and reviews food and drug ingredients, including pesticide residues, to determine if they pose health hazards.

U.S. Geological Survey (USGS): The USGS, part of the U.S. Department of the Interior, identifies the nation's land, water, mineral and energy resources. USGS conducts research, prepares topographic maps and collects and interprets data on mineral and water resources.

World Health Organization (WHO): WHO, an agency of the United Nations, carries out public and environmental health programs throughout the world. For example, WHO trains health personnel and assists countries to provide primary health care, prevent communicable diseases and combat malnutrition. WHO has developed international guidelines for pesticide residues in foods and chemicals in drinking water.

Chapter 72

Environmental Agencies and Advocate Groups

Following is a list of agencies and advocate groups serving those seeking help or information about the environment and it's effect on their health.

Action on Smoking and Health (ASH)
2013 H Street, NW
Washington, DC 20003
Tel: 202-659-4310
Internet: http://ash.org

Agency for Toxic Substances and Disease Registry (ATSDR)
1600 Clifton Road E-28
Atlanta, GA 30333
Toll Free: 888-422-8737
Tel: 404-639-0727
Fax: 404-498-0057
Internet: http://www.atsdr.cdc.gov
E-mail: ATSDRIC@cdc.gov

American Red Cross
431 18th Street, NW
Washington, DC 20006
Toll Free: 877-272-7337
Tel: 202-639-3520
Internet: http://www.redcross.org

American Lung Association
61 Broadway, 6th Floor
New York, NY 10006
Tel: 212-315-8700
Internet: http://www.lungusa.org

Americans for Nonsmokers Rights
2530 San Pablo Ave., Suite J
Berkeley, CA 94702
Tel: 510-841-3032
Fax: 510-841-3071
Internet: http://www.no-smoke.org
E-mail: anr@no-smoke.org

Americans with Disabilities Act Hotline
1331 F Street NW, Suite 1000
Washington, DC 20004-1111
Toll Free: 800-USA-ABLE
Tel: 202-272-5435
TDD: 202-653-7834
Fax: 202-272-5447
E-mail: info@access-board.gov
Internet: www.access-board.gov

Catholic Charities USA
1731 King Street
Alexandria, VA 22314
Tel: 703-549-1390
Fax: 703-549-1656
Internet: http://www.catholic
charitiesusa.org

Centers for Disease Control (CDC)
1600 Clifton Road
Atlanta, GA 30333
Toll Free: 800-311-3435
Tel: 404-639-3311
Internet: http://www.cdc.gov

Chemical Injury Information Network
P.O. Box 301
White Sulphur Springs, MT 59645
Tel: 406-547-2255
Fax: 406-547-2455
Internet: http://www.ciin.org

Chemically Sensitive Living
377 Wilbur Avenue, Suite 213
Swansea, MA 02777
Tel: 508-678-7293 (voice and fax)
Internet: http://
www.chemsenlvng. com

Environmental Defense Fund
257 Park Ave. South
New York, NY 10010
Tel: 212-505-2100
Fax: 212-505-2375
Internet: http://
www.environmentaldefense.org
E-mail: members@
environmentaldefense.org

Environmental Health Network (of California)
P.O. Box 1155
Larkspur, CA 94977
Tel: 415-541-5075
Internet: http://www.ehnca.org
E-mail: wilworks@lanminds.com

Environmental Protection Agency (EPA)
Ariel Rios Building
1200 Pennsylvania Ave, NW
Mail Code 3213A
Washington, DC 20460
Tel: 202-260-2090
Internet: http://www.epa.gov

Food and Drug Administration
Freedom of Information Office
5600 Fishers Lane, Room 12A-30
Rockville, MD 20587
Tel: 301-443-6310
Internet: http://www.fda.gov

Greenpeace, U.S.A.
702 H Street NW, Suite 300
Washington, DC 20001
Toll Free: 800-326-0959
Tel: 202-319-2444
Internet: http://
www.greenpeaceusa.org

Household Hazardous Waste Project
1031 E. Battlefield
Springfield, MO 65807
Tel: 417-889-5000
E-mail: owm@missouri.edu

Industrial/Environmental Toxicology Project
Industrial Workers of the World:
Advocates for MCS Sufferers
P.O. Box 20402
Seattle, WA 98102
Tel: 206-367-0477

MCS Referral and Resources
508 Westgate Rd.
Baltimore, MD 21229
Tel: 410-362-6400
Fax: 410-362-6401
Internet: http://www.mcsrr.org.

National Academy of Sciences
500 Fifth Street NW
Washington, DC 20001
Internet: http://
www4.nationalacademies.org/
nas/nashome.nsf

National Center for Environmental Health Strategies (NCEHS)
1100 Rural Ave.
Voorhees, NJ 08043
Tel: 856-429-5358
Internet: http://www.ncehs.org
E-mail: info@ncehs.org

National Coalition Against the Misuse of Pesticides
701 E Street SE, Suite 200
Washington, DC 20003
Tel: 202-543-5450
Fax: 202-543-4791
Internet: http://www.
beyondpesticides.org/main.html
E-mail: info@beyondpesticides.org

National Health Information Center
P.O. Box 1133
Washington, DC 20013-1133
Toll Free: 800-339-4797
Tel: 301-565-4167
Fax: 301-984-4256
Internet: http://www.health.gov/
nhic

National Hospice Association (HOSPICE)
1700 Diagonal Rd., Suite 625
Alexandria, VA 22314
Toll Free: 800-646-6460
Tel: 703-837-1500
Fax: 703-837-1233
Internet: http://www.nhpco.org
E-mail: nhpca_info@nhpco.org

National Institute for Occupational Safety and Health (NIOSH)
4676 Columbia Parkway
Cincinnati, OH 45226
Toll Free: 800-356-4674
Fax: 513-3-533-8573
Internet: http://www.cdc.gov/
niosh/homepage.html

National Institutes of Health
9000 Rockville Pike
Bethesda, MD 20892
Tel: 301-496-4000
Internet: http://www.nih.gov/
E-mail: NIHInfo@OD.NIH.GOV

National Organic Farmers Association Vermont (NOFA)
P.O. Box 697
Richmond, VT 05477
Tell: 802-434-4122
Internet: http://www.nofavt.org
E-mail: info@nofavt.org

National Pesticide Information Center
Oregon State University
333 Weniger Hall
Corvallis, Oregon 97331-6502
Toll Free: 800-858-7378
Fax: 541-737-0761
Internet: http://npic.orst.edu/
E-mail: npic@ace.orst.edu

New York: Citizens' Environmental Coalition (CEC)
33 Central Ave.
Albany, NY 12210
Tel: 518-462-5527
Fax: 518-465-8349
Internet: http://www.crisny.org/
not-for-profit/cectoxic
E-mail: cecanne@igc.org

New York Coalition for Alternatives to Pesticides (NYCAP)
353 Hamilton St.
Albany, NY 12210-1709
Tel: 518-426-8246
Fax: 518-426-3052
Internet: http://www.crisny.org/
not-for-profit/nycap
E-mail: nycap@crisny.org

New York: Division of Veterans Affairs
Dioxin Outreach Program
194 Washington Ave.
Albany, NY 12210
Tel: 518-474-6784

Occupational Safety and Health Administration (OSHA)
200 Constitution Ave. NW
Washington, DC 20210
Toll Free: 800-321-OSHA
TDD: 877-889-5627
Internet: http://www.osha.gov

Pesticide Registry of Washington
Washington State Department of Agriculture
P.O. Box 42560
Olympia, WA 98504-2560
Tel: 206-902-2040

Salvation Army, East U.S. Headquarters
440 West Nyack Rd.
West Nyack, NY 10994-1739
Tel: 845-620-7200
Fax: 845-620-7766
Internet: http://
www1.salvationarmy.org

Smoking Control Advocacy Resource Center (SCARC)
1707 L Street NW, Suite 400
Washington, DC 20036
Tel: 202-659-8475
Fax: 202-659-8484
Internet: http://
www.globalink.org/tobacco/docs/
na-docs/aa990407.shtml

U.S. Department of Housing and Urban Development (HUD)
451 7th St. SW
Washington, DC 20410
Tel: 202-708-1112
TDD: 202-708-1455
Internet: http://www.hud.gov

U.S. Social Security Administration
Windsor Park Building
6401 Security Blvd.
Baltimore, MD 21235
Toll Free: 800-772-1213
Internet: http://www.ssa.gov

U.S. Surgeon General
5600 Fishers Lane
Room 18-66
Rockville, MD 20857
Internet: http://
www.surgeongeneral.gov

Chapter 73

Environmental Resources on the Internet

Following is a list of Internet resources that contain information on various environmentally induced injuries and diseases.

Children

Association of Birth Defect Children
http://www.birthdefects.org

Children's Environmental Health Network
http://www.cehn.org

Children's Health Environmental Coalition Network
http://checnet.org

Learning Disabilities Association of America
http://www.ldanatl.org

Chronic Fatigue and Immune Dysfunction Syndrome (CFIDS)

CFIDS Association of America
http://www.cfids.org

The National CFIDS Foundation
http://www.cfidsfoundation.org

Environmental Groups

Californians for Alternatives to Toxics
http://www.reninet.com/catz

The internet resources listed in this chapter were compiled from many different sources. All resources were verified in February 2003.

Earth Island Institute
http://www.earthisland.org

Ecology Center of Ann Arbor
http://www.hvcn.org/info/ecaa

EDF (Environmental Defense Fund) Scorecard
http://www.scorecard.org

Environmental Defense Fund
http://www.edf.org

Environmental Health Coalition
http://www.environmentalhealth.org

Environmental Research Foundation
http://www.rachel.org

Friends of the Earth
http://www.foe.org

Greenpeace, U.S.A
http://www.greenpeaceusa.org

Health & Environment Resource Center
http://members.aol.com/Enviroknow/index.html

International Ozone Association
http://int-ozone-assoc.org

London Hazards Centre
http://www.lhc.org.uk

National Wildlife Federation
http://www.nwf.org

Natural Resources Defense Council
http://www.nrdc.org

Orion Society, The
http://www.orionsociety.org

Right-to-Know Network
http://www.rtk.net

Sierra Club
http://www.sierraclub.org

U.S. Public Interest Research Group
http://www.pirg.org

Fibromyalgia

American Fibromyalgia Syndrome Association
http://www.afsafund.org

Fibromyalgia Network
http://www.fmnetnews.com

Oregon Fibromyalgia Foundation
http://www.myalgia.com

Food

Mothers for Natural Law
http://www.safe-food.org/welcome.html

Pure Food Campaign
http://www.purefood.org

Truth in Labeling Campaign
http://www.truthinlabeling.org

Gulf War Syndrome

American Gulf War Veterans Association
http://www.gulfwarvets.com

Multiple Chemical Sensitivities (MCS)/ Environmental Illness (EI)

Chemical Injury Resource Association of Minnesota
http://www.mtn.org/~cira

EI/MCS Support Group of Louisville
http://users.adept.net/~mcsinfo

Environmental Health Network of California
http://www.ehnca.org

Human Ecology Action League
http://members.aol.com/Healnatnl/index.html

MCS Primer
http://www.geocities.com/HotSprings/Spa/4415/index.html

North Carolina Chemical Injury
http://ncchem.com

Rocky Mountain Environmental Health Association
http://www.rmeha.org

Support Network for the Aldehyde and Solvent Affected
http://www.ncchem.com/supald.htm

Other Health Issues

Action on Smoking and Health
http://ash.org

Allergy to Latex Education and Resource Team
http://www.execpc.com/~alert

Breast Cancer Action
http://bcaction.org

Citizens For Health
http://www.citizens.org

Citizens United to Reduce Emissions of Formaldehyde Poisoning Association
http://www.social.com/health/nhic/data/hr1700/hr1711.html

Maine Injured Workers Association
http://www.miwa.org

Potomac Latex Allergy Association
http://www.angelfire.com/md/plaa

Share, Care and Prayer, Inc.
http://www.sharecareprayer.org

Well Mind Association
http://www.speakeasy.org/~wma

White Lung Association
http://www.whitelung.org

Pesticide

National Coalition Against the Misuse of Pesticides
http://www.beyondpesticides.org

Northwest Coalition for Alternatives to Pesticides
http://www.efn.org/~ncap

Pesticide Action Network
http://www.panna.org/panna

Chapter 74

Environmental Hotlines

Acid Rain Hotline
Tel: 202-564-9620
Fax: 202-564-9620

The Acid Rain Hotline records questions and document requests covering all areas of the Acid Rain Program. The Hotline assists callers who have specific technical or policy questions by forwarding those inquiries to experienced EPA Acid Rain Division personnel, who review them and respond to the caller, typically within 24 hours. Utilities may find the Hotline especially useful for obtaining information that may help them comply with the acid rain regulations. Order Process: Dial the main hotline phone number. Listen to categories. Leave technical questions in the mail box; request documents from a menu, if desired. All documents are free and will be mailed promptly.

Aerometric Information Retrieval System (AIRS)—Airs Quality Subsystem (AQS)—Hotline
Toll Free: 800-334-2405

AIRS is an information management system which is the national repository for data about airborne pollution in the United States, and to a limited extent, in various other countries. As with many systems, the completeness of the data in this data base depends on what data

"Hotlines," an undated fact sheet produced by the U.S. Environmental Protection Agency (EPA). Available online at http://www.epa.gov/epahome/ hotline.htm. Cited February 2003. Resources verified February 2003.

has been submitted. AIRS comprises three major subsystems. This hotline is dedicated to AQS and GCS systems: AQS—Air Quality Subsystem—measurements of ambient concentrations of air pollutants and associated meteorological and monitoring site data; and GCS—Geo-Common Subsystem—reference information that is used with all of the AIRS subsystems. Reference information includes codes and code descriptions to identify places, pollutants, processes, geo-political entities, etc. The EPA compiles and maintains this information.

Aerometric Information Retrieval System (AIRS)—AIRS Facility Subsystem (AFS)—Helpline
Toll Free: 800-367-1044

AIRS is an information management system which is the national repository for data about airborne pollution in the United States, and to a limited extent, in various other countries. As with many systems, the completeness of the data in this data base depends on what data has been submitted. AIRS comprises three major subsystems. This hotline is dedicated to the AFS subsystem. AFS—The AIRS Facility Subsystem contains estimates of aerometric emissions, regulatory compliance data, and permit tracking data on point sources in the U. S.

Air Risk Information Center Hotline (Air RISC)
Tel: 919-541-0888
Fax: 919-541-1818

The Air RISC provides technical assistance and information in areas of health, risk, and exposure assessment for toxic and criteria air pollutants. Services include: the hotline for direct access to EPA experts; detailed technical assistance for more in-depth evaluations or information; and general technical guidance in the form of documents, reports and training materials related to health, risk and exposure assessment.

Antimicrobial Information Hotline
Tel: 703-308-0127
Fax: 703-308-6467

The Antimicrobials Information Hotline provides direct answers to questions concerning current antimicrobial issues. Please call during normal business hours (Monday-Friday 9 a.m. to 5 p.m.) or leave a message after hours. The information provided can cover issues relevant to any or all antimicrobial pesticides including health and safety issues, registration and re-registration issues, as well as information on pesticide laws, rules, and regulations relating to antimicrobials.

Asbestos Abatement/Management Ombudsman
Toll Free: 800-368-5888
Tel: 202-566-2822 (Washington, DC Area Local)
Fax: 202-566-0954

The assigned mission of the Asbestos Ombudsman is to provide to the public sector, including individual citizens and community services, information on handling, abatement, and management of asbestos in schools, the work place, and the home. Interpretation of the asbestos in schools requirements is provided. Publications to explain recent legislation are also available. Services are provided to private citizens, state agencies, local agencies, local public and private school systems, abatement contractors, and consultants.

Center for Exposure Assessment Modeling (CEAM) Help Desk
Tel: 706-355-8400

The Center for Exposure Assessment Modeling (CEAM) works to meet the scientific and technical exposure assessment needs of the EPA other state environmental and resource management agencies. CEAM provides proven predictive exposure assessment techniques for aquatic, terrestrial, and multimedia pathways for organic chemicals and metals and distributes environmental simulation model and database software for urban and rural nonpoint sources, conventional and toxic pollution of streams, lakes and estuaries, tidal hydrodynamics, geochemical equilibrium, and aquatic food chain bioaccumulation.

Clean Air Technology Center (CATC) Infoline
Tel: 919-541-0800 (English)
Tel: 919-541-1800 (Spanish)
Fax: 919-541-0242

The CATC provides technical support and assistance to state and local agencies and others in evaluating air pollution problems and pollution prevention and control technology applications at stationary air pollution sources. Specifically, hotline assistance provides quick access and consultation with appropriate EPA staff on air pollution technology questions. It also provides information on EPA's Reasonably Active Control Technology (RACT) / Best Available Control Technology

(BACT) / Lowest Achievable Emission Rate (LAER) Clearinghouse (RBLC), Federal Small Business Assistance Program (SBAP), and International Technical Information Center for Global Greenhouse Gases.

Clearinghouse for Inventories and Emission Factors (CHIEF) Help Desk
Tel: 919-541-5285

The Clearinghouse for Inventories and Emission Factors is a means of exchanging information regarding air pollutant emissions between state and local pollution control agencies, private citizens, universities, contractors, and foreign governments. It addresses criteria pollutants and toxic pollutants from both stationary and area sources. The Clearinghouse offers several electronic air emission estimation tools, including the Factor Information Retrieval (FIRE) database, TANKS database, and Air CHIEF CD-ROM.

Emergency Planning and Community Right-To-Know Act (EPCRA) Hotline
Toll Free: 800-424-9346 or 800-553-7672 (TDD)
Tel: 703-412-9810 (Washington, DC Area Local) or 703-412-3323 (TDD)

This hotline provides information about the regulations and programs implemented for the following environmental statutes:

- Resource Conservation and Recovery Act (RCRA)

- Comprehensive Environmental Response Compensation and Liability Act (CERCLA, or Superfund)

- Emergency Planning and Community Right-to-Know Act (EPCRA)/Superfund Amendments Reauthorization Act (SARA) Title III

This hotline also provides referrals for documents related to these programs. Translation is available for Spanish-speaking callers.

Endangered Species Hotline
Toll Free: 800-447-3813

This hotline provides an introduction to the Endangered Species Protection Program (ESPP) and its goals to protect endangered species from harmful pesticides and to minimize the impact of the Program on pesticide users. It answers questions related to the ESPP and the Endangered Species Act.

Energy Star
Toll Free: 888-STAR-YES, (888-782-7937)
Tel: 202-775-6650 (Washington, DC Area Local)

ENERGY STAR was a voluntary labeling program designed to identify and promote energy-efficient products, in order to reduce carbon dioxide emissions. EPA partnered with the U.S. Department of Energy in 1996 to promote the ENERGY STAR label, with each agency taking responsibility for particular product categories. ENERGY STAR has expanded to cover new homes, most of the buildings sector, residential heating and cooling equipment, major appliances, office equipment, lighting, consumer electronics, and more product areas. Call to receive helpful information regarding your household products.

Environmental Financing Information Network (EFIN)
Tel: 202-564-4994

The EFIN Center operates an infoline that provides callers with referrals, assistance with accessing and searching the EFIN database, and a point of contact for ordering documents.

Environmental Justice Hotline
Toll Free: 800-962-6215

Established to receive calls from concerned citizens about justice issues in their communities, the purpose of the Hotline is to make information easily accessible to the public and to the media, and to assist in the resolution of environmental justice issues. The Hotline is answered by the staff of the Office of Environmental Justice (OEJ). A procedure has been established to ensure thorough follow-up. A brochure describing the Hotline (in both English and Spanish) is available.

EPA Enforcement Economic Models Helpline
Toll Free: 888-ECONSPT, (888-326-6778)

EPA Enforcement Economic Models helpline offered by OECA provides information and assistance with enforcement financial computer models that calculate an individual's, municipality's or corporation's financial ability to pay environmental penalties. This service is primarily targeted at local state, and federal agency employees. This service is staffed by a agency contractor.

EPA Grants and Fellowships Hotline (National Center for Environmental Research Hotline)
Toll Free: 800-490-9194

This hotline provides easy access to research funding opportunities—grants and fellowships as well as past and present research projects and programs.

EPA Imported Vehicles and Engines Public Help Line
Tel: 202-564-9660 (Automated Voice)

The EPA Imported Vehicles and Engines Public Help Line is an automated telefax system which lets callers order documents about the importation of vehicles. Additional information can be found on the EPA Office of Transportation and Air Quality's (OTAQ) website at http://www.epa.gov/otaq/imports/imptop.htm and the U.S. Customs Service's website at http://www.customs.ustreas.gov/imp-exp2/informal/car.htm. The Importation Section of the EPA Vehicle Programs and Compliance Division, which can be reached at 202-564-9240 during business hours (Eastern Standard Time), may also be helpful.

Federal Facilities Docket Hotline
Toll Free: 800-548-1016

The Federal Agency Hazardous Waste Compliance docket is a key component in identifying and resolving environmental problems at federal facilities that engage in hazardous waste activity or have the potential to release hazardous substances into the environment. The docket contains information submitted by federal agencies to EPA under Sections 3005, 3010, and 3016 of the Resource Conservation and Recovery Act (RCRA) and under Section 103 of CERCLA.

Indoor Air Quality Information Clearinghouse (IAQINFO)
Toll Free: 800-438-4318

The IAQ INFO provides access to public information on indoor environments through a range of services including: an operator-assisted hotline; distribution of relevant EPA publications at no charge; literature searches on a topic for further reference; referrals to appropriate government agencies, research, public interest, and industry representatives; and information about training courses and materials.

Inspector General Hotline
Toll Free: 888-546-8740

Tel: 202-566-2476 (Washington, DC Area Local)
Fax: 202-401-1895

The Inspector General Hotline was established to receive and control complaints alleging fraud, waste, abuse, or mismanagement within the Environmental Protection Agency.

Integrated Risk Information System (IRIS) Hotline
Tel: 301-345-2870

IRIS is a database of human health effects that may result from exposure to various substances found in the environment. The hotline can assist you in using IRIS and understanding the methods used by the EPA for deriving values and the limitations of use.

Local Government Reimbursement Program Helpline
Toll Free: 800-431-9209

In 1987, Congress established the Local Government Reimbursement program under Superfund. The purpose of this program is to help defray expenses incurred by local municipalities in responding to hazardous substance threats such as chemical fires and explosions, tire fires, or fires at landfills. The reimbursement limit is $25,000 per response. The Agency employed its major contractor to help inform local governments about the program.

Methods Information Communication Exchange Service (MICE)
Tel: 703-676-4690
Fax: 703-318-4682

The Methods Information Communication Exchange (MICE) Service provides answers to questions and takes comments over the telephone on technical issues regarding the EPA Office of Solid Waste's methods manual known as "Test Methods for Evaluating Solid Waste: Physical/ Chemical Methods" or SW-846. Questions regarding the status of the methods, organic analyses, inorganic analyses, characteristics tests, and quality control issues are answered by chemists, groundwater monitoring specialists, and sampling experts who are experienced and knowledgeable in SW-846 procedures.

Mexico Border Hotline
Toll Free: 800-334-0741 (English/Spanish)

This hotline answers questions concerning the U.S.-Mexico Border XXI Program. This bi-national effort is working to ensure sustainable development through protection of human health and the environment and proper management of natural resources in both countries.

National Alternative Fuels Hotline

Toll Free: 800-423-1363
Tel: 703-934-3069 (Washington, DC Area Local)

Many alternative fuels are being used today in place of fossil fuels like oil. The U.S. Department of Energy classifies the following fuels as alternatives to gasoline: biodiesel, electric fuel, ethanol, hydrogen, methanol, natural gas, propane, p-series, and solar fuel. This hotline, offered by DOE, provides information on these fuels, as well as other related resources with more detailed information.

National Service Center for Environmental Publications (NSCEP)

Toll Free: 800-490-9198

The National Service Center for Environmental Publications maintains and distributes EPA publications in hardcopy, CD ROM and other multimedia formats. The publication inventory includes over 7,000 titles. NSCEP also develops and distributes the annual EPA National Publications Catalog.

National Hispanic Indoor Air Quality Hotline

Toll Free: 800-SALUD-12 (800-725-8312) (Spanish/English)

The National Hispanic Indoor Air Quality Hotline provides bilingual (Spanish/English) information about indoor air pollutants that consumers may find inside their homes, offices or schools.

National Lead Information Center Hotline

Toll Free: 800-424-LEAD (800-424-5323)

The Environmental Health Center (EHC) of the National Safety Council manages the National Lead Information Center (NLIC) under a cooperative agreement with the Environmental Protection Agency. The Hotline distributes a basic information packet on lead that includes the EPA brochure "Lead Poisoning and Your Children," three fact sheets, and a list of state and local contacts for additional information.

National Pesticide Information Center

Toll Free: 800-858-7378
Fax: 541-737-0761

A cooperative effort of Oregon State University and the EPA, this hotline offers science-based information about a wide variety of pesticide-related subjects and serves as a source of factual chemical, health, and environmental information about more than 600 pesticide active ingredients incorporated into over 50,000 different products registered for use in the United States since 1947.

National Poison Control Hotline
Toll Free: 800-222-1222 (emergency only)
Tel: 202-362-3867 (for administrative and materials requests)
TDD: 202-362-8563

The National Poison Control Hotline was established to respond to emergency calls from concerned citizens about poison prevention. Housed in The National Capital Poison Center in Washington, DC, this hotline is manned 24 hours a day/7 days a week by registered nurses or pharmacists with backgrounds in critical care. All specialists have passed a national certification exam in toxicology. The Poison Center staff has access to a 24 hour interpreter service, with over 140 languages available, so callers who do not speak English are able to receive immediate help for emergency calls.

National Radon Hotline
Toll Free: 800-SOS-RADON (800-767-7236)
Toll Free Helpline: 800-55-RADON
Tel: 202-293-2270
Fax: 202-293-0032

Run by the National Health Center of the National Safety Council, this hotline provides answers to questions regarding radon. Their website also offers fact sheets, educational materials, and activity reports.

National Response Center Hotline
Toll Free: 800-424-8802
Tel: 202-267-2675 (Washington, DC Area Local)

The National Response Center is the federal government's national communications center, which is staffed 24 hours a day by U.S. Coast Guard officers and marine science technicians. The NRC receives all reports of releases involving hazardous substances and oil that trigger the federal notification requirements under several laws. Reports to the NRC activate the National Contingency Plan and the federal government's response capabilities.

National Small Flows Clearinghouse Hotline
Toll Free: 800-624-8301
Tel: 304-293-4191 (West Virginia Local)

Managed by West Virginia University, the National Small Flows Clearinghouse provides information and technical assistance to help small communities and homeowners reach practical, affordable solutions to their waste water treatment problems.

Ozone Protection Hotline
Toll Free: 800-296-1996
Fax: 301-231-6377

The Stratospheric Ozone Information Hotline offers consultation on ozone protection regulations and requirements under Title VI of the Clean Air Act Amendments (CAAA) of 1990. Title VI covers the following key aspects of the production, use, and safe disposal of ozone-depleting chemicals: 1) production phase out and controls; 2) servicing of motor vehicle air conditioners; 3) recycling and emission reduction; 4) technician and equipment certification; 5) approval of alternatives; 6) a ban of nonessential uses; 7) product labeling; and 8) federal procurement. The hotline also sends out publications: Title VI of CAAA and all published rules, Federal Register notices, science and policy reports, and Fact Sheets.

Pay-As-You-Throw (PAYT) Helpline
Toll Free: 888-EPA-PAYT (888-372-7298)

In communities with pay-as-you-throw programs (also known as unit pricing or variable-rate pricing), residents are charged for the collection of municipal solid waste-ordinary household trash-based on the amount the throw away. This creates a direct economic incentive to recycle more and to generate less waste. EPA supports this new approach to solid waste management because it encompasses environmental sustainability, economic sustainability, and equity. The hotline provides information and tools to support this ongoing effort.

Pollution Prevention Information Clearinghouse (PPIC)
Tel: 202-566-0799
Fax: 202-566-0794

The Pollution Prevention Information Clearinghouse (PPIC) is a free, nonregulatory service of the U.S. EPA. PPIC is dedicated to reducing or eliminating industrial pollutants through technology transfer, education, and public awareness. A Reference and Referral Telephone Service is available to answer questions, take orders for documents distributed by PPIC, or refer callers to appropriate contacts.

RCRA, Superfund and EPCRA Hotline
Toll Free: 800-424-9346 or 800-553-7672 (TDD)
Tel: 703-412-9810 (Washington, DC Area Local), or 703-412-3323 (TDD)

The Resource Conservation and Recovery Act (RCRA) was enacted in 1976 to address the issue of how to safely manage and dispose of the huge volumes of municipal and industrial waste generated nationwide. The Emergency Planning and Community Right-to-Know Act (EPCRA) also known as SARA Title III, was enacted in November 1986. This law provides an infrastructure at the state and local levels to plan for chemical emergencies. This hotline is dedicated to providing information and fielding requests to the appropriate office.

Safe Drinking Water Hotline
Toll Free: 800-426-4791
Fax: 703-412-3333

The SDW Hotline provides information about EPA's drinking water regulations and other related drinking water and ground water topics to the regulated community, State and local officials, and the public. Specifically, the Hotline clarifies drinking water regulations, provides appropriate 40 CFR and Federal Register citations, explains EPA-provided policies and guidelines and gives update information on the status of regulations. The Hotline can also provide State and local contacts.

Small Business Ombudsman Hotline
Toll Free: 800-368-5888
Tel: 202-566-2822 (Washington, DC Area Local)
Fax: 202-566-0954

The mission of the EPA Small Business Ombudsman Clearinghouse/ Hotline is to provide information to private citizens, small communities, small business enterprises, and trade associations representing the small business sector regarding regulatory activities. Mailings are made to update the audience on recent regulatory actions. Special attention is directed to apprising the trade associations representing small business interests with current regulatory developments. Technical questions are answered following appropriate contacts with program office staff members. Questions addressed cover all media program aspects within EPA.

STORET Water Quality System Hotline
Toll Free: 800-424-9067

The EPA maintains two data management systems containing water quality information: the Legacy Data Center (LDC) and STORET (STOrage and RETrieval). STORET contains data collected beginning in 1999, along with older data that has been properly documents and migrated from the LDC. Both systems contain raw biological, chemical and physical data on surface and ground water collected by federal, state and local agencies, Indian Tribes, volunteer groups, academics, and other. All 50 States, territories, and jurisdictions of the U.S., along with portions of Canada and Mexico are represented in these systems.

Tools for Schools (IAQ) Technical Assistance Hotline
Toll Free: 866-837-3721

A Technical assistance information hotline for users of the IAQ Tools for Schools Kit, the Tools for Schools Technical Assistance Hotline provides information and answers questions on topics including mechanical systems, ventilation, pollutant sources, and application of the Kit. The hotline can be accessed weekdays from 8:30 a.m. to 4:30 p.m. central time through their toll-free telephone number.

Toxic Release Inventory—User Support Service
Tel: 202-566-0250

TRI-US offers specialized assistance to individuals seeking Toxics Release Inventory (TRI) data collected by EPA under Section 313 of EPCRA (Emergency Planning and Community Right-To-Know Act). It provides comprehensive search assistance for the TRI on-line and CD-ROM databases. In addition to access, user support and search assistance, TRI-US conducts training and demonstrations for both the TRI CD-ROM and the National Library of Medicine/ TOXNET databases.

Toxic Release Inventory—Community Right-To-Know— EPCRA Hotline
Toll Free: 800-424-9346 or 800-553-7672 (TDD)
Tel: 703-412-9810 (Washington, DC Area Local) or 703-412-3323 (TDD)

The Toxics Release Inventory (TRI) is a source of information concerning waste management activities and toxic chemicals that are being used, manufactured, treated, transported, or released into the environment. Two statutes, Section 313 of the Emergency Planning and Community Right-To-Know Act (EPCRA) and section 6607 of the Pollution Prevention Act (PPA), mandate that a publicly accessible toxic chemical database be developed and maintained by U.S. EPA.

Toxic Substances Control Act (TSCA) Hotline
Tel: 202-554-1404
Fax: 202-554-5603

The TSCA Assistance Information Service (TAIS) provides technical assistance and information about programs implemented under TSCA, the Asbestos School Hazard Abatement Act (ASHAA), the Asbestos Hazard Emergency Response Act (AHERA), the Asbestos School Hazard Abatement Reauthorization Act (ASHARA), the Residential Lead-Based Paint Hazard Reduction Act (Title X of TSCA), and EPA's 33/50 program.

WasteWise Helpline
Toll Free: 800-EPA-WISE (800-372-9473)
Fax: 703-308-8686

WasteWise is a free, voluntary, EPA program through which organizations eliminate costly municipal solid waste, benefiting their bottom line and the environment. WasteWise provides free technical assistance to help you develop, implement, and measure your waste reduction activities. WasteWise offers publicity to organizations that are successful in reducing waste through EPA publications, case studies, and national and regional events.

Wetlands Information Hotline
Toll Free: 800-832-7828
Tel: 202-566-1730 (Washington, DC Area Local)
Fax: 202-566-1736

The EPA Wetlands Helpline is a contractor-operated, toll-free telephone service and e-mail correspondent, which answers requests for information about wetlands regulation, legislation and policy pursuant to Section 404 of the Clean Water Act, wetlands values and functions, and wetlands agricultural issues.

Chapter 75

Environmental Protection Agency (EPA) Compliance and Enforcement Information

The Office of Enforcement and Compliance Assurance (OECA), working in partnership with EPA Regional Offices, State Governments, Tribal Governments and other Federal agencies, ensures compliance with the nation's environmental laws. Employing an integrated approach of compliance assistance, compliance incentives and innovative civil and criminal enforcement, OECA and its partners seek to maximize compliance and reduce threats to public health and the environment.

Compliance and Enforcement information is provided through nine broad topic areas. Information about each topic area is found at the following Internet sites:

Planning and Results
http://www.epa.gov/compliance/planning/index.html

Provides overall program direction and results of the enforcement and compliance assurance program. This site also provides reports on enforcement trends and progress and identifies measures and checklists used to evaluate program accomplishments. The national compliance data systems, which are the basis for the reports and analysis, and State and tribal activities in the enforcement and compliance area are also found on this site.

"Compliance and Enforcement," an undated fact sheet produced by the U.S. Environmental Protection Agency. Available online at http://www.epa.gov/compliance/index.html. Cited February 2003. Resources verified February 2003.

Compliance Assistance

http://www.epa.gov/compliance/assistance/index.html

Helps the regulated community understand and meet their environmental obligations. Statute-specific assistance includes compliance assistance activities or tools related to specific EPA statutes or regulations. Sector-oriented assistance addresses compliance issues or needs across particular business and industry sectors, or to government sectors.

Compliance Incentives and Auditing

http://www.epa.gov/compliance/incentives/index.html

Provides information on innovative enforcement and compliance approaches through policies and programs that eliminate, reduce or waive penalties under certain conditions for business, industry, and government facilities.

Compliance Monitoring

http://www.epa.gpv/compliance/monitoring/index.html

Provides information related to assuring compliance by the regulated community with environmental laws/regulations through effective monitoring and compliance assessment.

Civil Enforcement

http://www.epa.gov/compliance/civil/index.html

Provides information on the investigations and cases brought to address the most significant violations, and includes EPA administrative actions and judicial cases referred to the Department of Justice. EPA works closely with states to implement federal programs, as well as with tribes and federal agencies.

Clean Up Enforcement

http://www.epa.gpv/compliance/cleanup/index.html

Provides information related to environmental cleanup under the Comprehensive, Environmental Response, Compensation and Liability Act (CERCLA or Superfund), the Resource Conservation and Recovery Act (RCRA), including the Underground Storage Tank (UST) Program and the Oil Pollution Act (OPA) under the Clean Water Act.

Environmental Justice

http://www.epa.gov/compliance/environmentaljustice/index.html

Provides access to information regarding the fair treatment and meaningful involvement of all people regardless of race, color, national origin, or income with respect to the development, implementation, and enforcement of environmental laws, regulations, and policies.

Criminal Enforcement
http://www.epa.gov/compliance/criminal/index.html

Provides information on the multi-media criminal enforcement program and its role in identifying, apprehending, and assisting prosecutors in successfully convicting those who are responsible for the most significant and egregious violations of environmental law that pose substantial risks to human health and the environment.

The National Environmental Policy Act (NEPA)
http://www.epa.gov/compliance/nepa/index.html

Requires federal agencies to integrate environmental values into their decision making processes by considering the environmental impacts of their proposed actions and reasonable alternatives to those actions. To meet this requirement, federal agencies prepare a detailed statement known as an Environmental Impact Statement (EIS), which is available along with other related information from this site.

Index

Index

Page numbers followed by 'n' indicate table or illustration.

A

"About Cancer Clusters" (CDC) 29n
absorption, defined 585
AC *see* alternating current
acaricides, described 285
ACGIH *see* American Conference of Governmental Industrial Hygienists
acid rain
  nitrogen oxides 153, 158, 159
  overview 157–62
  sulfur dioxide 155, 158, 159
"Acid Rain" (EPA) 157n
Acid Rain Hotline 605
acrylamide
  drinking water 215
  drinking water regulation *204*
actinolite 95
Action on Smoking and Health (ASH)
  contact information 595
  Web site address 603
acute
  versus chronic *314*
  defined 585

advanced oxidation, described 228
Advanced Research Cooperation in Environmental Health (ARCH program) 576–77
Aerometric Information Retrieval System (AIRS) Hotline 605
African-Americans
  hypertension 563
  lung cancer 564
AFS *see* AIRS Facility Subsystem
age factor, health threats 555–56
Agency for Toxic Substances and Disease Registry (ATSDR)
  asbestos publication 95n
  contact information 595
  described 592
Agent Orange 263, 265
agricultural workers, environmental health 558–59
Ah receptors, dioxins 264
air conditioned spaces, mold control 128
air duct cleaning, indoor air quality 133–47
air exchange rate, described 92
air pollution, overview 5–6
  see also indoor air quality; outdoor air quality

625

air quality index (AQI)
  carbon monoxide *184*
  color scale *177*
  nitrogen dioxide *186*
  overview 175–87
  ozone *180*
  particulate matter *182*
  sulfur dioxide *185*
"Air Quality Index" (EPA) 175n
"Air Quality Where You Live" (EPA) 149n
Air RISC *see* Air Risk Information Center Hotline
Air Risk Information Center Hotline (Air RISC) 606
AIRS *see* Aerometric Information Retrieval System
AIRS Facility Subsystem (AFS) Helpline 606
AIRS Quality Subsystem (AQS) Hotline 605
air stripping, described 228
alachlor
  drinking water 215
  drinking water regulation *204*
Alchemy Environmental Laboratories, Inc., drinking water chlorination publication 219n
aldehydes, indoor air quality 104, 108
algicides, described 284
allergens
  asthma 27–28
  mold 123, 124–25
allergies
  air ducts 133–34
  bioengineering 516–17
  chemicals 315
  diagnosis 62
  environmental hazards 17
  formaldehyde 116
  smallpox vaccine 444
  see also multiple chemical sensitivity syndrome
"Allergies - Multiple Chemical Sensitivity" (NIEHS) 327n
Allergy to Latex Education and Resourse Team, Web site address 603
alpha particles, drinking water regulation *208*, 214

alternating current (AC), described 372–73
alternative energy, acid rain 160
aluminum, drinking water regulation *211*
ambient, defined 585
American Conference of Governmental Industrial Hygienists (ACGIH), described 591–92
American Fibromyalgia Syndrome Association, Web site address 602
American Gulf War Veterans Association, Web site address 603
American Lung Association, contact information 595
American Red Cross, contact information 595
Americans for Nonsmokers Rights, contact information 595
Americans with Disabilities Act Hotline, contact information 596
American Water Works Association, contact information 222
americium 363
ammonia
  defined 221
  formaldehyde 121
amnesic shellfish poisoning 495–97
amosite 95
amoxicillin 419
analyte, defined 585
aniline dyes 535
anthophyllite 95
anthrax, overview 409–23
antibiotic medications
  anthrax 418–22
  bioengineering 517
  pneumonic plague 436
  tularemia 445, 447
antifouling agents, described 284
Antimicrobial Information Hotline 606
antimicrobial pesticides, described 286–87
antimicrobials
  anthrax 418
  described 284
antimony
  drinking water 215
  drinking water regulation *201*

apoptosis, described 71
AQI *see* air quality index
AQS *see* AIRS Quality Subsystem
aquifers
  defined 255, 586
  water quality 192–93
ARCH program *see* Advanced Research Cooperation in Environmental Health
"Are Bioengineered Foods Safe?" (Thompson) 513n
arenaviruses, described 449–50
arsenic
  drinking water 194, 214
  drinking water regulation *201*
asbestos
  drinking water 215
  drinking water regulation *201*
  questions and answers 95–98
Asbestos Abatement/Management Ombudsman, contact information 607
asbestosis, described 96–97
ASH *see* Action on Smoking and Health
Association of Birth Defects Children, Web site address 601
asthma
  children 91
  environmental triggers 25–28
  formaldehyde 116
  mold 123
  ozone 165, 181
  research 559–62
  statistics 9–10
  sulfur dioxide 155
"Asthma Facts" (EPA) 25n
Atomic Energy Act
  described 56
  hazardous waste 38
atrazine
  drinking water 215
  drinking water regulation *204*
ATSDR *see* Agency for Toxic Substances and Disease Registry
attractants, described 284
autoimmune diseases, women 548
azinphos-methyl *532*

B

Bacillus anthracis 409–21
Bacillus thuringiensis 287, 290–91, 300, 515
backflow, defined 255
background level, defined 586
bacteria
  defined 255
  swimming water *259*
  well water 245
Bailey, John E. 504–6
barium
  drinking water 215
  drinking water regulation *201*
Barlow, Janice 549
Barrett, J. Carl 68
"Basic Principles of the Worker Protection Standard" (EPA) 295n
BEACH *see* Beaches Environmental Assessment and Coastal Health Act
Beaches Environmental Assessment and Coastal Health Act (BEACH; 2000) 257
bedrock, defined 586
beef tapeworm 475–77
"Before You Go to the Beach ..." (EPA) 257n
Benz, Chris 549
benzene
  drinking water 216
  drinking water regulation *204*
benzopyrene
  drinking water 215
  drinking water regulation *204*
beryllium
  drinking water 215
  drinking water regulation *202*
BEST *see* Bridging Education, Science and Technology Program
beta particles, drinking water regulation *208*, 214
biocides
  air ducts 143–45
  described 284
bioengineered food safety, overview 513–20
biological monitoring, defined 586

biopesticides, described 287–89
birth defects, environmental hazards 17–18
body burden, defined 586
"Botulism" (CDC) 425n
botulism, overview 425–28
breast cancer 546–47, 548–50, 568–70
Breast Cancer Action, Web site address 603
Brenner, Keri 545n
brevetoxins 495
Bridging Education, Science and Technology Program (BEST) 580
bromate
    drinking water 217
    drinking water regulation *200*
bronchitis, ozone 165
"Brucellosis" (CDC) 429n
brucellosis, overview 429–32
bubonic plague, described 434
Buffler, Patricia 549
bunyaviruses, described 449–50

C

cadmium
    drinking water 215
    drinking water regulation *202*
    osteoporosis 547
CAFO *see* concentrated animal feeding operations
Californians for Alternatives to Toxics, Web site address 601
cancer
    airborne particles 108
    asbestos 97
    DEET 305–6
    dioxins 265
    drinking water 194, 214
    electric and magnetic fields 375–79
    environmental hazards 18
    environmental tobacco smoke 131
    ozone 166–67
    radiation 335–37
    toxic chemicals 316–17
    women 546–47
cancer clusters, described 29–31

carbofuran
    drinking water 215
    drinking water regulation *204*
carbon monoxide (CO)
    air quality index 183–85, *184*
    charcoal grills 105
    described 152–53
    detectors 61, 101
    environmental tobacco smoke 131
    indoor air quality 107
    overview 99–101
    treatment 108–9
"Carbon Monoxide" (NSC) 99n
carbon tetrachloride
    drinking water 216
    drinking water regulation *204*
carcinogens, described 317
Carson, Rachel 4
case control study, defined 586
CASTNET *see* Clean Air Status and Trends Network
CATC *see* Clean Air Technology Center
Catholic Charities USA, contact information 596
CDC *see* Centers for Disease Control and Prevention
CDRH (Center for Devices and Radiological Health) *see* US Food and Drug Administration
CEAM *see* Center for Exposure Assessment Modeling
CEC *see* Citizens' Environmental Coalition of New York
"Cell Phone Facts: Consumer Information on Wireless Phones, Questions and Answers" (FDA) 391n
cellular telephones
    electric and magnetic fields 389
    safety concerns 391–406
Center for Devices and Radiological Health (CDRH) *see* US Food and Drug Administration
Center for Exposure Assessment Modeling (CEAM) Help Desk 607
Center for Food Safety and Applied Nutrition (CFSAN) *see* US Food and Drug Administration

Centers for Disease Control and Prevention (CDC)
  contact information 596
  described 592
  publications
    anthrax 409n
    botulism 425n
    brucellosis 429n
    cancer clusters 29n
    Escherichia coli 479n
    pneumonic plague 433n
    salmonellosis 483n
    shigellosis 489n
    smallpox 439n
    tularemia 445n
    viral hemorrhagic fevers 449n
central nervous system (CNS), defined 586
CERCLA *see* Comprehensive Environmental Response, Compensation, and Liability Act
CESQG *see* conditionally exempt small quantity generators
CFC *see* chlorofluorocarbons
CFIDS (chronic fatigue and immune dysfunction syndrome) Association of America, Web site address 601
CFR *see* Code of Federal Regulations
CFSAN (Center for Food Safety and Applied Nutrition) *see* US Food and Drug Administration
"Chapter 8: Environmental Health" (DHHS) 3n
charcoal grills, indoor air quality 105
chemical biocides, air ducts 143–45
Chemical Injury Information Network, contact information 596
Chemical Injury Resource Associaton of Minnesota, Web site address 603
Chemically Sensitive Living, contact information 596
Chemical Manufacturers Association, Responsible Care Initiative, contact information 222
chemicals, workplace hazards 309–26
CHIEF*see* Clearinghouse for Inventories and Emission Factors

children
  asbestos 97–98
  asthma 26
  drinking water safety 193–94
  electric and magnetic fields 375–77
  environmental health 523–41, 565–67
  environmental tobacco smoke 132
  indoor air quality 90–91, 104
  Internet resources 601
  lead poisoning 9, 62–63, 155–56, 267–74, 543–44, 562–63
  mercury poisoning 379
  nitrogen dioxide 187
  nitrogen dioxide exposure 107
  ozone 180
  radiation exposure 336
  Salmonella 486
  sulfur dioxide 185
"Children's Environmental Exposures" (EPA) 523n
Children's Environmental Health Network, Web site address 601
Children's Health Environmental Coalition Network, Web Site address 601
chloramination, defined 221
chloramines
  defined 221
  drinking water regulation *201*
chlordane
  drinking water 215
  drinking water regulation *204*
chloride, drinking water regulation *211*
chlorination
  defined 221
  drinking water 219–22
"Chlorination of Drinking Water" (Alchemy Environmental Laboratories, Inc.) 219n
chlorine
  defined 221
  drinking water 216
  drinking water regulation *201*
Chlorine Chemistry Council, contact information 222
chlorine dioxide, drinking water 217
Chlorine Institute, Inc., contact information 222

chlorite
  drinking water 217
  drinking water regulation *200*
chlorobenzene
  drinking water 216
  drinking water regulation *204*
chlorofluorocarbons (CFC), described
  168
chlorpynifos *532*
cholinesterase inhibitors, described
  275–76
choramine, drinking water 217
chromium
  drinking water 215
  drinking water regulation *202*
chronic
  versus acute *314*
  defined 586
chronic fatigue and immune dysfunction syndrome (CFIDS), Internet resources 601
chrysolite 95
Cipro *see* ciprofloxacin
ciprofloxacin (Cipro) 418–22
cis-1,2-dichloroethylene
  drinking water 216
  drinking water regulation *205*
Citizens' Environmental Coalition of New York (CEC), contact information 598
Citizens For Health, Web site address 603
"Citizen's Guide to Radon: The Guide to Protect Yourself and Your Family from Radon" (EPA) 341n
Citizens United to Reduce Emissions of Formaldehyde Poisoning Association, Web site address 603
Clarke, Tina 549
Clean Air Act
  enforcement 620
  MTBE 231
  national ambient air quality standards 149
Clean Air Act Amendments (1990) 86
Clean Air Status and Trends Network (CASTNET) 158
Clean Air Technology Center (CATC) Infoline 607

cleaning products, indoor air quality 92
Clean Water Act
  described 56
  hazardous waste 38
  regulation 56
Clearinghouse for Inventories and Emission Factors (CHIEF) Help Desk 608
Clostridium botulinum 425–28
clotrimazole 422
CNS *see* central nervous system
CO *see* carbon monoxide
coal
  acid rain 159
  sufur dioxide 185
coal stoves, maintenance schedule *113*
coated paper products, formaldehyde 118
coatings, formaldehyde 118
Code of Federal Regulations (CFR)
  emergency planning 78
  waste management regulations 35
cohort study, defined 586
coliforms, drinking water *198*, 213
color, drinking water regulation *211*
color additives, described 503–11
"Color Additives Fact Sheet" (FDA) 503n
combustion appliances, indoor air pollution 103–14
community, hazardous waste regulations 48–50
community health
  overview 7
  research 571–82
Community Right-to-Know requirements *see* Emergency Planning and Community Right-to-Know Act
"Compliance and Enforcement" (EPA) 619n
composite sample, defined 586
Comprehensive Environmental Response, Compensation, and Liability Act (CERCLA; Superfund) 34, 56, 591
computers, electric and magnetic fields 387–88
concentrated animal feeding operations (CAFO), well water 245

concentration, defined 586
condensation
air ducts 141–42
mold control 129
conditionally exempt small quantity generators (CESQG), described 40
confining layer, defined 255
Consumer Product Safety Commission *see* US Consumer Product Safety Commission
contaminants
defined 255, 587
drinking water 192–94
copper
drinking water 215
drinking water regulation *202, 211*
corrosivity
described 36
drinking water regulation *211*
cosmetics, formaldehyde 118
CPSC *see* US Consumer Product Safety Commission
crocidolite 95
cross-connection, defined 255
Crutzen, Paul 168
cryptosporidiosis
described 469–71
statistics 6
Cryptosporidium, drinking water 193, *198*, 214, 233–36
Cryptosporidium parvum, foodborne illness 469–71
"Current Drinking Water Standards" (EPA) 197n
curtains, formaldehyde 118
cutaneous anthrax, described 410
cyanide
drinking water 215
drinking water regulation *202*
Cyclospora cayetanensis, foodborne illness 471–72
cyclosporiasis, described 471–72
cysticercosis, described 475–77

D

dalapon
drinking water 215
drinking water regulation *204*

DBCP *see* 1,2-dibromo-3-chloropropane
DBPS *see* disinfection byproducts
DC *see* direct current
DEET (N,N-diethyl-meta-toluamide), overview 303–8
"DEET: General Fact Sheet" (NPIC) 303n
defoliants, described 285
dental fluorosis, described 215
deoxyribonucleic acid (DNA)
electric and magnetic fields 382
research 67–71
Department of Agriculture *see* US Department of Agriculture
Department of Energy *see* US Department of Energy
Department of Health and Human Services *see* US Department of Health and Human Services
Department of Housing and Urban Development *see* US Department of Housing and Urban Development
Department of Labor *see* US Department of Labor
dermal, defined 587
dermatitis, environmental hazards 18
desiccants, described 285
detection limit, defined 587
detoxification, described 71
DHHS *see* US Department of Health and Human Services
di 2-ethylhexyl adipate
drinking water 215
drinking water regulation *205*
di 2-ethylhexyl phthalate
drinking water 216
drinking water regulation *205*
diarrheic shellfish poisoning 495–97
Diazinon *532*
dibromochloropropane, drinking water 216
dichloromethane
drinking water 216
drinking water regulation *205*
diet and nutrition
children 525–27
family environmental health 64
Dine College, environmental research 578

dinoflagellates 495
dinophysis toxins 495
dinoseb
  drinking water 216
  drinking water regulation *205*
"Dioxin Research at the National Institute of Environmental Health Sciences (NIEHS)" (NIEHS) 263n
dioxins
  drinking water 216
  drinking water regulation *205*
  overview 263–66
diphenoxylate 490
diquat
  drinking water 216
  drinking water regulation *205*
direct current (DC), described 372–73
disinfectants, described 284
disinfection byproducts (DBPS)
  chlorination 220
  defined 221
  drinking water 194, 233–39
  drinking water regulation *200–201*
disposal facilities, described 41
DNA *see* deoxyribonucleic acid
DNA polymorphism, described 68
DOE *see* US Department of Energy
DOL *see* US Department of Labor
domoic acid 495
dose, defined 587
doxycycline 419, 421, 432
draperies, formaldehyde 118
drinking water
  chlorination 219–22
  contaminants 213–18
  disinfection byproducts 194, 233–39
  lead contamination 223–25
  malathion 276
  MTBE 227–32
  overview 191–96
  see also water quality
"Drinking Water and Health: What You Need to Know!" (EPA) 191n
"Drinking Water Contaminants" (EPA) 213n
"Drinking Water from Household Wells" (EPA) 241n

"Drinking Water Priority Rulemaking: Microbial and Disinfection Byproduct Rules" (EPA) 233n
duct cleaning, indoor air quality 133–47
durable-press fabrics, formaldehyde 118
Durham Technical Community College, environmental research 579

E

early detection, cancer 31
Earth Island Institute, Web site address 602
Ebola hemorrhagic fever 451
Ecology Center of Ann Arbor, Web site address 602
EDF (Environmental Defense Fund) Scorecard, Web site address 602
EFIN *see* Environmental Financing Information Network
EGP *see* Environmental Genome Project
EI/MCS Support Group of Louisville, Web site address 603
electric and magnetic fields (EMF), overview 369–90
electric power substations, electric and magnetic fields 385–86
electromagnetic energy, described 391–92
Emergency Planning and Community Right-to-Know Act (EPCRA; 1980) 50, 56, 77–86, 608
"Emergency Planning and Community Right-to-Know Act" (EPA) 77n
EMF *see* electric and magnetic fields
"EMF: Electric and Magnetic Field Associated with the Use of Electric Power, Questions and Answers" (NIEHS) 369n
EMF RAPID Program 369–70
emphysema
  environmental hazards 18
  ozone 165

Endangered Species Hotline 608
endometriosis
  dioxins 265
  environmental health 547
endothall
  drinking water 216
  drinking water regulation *205*
endrin
  drinking water 216
  drinking water regulation *205*
Energy Star, contact information 609
enteric viruses, drinking water *198*
environment
  described 3
  health hazards overview 3–16
Environmental Defense Fund
  contact information 596
  Web site address 602
"Environmental Diseases from A to Z"
  (NIEHS) 17n
Environmental Financing Information Network (EFIN), contact information 609
Environmental Genome Project
  (EGP)
  described 67–71
  minority populations 564–65
environmental groups, Internet resources 601–2
Environmental Health Coalition, Web
  site address 602
Environmental Health Network (California), contact information 596
Environmental Health Network of
  CA, Web site address 603
environmental health research evaluation 576–77, 578, 579
environmental illnesses (EI), Internet
  resources 603
Environmental Justice Hotline 609
environmentally responsive genes,
  described 69, 70–71
Environmental Protection Agency *see*
  US Environmental Protection
  Agency
environmental public health tracking
  program, described 73–75
Environmental Research Foundation,
  Web site address 602

environmental tobacco smoke (ETS),
  indoor air quality 131–32
"Environmental Tobacco Smoke"
  (NSC) 131n
EPA *see* US Environmental Protection Agency
EPCRA *see* Emergency Planning and
  Community Right-to-Know Act
epichlorohydrin
  drinking water 216
  drinking water regulation *205*
epidemiology
  defined 587
  electric and magnetic fields 375
  research 67
"*Escherichia Coli* O157:H7" (CDC)
  479n
Eschericia coli
  drinking water *198*
  foodborne illness 479–82
ethanol 535
ethnic factors
  air quality demographics *11–12*
  HIV infection 531
  see also racial factor
ethylbenzene
  drinking water 216
  drinking water regulation *205*
ethylene dibromide
  drinking water 216
  drinking water regulation *206*
exercise, heat cautions 63
exposure, defined 587
exposure assessment, defined 587
exposure-disease paradigm, described
  69–70

F

factory farms, described 245
"Facts about Lead in Drinking Water"
  (SCDHEC) 223n
"Facts about Pneumonic Plague"
  (CDC) 433n
"Facts about Tularemia" (CDC) 445n
"Family Guide: 20 Easy Steps to Per-
  sonal Environmental Health NOW"
  (NIEHS) 59n

family issues
anthrax 414
asbestos exposure 97–98
environmental health guide 59–66
lead poisoning 247–74
well water safety 241
"FAQs about Anthrax" (CDC) 409n
FDA *see* US Food and Drug Administration
feasibility study (FS), defined 587
fecal coliform, drinking water *198*, 213
Federal Facilities Docket Hotline 610
Federal Insecticide, Fungicide, and Rodenticide Act 56
fertility, environmental hazards 18–19
fertilizers, well water 245–46
fiberglass, air ducts 143, 145–46
fibromyalgia, Internet resources 602
Fibromyalgia Network, Web site address 602
filoviruses, described 449–50
"Finding Causes of Breast Cancer" (Brenner) 545n
fireplaces, indoor air quality *106*
Firman, James 555
flaviviruses, described 449–50
flu-like symptoms
anthrax 411, 412
carbon monoxide 107
cryptosporidiosis 469
cyclosporiasis 471
foodborne illness 458
formaldehyde 116
giardiasis 468
toxoplasmosis 473
fluoride
drinking water 215
drinking water regulation *202*, *211*
well water 245
fluoroquinolones 422, 436
foaming agents, drinking water regulation *211*
Food, Drug, and Cosmetic Act (1938) 506, 509
Food and Drug Administration *see* US Food and Drug Administration

foodborne illness
Eschericia coli 479–82
parasites 457–58, 467–77
prevention 457–65
Foodborne Pathogenic Microorganisms and Natural Toxins Handbook: The Bad Bug Book (FDA) 495n
food labels, chemicals 60
formaldehyde
allergic reaction 315–16
environmental tobacco smoke 131
indoor air quality 115–21
Francisella tularensis 445–47
Franzi, Anita 549
"Frequent Questions: Indoor Air" (EPA) 89n
"Frequenty Asked Questions (FAQ) about Plague" (CDC) 433n
"Frequenty Asked Questions (FAQ) about Tularemia" (CDC) 445n
Friends of the Earth, Web site address 602
FS *see* feasibility study
fuel oxygenates, described 227
fumigants, described 284
fungicides, described 284
furnaces
air duct cleaning 133–47
indoor air quality 91, *106*
maintenance schedule *113*
furniture, formaldehyde 120

G

GAC *see* granular activated carbon
gastrointestinal anthrax, described 410
genetic factors
radiation exposure 338
research 67–71
toxic chemicals 317–18
see also heredity
Giardia lamblia, drinking water *198*, 214, 234–35
Giarida duodenalis, foodborne illness 468–69
gigahertz (GHz), described 392
global environmental health, overview 8–9

glyphosate
  drinking water 216
  drinking water regulation *206*
goiter, environmental hazards 19
gradient, defined 587
granular activated carbon (GAC), described 228
Greenpeace, USA
  contact information 596
  Web site address 602
ground water
  hazardous waste regulations 50–51
  pollution 242–50
Gulf War syndrome, Internet resources 603
gypsum board
  formaldehyde 118
  mold control 128

H

haloacetic acids
  drinking water 217
  drinking water regulation *200*
hand washing, family environmental health 64
hantavirus pulmonary syndrome (HPS) 451
Hartwell, Leland H. 68
Hazard Evaluation System and Information Service (HESIS), chemical hazards publication 309n
Hazardous and Solid Waste Amendments (1984) *see* Resource Conservation and Recovery Act
Hazardous Materials Transportation Act 56
hazardous substances
  health risk evaluations 4
  versus toxicity 310
hazardous waste
  characteristics, described 36
  control overview 39–51
  described 35–39
  risk reduction overview 33–57
hazardous wastes, industry-generated *38*

hazardous waste sites, cleanup efforts 4
hazardous waste treatment technologies *45*
Health and Environment Resource Center, Web site address 602
health assessment for contaminated sites, defined 587–88
"Health Disparities Research" (NIEHS) 557n
health effects studies related to contaminants, defined 588
health registry, defined 588
Healthy People 2010 (DHHS) 3n
hearing loss, loud noise 60–61
heart disease, environmental hazards 19
heart rate, electric and magnetic fields 380
heavy metals
  defined 255
  osteoporosis 547
  well water 245
helminths, described 467, 475
hemorrhagic fever with renal syndrome (HFRS) 451
Henkel, John 511
Henny, Jane E. 514–20
HEPA *see* high-efficiency particle air filters
"Hepatitis A Virus" (FDA) 499n
hepatitis A virus, foodborne illness 499–501
heptachlor, drinking water 216
heptachlor eposide, drinking water 216
hepthachlor, drinking water regulation *206*
hepthachlor epoxide, drinking water regulation *206*
herbicides
  bioengineering 515–16
  described 284
  dioxins 263
heredity
  dioxins 264
  environmental susceptibilities 68–69
hertz (Hz), described 392

HESIS *see* Hazard Evaluation
System and Information
Service
heterotrophic plate count (HPC),
drinking water *198*
hexachlorophene 535
hexachlrocyclopentadiene, drinking
water 216
hexaghlorobenzene
drinking water 216
drinking water regulation *206*
HFRS *see* hemorrhagic fever with renal syndrome
HGP *see* Human Genome Project
high efficiency particle air filters
(HEPA)
air ducts 138
ozone 171
vacuum cleaners 141
Hispanics, air quality demographics
11–12
HIV *see* human immunodeficiency
virus
hormones
autoimmune diseases 548
electric and magnetic fields 380
environmental health 570–71
HOSPICE *see* National Hospice Association
"Hotlines" (EPA) 605n
household air pollution, described
90–93
household chemicals, environmental
safety 60, 61
household hazardous waste, regulation 53
Household Hazardous Waste Project,
contact information 597
"How Carbon Monoxide Affects the
Way We Live and Breathe" (EPA)
149n
"How Ground-Level Ozone Affects the
Way We Live and Breathe" (EPA)
149n
"How Lead Affects the Way We Live
and Breathe" (EPA) 149n
"How Nitrous Oxides Affects the
Way We Live and Breathe" (EPA)
149n

"How Particulate Matter Affects the
Way We Live and Breathe" (EPA)
149n
"How Sulfur Dioxide Affects the Way
We Live and Breathe" (EPA) 149n
HPS *see* hantavirus pulmonary syndrome
HUD *see* US Department of Housing
and Urban Development
human DNA polymorphism, research
67–71
Human Ecology Action League, Web
site address 603
Human Genome Project (HGP), described 68
human genome sequencing, described
68
human immunodeficiency virus
(HIV), children 531
hydrocarbons, indoor air quality 104,
108
hydrocortisone 536
hydrolysis, defined 221
hypochlorous acid, defined 222

I

IAQINFO *see* Indoor Air Quality
Information Clearinghouse
"IAQ Tools for Schools Kit - IAQ
Coordinator's Guide, Appendix H -
Mold and Moisture" (EPA) 123n
IARC *see* International Agency for
Research on Cancer
ignitability, described 36
immune deficiency diseases, environmental hazards 19
Imodium (loperamide) 490
"Indoor Air: Frequent Questions"
(EPA) 89n
indoor air quality
air ducts 133–47
combustion appliances 103–14
environmental tobacco smoke 131–32
formaldehyde 115–21
mold 123–29
overview 89–93
see also air pollution

"Indoor Air Quality" (NSC) 89n
Indoor Air Quality Information Clearinghouse (IAQINFO), contact information 610
Industrial/Environmental Toxicology Project, contact information 597
industrial wastes
  regulation 52
  well water 246–47
ingestion, defined 588
inhalation, defined 588
inhalation anthrax, described 410
inorganic chemicals, drinking water regulation *201–3*
insect growth regulators, described 285
insecticides, described 285
Inspector General Hotline 610–11
insulation
  indoor air quality 115
  mold control 126
Integrated Risk Information System (IRIS) Hotline 611
Interim Remedial Measure (IRM), defined 588
International Agency for Research on Cancer (IARC), described 592
International Ozone Association, Web site address 602
inversion, described 164
ionization, described 392
IRIS *see* Integrated Risk Information System
IRM *see* Interim Remedial Measure
iron, drinking water regulation *211*

J

job-related illnesses, environmental hazards 19–20

K

kidney diseases
  environmental hazards 20
  lead contamination 563
kilohertz (kHz), described 392
Kotelchuck, David 551n

L

labels, chemicals 60
land disposal restrictions, described 43
landfill sites
  described 43
  ground water contamination 51
land treatment, described 44
large quantity generators (LQG), described 40
larvicides, mosquito control 289–94, 300–301
"Larvicides for Mosquito Control" (EAP) 283n
latency period
  defined 588
  described 313–14
leachate, described 50
leaching, defined 588
leaching field, defined 255
lead
  drinking water 215, 223–25
  drinking water regulation *203*
  osteoporosis 548
  overview 267–74
lead contamination
  children 9, 62–63, 155–56, 267–74, 543–44, 562–63
  described 155–56
  environmental hazards 20
  statistics 9
"Lead in Paint, Dust, and Soil: Basic Information" (EPA) 267n
leaking underground storage tanks (LUST) 232
Learning Disabilities Association of America, Web site address 601
Legionella, drinking water *198*
leiomyomas 547
LEPC *see* Local Emergency Planning Committees
levofloxacin 422
lime, acid rain 160–61
lindane
  drinking water 216
  drinking water regulation *206*

Local Emergency Planning Committees (LEPC)
  described 79–80, 85
  hazardous substances 78–79
Local Government Reimbursement Program Hotline 611
Lomotil (diphenoxylate) 490
London Hazards Centre, Web site address 602
loperamide 490
low birth weight, lead contamination 562–63
LQG *see* large quantity generators
lung cancer
  biomarkers 564
  radon 341, *350, 351*
lung diseases
  ozone 165–66, 181
  pneumonic plague 433–37
lupus 548, 567
LUST *see* leaking underground storage tanks

M

magnetic fields *see* electric and magnetic fields
Maine Injured Workers Association, Web site address 603
malathion
  health hazards 275–77
  mosquito control 301
"Malathion Summary" (EPA) 275n
"Managing Radioactive Materials and Waste" (EPA) 353n
manganese, drinking water regulation *211*
Marburg hemorrhagic fever 451
Marine Protection, Research, and Sanctuaries Act 56
material safety data sheets (MSDS)
  described 80–82, 85
  workplace safety 314, 322, 325
Maximum Contaminant Level (MCL), defined 208
maximum contaminant level (MCL), defined 588–89

maximum contaminant level goal (MCLG), defined 208
maximum residual disinfectant level (MRDL), defined 208
maximum residual disinfectant level goal (MRDLG), defined 208–9
MCL *see* Maximum Contaminant Level
MCLG *see* maximum contaminant level goal
MCS *see* multiple chemical sensitivity syndrome
MCS Primer, Web site address 603
MCS Referral and Resources, contact information 597
MDF *see* medium density fiberboard
mechanical ventilation devices, described 92
media, defined 589
Medical Waste Tracking Act (1988) 34
medium density fiberboard (MDF), indoor air quality 115, 120
megahertz (MHz), described 392
melatonin, electric and magnetic fields 380–81
mercury
  drinking water 215
  drinking water regulation *203*
  environmental hazards 20
  health hazards 279–81
"Mercury Health Hazards" (ORS) 279n
metabolism, defined 589
Methods Information Communication Exchange Service (MICE), contact information 611
methoprene, described 291–92
methoxychlor
  drinking water 216
  drinking water regulation *206*
methyl-mercury *see* mercury
methyl-*tert*-butyl ether (MTBE)
  drinking water 217–18, 227–32
Mexico Border Hotline 611
MICE *see* Methods Information Communication Exchange Service
microbial larvicides, described 290–91
microbial pesticides, described 285, 287

microorganisms
   defined 255
   pesticides 283
   well water 244
"Microwave Oven Radiation" (FDA)
   357n
microwave radiation, overview 357–
   62
minerals, drinking water 194
Minority Worker Training Program
   (MWTP) 579–80
miticides, described 285
moisture control
   air ducts 133, 141–42
   mold 123–29
mold
   air ducts 133
   indoor air quality 123–29
Molina, Mario 168
molluscicides, described 285
monomolecular films, described 293
morbidity, defined 589
Morehouse College Public Health
   Science Institute, environmental
   research 578
Morehouse School of Medicine, environmental research 579
mosquito control, larvicides 289–94
Mothers for Natural Law, Web site
   address 602
motor vehicles
   acid rain 159–60
   air pollution 6
   carbon monoxide 152
   lead contamination 155
   ozone 169
MRDL see maximum residual disinfectant level
MRDLG see maximum residual disinfectant level goal
MSDS see material safety data sheets
MTBE see methyl-*tert*-butyl ether
"MTBE in Drinking Water" (EPA)
   227n
mucus, described 25
multiple chemical sensitivity syndrome (MCS)
   Internet resources 603
   overview 327–29

municipal solid waste, regulation 51–
   53
mutagens, described 318
MWTP see Minority Worker Training
   Program
Myerhoff Program 580

N

NADCA see National Air Duct Cleaners Association
NAIMA see North American Insulation Manufacturers Association
National Academy of Sciences, contact information 597
National Air Duct Cleaners Associa-
   tion (NADCA), indoor air quality
   136–38, 143, 146–47
National Alternative Fuels Hotline
   612
national ambient air quality stan-
   dards, described 149
National Atmospheric Deposition
   Program 158
National Center for Environmental
   Health Strategies (NCEHS), contact
   information 597
National CFIDS Foundation, Web site
   address 601
National Coalition Against the Mis-
   use of Pesticides
   contact information 597
   Web site address 604
National Drinking Water Advisory
   Council (NDWAC), described 199–
   200
National Environmental Policy Act
   (NEPA; 1969) 394
National Ground Water Associa-
   tion (NGWA), contact informa-
   tion 253
National Health Information Center,
   contact information 597
National Hispanic Indoor Air Quality
   Hotline 612
National Hospice Association
   (HOSPICE), contact information
   597

National Institute for Occupational
Safety and Health (NIOSH)
contact information 597
described 593
National Institute of Environmental
Health Sciences (NIEHS)
described 592–93
minority health issues 557–82
publications
dioxins 263n
electric fields 369n
environmental diseases list 17n
environmental health for families
59n
magnetic fields 369n
minorities' environmental health
557n
multiple chemical sensitivity syndrome 263n
ozone 163n
women's health 545n
National Institutes of Health (NIH)
contact information 598
described 593
mercury hazards publication 279n
National Lead Information Center
Hotline 612
National Organic Farmers Association Vermont (NOFA), contact information 598
National Pesticide Information Center (NPIC)
contact information 598, 612
DEET publication 303n
National Poison Control Hotline 613
National Primary Drinking Water
Regulations (NPDWR) 199–211
National Priority List (NPL), defined
589
National Radon Hotline 613
National Response Center Hotline
613
National Safety Council (NSC), publi-
cations
carbon monoxide 99n
environmental tobacco smoke 131n
indoor air quality 89n
National Secondary Drinking Water
Regulations (NSDWR) 199, 211

National Service Center for Environ-
mental Publications (NSCEP) 612
National Small Flows Clearinghouse
Hotline 614
National Wildlife Federation, Web
site address 602
Natural Resources Conservation Ser-
vice (NRCS) 254
Natural Resources Defense Council,
Web site address 602
NCEHS *see* National Center for Envi-
ronmental Health Strategies
NDWAC *see* National Drinking Water
Advisory Council
nematicides, described 285
nervous system disorders, environ-
mental hazards 21
neurotoxic shellfish poisoning 495–97
"New Aging Initiative to Protect
Older Persons from Environmental
Health Threats" (EPA) 555n
New York Coalition for Alternatives
to Pesticides (NYCAP), contact information 598
New York Division of Veterans Affairs,
contact information 598
NIEHS *see* National Institute of Environmental Health Sciences
NIH *see* National Institutes of Health
NIOSH *see* National Institute for Occupational Safety and Health
nitrates
defined 255
drinking water 215
drinking water regulation *203*
well water 244, 245
nitrites
drinking water 215
well water 244
nitrogen dioxide (NO2)
air quality index *186*, 186–87
indoor air quality 107
ozone 164
nitrogen oxides (NOx)
acid rain 158, 159
described 153–54
NOFA *see* National Organic Farmers
Association (Vermont)
"Noise Hazards" (Kotelchuck) 551n

nonhazardous waste, regulation 52
non-stochastic health effects, radionuclides 334, *335*
North American Insulation Manufacturers Association (NAIMA), indoor
air quality 137–38, 143, 146–47
North Carolina Chemical Injury, Web
site address 603
Northwest Coalition for Alternatives
to Pesticides, Web site address 604
NPDWR *see* National Primary Drink-
ing Water Regulations
NPIC *see* National Pesticide Informa-
tion Center
NPL *see* National Priority List
NRCS *see* Natural Resources Conser-
vation Service
NSC *see* National Safety Council
NSCEP *see* National Service Center
for Environmental Publications
NSDWR *see* National Secondary
Drinking Water Regulations
NYCAP *see* New York Coalition for
Alternatives to Pesticides

O

OAR *see* Office of Air and Radiation
Occupational Safety and Health Act 57
Occupational Safety and Health Administration (OSHA)
asbestos exposure 98
chemical accident prevention 86
contact information 598
described 593
OCHP (Office of Children's Health
Protection) *see* US Environmental
Protection Agency
o-dichlorobenzene
drinking water 216
drinking water regulation *204*
odor, drinking water regulation *211*
odor threshold, defined 589
Office of Air and Radiation (OAR), air
duct publication 133n
Office of Children's Health Protection
(OCHP) *see* US Environmental Protection Agency

Office of Research Services (ORS),
mercury hazards publication 279n
ofloxacin 422
Oil Pollution Act (1990; OPA) 85, 620
oils, mosquito control 293–94
okadaic acid 495
Olden, Kenneth 548–49
1,1-dichloroethylene
drinking water 216
drinking water regulation *205*
1,1,1-trichloroethane
drinking water 216
drinking water regulation *207*
1,1,2-trichloroethane
drinking water 216
drinking water regulation *207*
1,2-dibromo-3-chloropropane
(DBCP), drinking water regulation
204
1,2-dichloroethane
drinking water 216
drinking water regulation *205*
1,2-dichloropropane
drinking water 216
drinking water regulation *205*
1,2,4-trichorobenzene
drinking water 216
drinking water regulation *207*
OPA *see* Oil Pollution Act
Oregon Fibromyalgia Foundation,
Web site address 602
organic, defined 589
organic chemicals, drinking water
regulation *203–7*
organophosphate insecticides
children *532*
described 275–76, 301
Orion Society, Web site address 602
ORS *see* Office of Research Services
OSHA *see* Occupational Safety and
Health Administration
osteoporosis
environmental hazards 21
women 547–48
outdoor air quality
children 531–33
overview 5–6, 149–56
see also air pollution
ovicides, described 285

oxamyl
drinking water 216
drinking water regulation *206*
Oxyfuel 230–32
oxygenates, described 227
ozone
air ducts 143–44
air quality index 179–81, *180*
described 64, 150–51
overview 163–74
ozone air fresheners 170–71
"Ozone Alerts" (NIEHS) 163n
ozone alert values *170–71*
Ozone Protection Hotline 614

P

pacemakers
electric and magnetic fields 388
microwave ovens 361
paints
formaldehyde 118
lead poisoning 267–74
paint strippers, indoor air quality 91
paralytic shellfish poisoning 495–97
parasites, foodborne illness 457–58,
467–77
"Parasites and Foodborne Illness"
(USDA) 467n
parathion *532*, 533
particleboard, indoor air quality 115,
120
particles, indoor air quality 107–8
see also alpha particles; beta particles
particulate matter
air quality index 181–83, *182*
described 151–52
Pay-As-You-Throw (PAYT) Helpline
614
PAYT *see* Pay-As-You-Throw
PCB *see* polychlorinated biphenyls
PCDD *see* polychlorinated
dibenzodioxins
PCDF *see* polychlorinated
dibenzofurans
p-dichlorobenzene
drinking water 216
drinking water regulation *205*

pectenotoxins 495
pentachlorophenol
drinking water 216
drinking water regulation *206*
permeability, defined 589
permethrin 301
permitting system, described 46–47
persistence, defined 589
PESP *see* Pesticide Environmental
Stewardship Program
pest control devices, described 285
Pesticide Action Network, Web site
address 604
Pesticide Environmental Stewardship
Program (PESP) 288
Pesticide Registry of Washington,
contact information 598
pesticides
bioengineering 515–16
cautions 64
children 531, *532*, 543–44
drinking water 194
indoor air quality 92
Internet resources 604
mosquito control 299–302
overview 283–94
statistics 8
well water 245–46
worker safety 295–97
"Pesticides and Mosquito Control"
(EPA) 299n
phenolic disinfectants 535
PHEPR (Public Health Emergency
Preparedness and Response) *see*
Centers for Disease Control and
Prevention
pheromones, described 285
phosmet *532*
photon emitters, drinking water regulation *208*, 214
picloram
drinking water 216
drinking water regulation *207*
plague 433–37
planktonic algae 495
plant growth regulators, described
285
plant incorporated protectants, described 287

pleural membranes, asbestos 96–97
plume, defined 590
pneumoconiosis, environmental hazards 21
pneumonic plague, overview 433–37
poison control centers, statistics 7
Pollution Prevention Act (1990) 57, 83
Pollution Prevention Information Clearinghouse (PPIC), contact information 614
polychlorinated biphenyls (PCB)
  described 263
  drinking water 216
  drinking water regulation *206*
polychlorinated biphenyls (PCB), Yusho poisoning 23–24
polychlorinated dibenzodioxins (PCDD), described 263
polychlorinated dibenzofurans (PCDF), described 263
polymorphism, research 67
Ponce University School of Medicine, environmental research 577
pork tapeworm 475–77
potentiation, described 315
Potomac Latex Allergy Association, Web site address 603
poverty levels
  air quality demographics *11–12*
  environmental health 557–58
power lines, electric and magnetic fields 385
PPIC *see* Pollution Prevention Information Clearinghouse
Preliminary Site Assessment (PSA), defined 589–90
prescription medications, environmental safety 61
pressed wood products, formaldehyde 116–18
programmed cell death, described 71
protocol, defined 590
protozoa
  defined 256
  described 467
  swimming water *259*
PSA *see* Preliminary Site Assessment

Public Health Emergency Preparedness and Response (PHEPR) *see* Centers for Disease Control and Prevention
Pure Food and Drugs Act (1906) 509
Pure Food Campaign, Web site address 602

Q

QA *see* quality assurance
QC *see* quality control
quality assurance (QA), defined 590
quality control (QC), defined 590
Queensland fever, environmental hazards 21

R

racial factor 557–71
  air quality demographics *11–12*
  HIV infection 531
  lead poisoning 62
  see also ethnic factors
radiation exposure
  health effects 333–39
  microwave ovens 357–62
  smoke detectors 363–64
  televisions 365–68
radioactive waste, overview 353–55
radio-frequency energy (RF), described 391–95
radionuclides
  defined 256
  drinking water 194
  drinking water regulation *208*
  health effects 333–34
  well water 244
radium 226; radium 228, drinking water regulation *208*, 214
radon
  defined 256
  drinking water 214
  overview 341–52
  tests 63
RCRA *see* Resource Conservation and Recovery Act

RCRA, Superfund and EPCRA
  Hotline 615
"RCRA: Reducing Risk from Waste"
  (EPA) 33n
reactivity, described 36
recharge area, defined 256
recovery and reuse *see* recycling
recycling, described 43
  see also waste minimization
reformulated gasoline (RFG) 230–31
Reiter's syndrome, described 490
relative humidity, described 124
Remedial Investigation (RI), defined
  590
remediation, defined 590
repellants, described 285
reproductive disorders, environmental hazards 22
reservoirs, drinking water 193
resmethrin 301
Resource Conservation and Recovery
  Act (RCRA; 1976)
  enforcement 620
  Hazardous and Solid Waste
    Amendements 34
  overview 33–56
RF *see* radio-frequency energy
RFG *see* reformulated gasoline
RI *see* Remedial Investigation
rifampin 432
Right-to-Know Network, Web site address 602
risk, defined 590
risk assessment, defined 590
risk management, defined 590–91
Rocky Mountain Environmental
  Health Association, Web site address 603
rodenticides, described 285
room heaters, indoor air quality *106*
route of exposure, defined 591
Rowland, F. Sherwood 168

S

safe, defined 591
Safe Drinking Water Act (1974)
  described 57

Safe Drinking Water Act (1974), continued
  drinking water quality 194, 197
  MTBE 229
  well water 247
Safe Drinking Water Amendments
  (1996) 233
Safe Drinking Water Hotline 228,
  615
"Safety and Health Topics: Multiple
  Chemical Sensitivites" (DOL) 327n
Salmonella, foodborne illness 483–87
"Salmonellosis" (CDC) 483n
salmonellosis, overview 483–87
Salvations Army, East US Headquarters, contact information 599
sanitizers, described 284
SAR *see* specific absorption rate
saturated zone, defined 256
saxitoxin 495
SCARC *see* Smoking Control Advocacy
  Resource Center
SCDHEC *see* South Carolina Department of Health and Environmental
  Control
sealants, air ducts 145–46
secondhand smoke *see* environmental
  tobacco smoke; tobacco use
segregation, described 43
selenium
  drinking water 215
  drinking water regulation *203*
Seoul virus 451
septicemic plague, described 434
SERC *see* State Emergency Response
  Commission
set-back thermostats, mold control
  127–28
"Setting Standards for Safe Drinking
  Water" (EPA) 197n
sexually transmitted diseases, family
  environmental health 65–66
Share, Care and Prayer, Inc., Web site
  address 604
Sheet Metal and Air Conditioning
  Contractors' National Association
  (SMACNA)
  indoor air quality 146
shellfish, toxins 495–97

Shigella, foodborne illness 489–94
"Shigellosis" (CDC) 489n
shigellosis, overview 489–94
"Should You Have the Air Ducts in Your Home Cleaned?" (OAR) 133n
Sierra Club, Web site address 602
Silent Spring (Carson) 4
silver, drinking water regulation *211*
silvex
  drinking water 215
  drinking water regulation *207*
simazine
  drinking water 216
  drinking water regulation *207*
site inspection, defined 591
skin cancer, environmental hazards 22
sleep electrophysiology, electric and magnetic fields 380
SMACNA *see* Sheet Metal and Air Conditioning Contractors' National Association
Small Business Ombudsman Hotline 615
smallpox, overview 439–44
"Smallpox Fact Sheet: Smallpox Overview" (CDC) 439n
"Smallpox Fact Sheet: Vaccine Overview" (CDC) 439n
small quantity generators (SQG), described 40
smog, described 164
smoke detectors, radiation 363–64
"Smoke Detectors and Radiation" (EPA) 363n
Smoking Control Advocacy Resource Center (SCARC), contact information 599
SO2 *see* sulfur dioxide
Social Security Administration *see* US Social Security Administration
soil consumption, children 528–30
solid waste, described 37
Solid Waste Disposal Act (1965) 33
solubility, defined 591
solvents
  drinking water 194
  indoor air quality 91
source separation, described 43

South Carolina Department of Health and Environmental Control (SCDHEC), lead in drinking water publication 223n
space heaters
  indoor air quality 91
  maintenance schedule *113*
specific absorption rate (SAR), cellular telephones 395–96
spores, mold 123
SQC *see* small quantity generators
SSA *see* US Social Security Administration
State Emergency Response Commission (SERC)
  described 79–80, 85
  hazardous substances 78–79
state responsibilities
  hazardous waste regulations 48
  waste management 35
stochastic health effects, radionuclides 333–34
storage facilities, described 41
STORET Water Quality System Hotline 616
stoves, indoor air quality 91, *106*
styrene
  drinking water 216
  drinking water regulation *207*
sulfate, drinking water regulation *211*
sulfur dioxide (SO2)
  acid rain 158, 159
  air quality index *185*, 185–86
  described 154–55
  indoor air quality 108
sumithrin 301
sunburn
  children 530
  environmental hazards 22
  family environmental health 66
  skin caner 169
Superfund, defined 591
  see also Comprehensive Environmental Response, Compensation, and Liability Act
superheated water, described 362
Support Network for the Aldehyde and Solvent Affected, Web site address 603

surface impoundments, described 43
Surface Mining Control and Reclamation Act 57
surface temperature dominated mold growth, described 126
Surgeon General *see* US Surgeon General
synergism, described 315

T

Taenia saginata, foodborne illness 475–77
taeniasis, described 475–77
Taenia solium, foodborne illness 475–77
tapeworms, described 475–77
target organ, defined 591
Taylor, Jack A. 68
TCDD *see* dioxins
TCLP *see* toxicity characteristic leaching procedure
telephones *see* cellular telephones
televisions, radiation 365–68
temephos, described 292–93
"Ten Tips to Protect Children from Pesticide and Lead Poisonings around the Home" (EPA) 543n
teratogenic mutations, described 337
teratogens, described 318
tests
    anthrax 416–17
    asbestos exposure 98
    botulism 426
    brucellosis 431
    Eschericia coli 481
    lead 224
    radon 342, 343–45
    Salmonella 484
    tularemia 447
    well water 243, 250–51, *252*
tetrachloroethylene
    drinking water 216
    drinking water regulation *207*
tetracycline 436
thallium
    drinking water 215
    drinking water regulation *203*

thermal bridges, mold control 128–29
Thompson, Larry 513n
thyroid, iodine concentrations 337, 535
tobacco use
    family environmental health 66
    formaldehyde 115
    indoor air quality 91, 104–5
    radon *350*
Tollefson, Linda 505
toluene, drinking water regulation *207*
Tools for Schools IAQ Technical Assistance Hotline 616
tooth decay, environmental hazards 22
total dissolved solids, drinking water regulation *211*
total trihalomethanes
    drinking water 217
    drinking water regulation *200*
toxaphene
    drinking water 216
    drinking water regulation *207*
"ToxFAQs for Asbestos" (ATSDR) 95n
toxicity
    described 36
    versus hazards 310
toxicity characteristic leaching procedure (TCLP), described 36
Toxic Release Inventory
    Community Right-To-Know - EPCRA Hotline 616
    User Support Service, contact information 616
Toxic Release Inventory (TRI), described 50, 82–83
Toxic Substance Control Act (TSCA) 57
    Hotline 617
toxic waste, overview 6–7
toxins, shellfish 495–97
Toxoplasma gondii, foodborne illness 472–74
toxoplasmosis, described 472–74
tracking system, described 45–46
trade secrets, legislation 83–84

trans-1,2-dichloroethylene
drinking water 216
drinking water regulation *205*
transporters, described 41
treatment facilities, described 41
treatment technique, defined 209
tremolite 95
TRI *see* Toxic Release Inventory
Trichinella spiralis, foodborne illness
474–75
trichinosis, described 474–75
trichloroethylene
drinking water 216
drinking water regulation *207*
Truth in Labeling Campaign, Web
site address 603
TSCA *see* Toxic Substances Control Act
tularemia, overview 445–48
turbidity, drinking water *198*, 213–14,
236
2,4-D
drinking water 215
drinking water regulation *204*
2,4,5-TP
drinking water 215
drinking water regulation *207*
2,3,7,8-tetrachlorodibenzo-p-dioxin
(TCDD) *see* dioxins

U

ultraviolet light, family environmental health 66
underground injection wells, described
44
underground storage tanks (UST)
MTBE 230–31
regulation 34, 620
"Understanding Radiation: Health
Effects" (EPA) 333n
*Understanding Toxic Substances: An
Introduction to Chemical Hazards
in the Workplace* (HESIS) 309n
University of Maryland at Baltimore
County, Meyerhoff Scholars Program
578
unsaturated zone, defined 256
unvented appliances, described 105

"Unwelcome Dinner Guest: Preventing Foodborne Illness" (FDA)
457n
"Update on Formaldehyde - 1997 Revision" (CPSC) 115n
uranium
drinking water regulation *208*
environmental hazards 22–23
Uranium Education Project 578
urea-formaldehyde insulation, indoor
air quality 115, 117–18, 120
US Consumer Product Safety Commission (CPSC)
described 592
publications
combustion appliances 103n
formaldehyde 115n
USDA *see* US Department of Agriculture
US Department of Agriculture
(USDA)
foodborne illnesses publication 467n
household wells 254
US Department of Energy (DOE)
described 593
Office of Health and Environmental
Research, contact information
222
US Department of Health and Human
Services (DHHS)
described 593–94
publications
environmental health 3n
radon 341n
US Department of Housing and Urban
Development (HUD)
contact information 599
formaldehyde 117
US Department of Labor (DOL), multiple chemical sensitivity syndrome
publication 327n
used oil management standards, described 44–45
US Environmental Protection Agency
(EPA)
compliance and enforcement information 619–21
contact information 596
described 593

US Environmental Protection Agency (EPA), continued
  EPA Enforcement Economic Models Helpline 609
  EPA Grants and Fellowships Hotline 610
  EPA Imported Vehicles and Engines Public Help Line 610
  EPA Safe Drinking Water Hotline, contact information 222
  publications
    acid rain 157n
    Aging Initiative 555n
    air quality index 175n
    asthma 25n
    compliance information 619n
    drinking water rules 233n
    drinking water safety 191n, 197n, 213n
    emergency plans 77n
    enforcement information 619n
    hazardous waste risks 33n
    hotlines 605n
    household wells 241n
    indoor air pollutants 149n
    indoor air quality 89n
    lead contamination 267n
    lead poisoning 543n
    malathion 275n
    mole 123n
    MTBE 227n
    overview 449–53
    pesticides 283n, 295n, 299n, 543n
    protecting children 523n, 543n
    radiation exposure 333n
    radioactive waste 353n
    radon 341n
    smoke detectors 363n
    swimming water hazards 257n
US Food and Drug Administration (FDA)
  contact information 596
  publications
    cellular telephones 391n
    color additives 503n
    foodborne illnesses 457n
    microwave ovens 357n
    shellfish toxins 495n, 499n
    television radiation 365n

US Geological Survey (USGS)
  described 594
  water quality 254
USGS *see* US Geological Survey
US Public Health Service Office of Air and Radiation, radon publication 341n
US Public Interest Research Group, Web site address 602
US Social Security Administration (SSA), contact information 599
US Surgeon General, contact information 599
UST *see* underground storage tanks
uterine fibroids 547, 567

V

vaccines
  anthrax 423
  plague 437
  smallpox 442–44
  tularemia 446, 448
vapor pressure, described 124
vapor pressure dominated mold growth, described 125–26
"Various Shellfish-Associated Toxins" (FDA) 495n
vented appliances, described 105
ventilation, indoor air quality 92–93
VHF *see* viral hemorrhagic fevers
vinyl chloride
  drinking water 216
  drinking water regulation *207*
"Viral Hemorrhagic Fevers" (CDC) 449n
viral hemorrhagic fevers (VHF), overview 449–53
viruses
  defined 256
  drinking water *198*
  swimming water *259*
vision problems, environmental hazards 23
vitamin supplements, family environmental health 65
VOC *see* volatile organic compound
volatile, defined 591

volatile organic compounds (VOC)
  defined 591
  formaldehyde 115
  nitrogen dioxide 187
  ozone 150
vydate
  drinking water 216
  drinking water regulation *206*

W

warfarin 535
waste minimization, described 42
waste piles, described 44
WasteWise Helpline 617
waterborne diseases
  environmental hazards 23
  family environmental health 62
water heaters
  indoor air quality *106*
  maintenance schedule *113*
water quality
  nitrogen oxides 153
  overview 6
  radon 346–47
  swimmers 257–60
  see also drinking water
watershed, defined 256
water table, defined 256
water vapor
  described 124
  indoor air quality 104–5
well cap, defined 256
well casing, defined 256
wellhead, defined 256
Well Mind Association, Web site address 604
wells
  drinking water 241–56
  water quality 191–93
Wetlands Information Hotline 617
"We Want You to Know about Television Radiation" (FDA) 365n
"What Are Antimicrobial Pesticides?" (EPA) 283n
"What Are Biopesticides?" (EPA) 283n
"What are the Six Common Air Pollutants?" (EPA) 149n

"What Is a Pesticide" (EPA) 283n
"What Society Can Do about Acid Deposition" (EPA) 157n
"What You Should Know about Combustion Appliances and Indoor Air Pollution" (CPSC) 103n
White Lung Association, Web site address 604
Whitman, Christie 555
WHO *see* World Health Organization
windows, mold control 129
wireless telephone base stations, described 397–98
wireless telephones, safety concerns 391–406
women, environmental health 545–50, 567–71
"Women's Health and the Environment" (NIEHS) 545n
woodstoves
  indoor air quality 110–12
  maintenance schedule *113*
"Worker Safety and Training: Who and What Are Covered?" (EPA) 295n
workplace
  asbestos exposure 96
  chemical hazards 309–26
  electric and magnetic fields 378–79, 386–87
  environmental tobacco smoke 132
  lead poisoning 269
  malathion 276
  mercury hazards 281
  noise hazards 551–53
  pesticide safety 295–97
workplace exposure, diseases 69
workplace safety, precautions 61
World Health Organization (WHO)
  chlorination 220
  described 594
worms, swimming water *259*

X

Xeroderma pigmentosa, environmental hazards 23

xylenes
  drinking water 216
  drinking water regulation *207*

Y

Yersinia pestis 433–37
yessotoxin 495
Yusho poisoning, environmental
  hazards 23–24

Z

zinc, drinking water regulation
  211
zinc deficiency, environmental
  hazards 24
zinc poisoning, environmental
  hazards 24

Health Reference Series
COMPLETE CATALOG

Adolescent Health Sourcebook

Basic Consumer Health Information about Common Medical, Mental, and Emotional Concerns in Adolescents, Including Facts about Acne, Body Piercing, Mononucleosis, Nutrition, Eating Disorders, Stress, Depression, Behavior Problems, Peer Pressure, Violence, Gangs, Drug Use, Puberty, Sexuality, Pregnancy, Learning Disabilities, and More

Along with a Glossary of Terms and Other Resources for Further Help and Information

Edited by Chad T. Kimball. 658 pages. 2002. 0-7808-0248-9. $78.

"It is written in clear, nontechnical language aimed at general readers. . . . Recommended for public libraries, community colleges, and other agencies serving health care consumers."
— *American Reference Books Annual, 2003*

"Recommended for school and public libraries. Parents and professionals dealing with teens will appreciate the easy-to-follow format and the clearly written text. This could become a 'must have' for every high school teacher." — *E-Streams, Jan '03*

"A good starting point for information related to common medical, mental, and emotional concerns of adolescents." — *School Library Journal, Nov '02*

"This book provides accurate information in an easy to access format. It addresses topics that parents and caregivers might not be aware of and provides practical, useable information." — *Doody's Health Sciences Book Review Journal, Sep-Oct '02*

"Recommended reference source."
— *Booklist, American Library Association, Sep '02*

■

AIDS Sourcebook, 3rd Edition

Basic Consumer Health Information about Acquired Immune Deficiency Syndrome (AIDS) and Human Immunodeficiency Virus (HIV) Infection, Including Facts about Transmission, Prevention, Diagnosis, Treatment, Opportunistic Infections, and Other Complications, with a Section for Women and Children, Including Details about Associated Gynecological Concerns, Pregnancy, and Pediatric Care

Along with Updated Statistical Information, Reports on Current Research Initiatives, a Glossary, and Directories of Internet, Hotline, and Other Resources

Edited by Dawn D. Matthews. 664 pages. 2003. 0-7808-0631-X. $78.

ALSO AVAILABLE: AIDS Sourcebook, 1st Edition. Edited by Karen Bellenir and Peter D. Dresser. 831 pages. 1995. 0-7808-0031-1. $78.

AIDS Sourcebook, 2nd Edition. Edited by Karen Bellenir. 751 pages. 1999. 0-7808-0225-X. $78.

"Highly recommended."
— *American Reference Books Annual, 2000*

"Excellent sourcebook. This continues to be a highly recommended book. There is no other book that provides as much information as this book provides."
— *AIDS Book Review Journal, Dec-Jan 2000*

"Recommended reference source."
— *Booklist, American Library Association, Dec '99*

"A solid text for college-level health libraries."
— *The Bookwatch, Aug '99*

Cited in *Reference Sources for Small and Medium-Sized Libraries, American Library Association, 1999*

■

Alcoholism Sourcebook

Basic Consumer Health Information about the Physical and Mental Consequences of Alcohol Abuse, Including Liver Disease, Pancreatitis, Wernicke-Korsakoff Syndrome (Alcoholic Dementia), Fetal Alcohol Syndrome, Heart Disease, Kidney Disorders, Gastrointestinal Problems, and Immune System Compromise and Featuring Facts about Addiction, Detoxification, Alcohol Withdrawal, Recovery, and the Maintenance of Sobriety

Along with a Glossary and Directories of Resources for Further Help and Information

Edited by Karen Bellenir. 613 pages. 2000. 0-7808-0325-6. $78.

"This title is one of the few reference works on alcoholism for general readers. For some readers this will be a welcome complement to the many self-help books on the market. Recommended for collections serving general readers and consumer health collections."
— *E-Streams, Mar '01*

"This book is an excellent choice for public and academic libraries."
— *American Reference Books Annual, 2001*

"Recommended reference source."
— *Booklist, American Library Association, Dec '00*

"Presents a wealth of information on alcohol use and abuse and its effects on the body and mind, treatment, and prevention." — *SciTech Book News, Dec '00*

"Important new health guide which packs in the latest consumer information about the problems of alcoholism." — *Reviewer's Bookwatch, Nov '00*

SEE ALSO Drug Abuse Sourcebook, Substance Abuse Sourcebook

Allergies Sourcebook, 2nd Edition

Basic Consumer Health Information about Allergic Disorders, Triggers, Reactions, and Related Symptoms, Including Anaphylaxis, Rhinitis, Sinusitis, Asthma, Dermatitis, Conjunctivitis, and Multiple Chemical Sensitivity

Along with Tips on Diagnosis, Prevention, and Treatment, Statistical Data, a Glossary, and a Directory of Sources for Further Help and Information

Edited by Annemarie S. Muth. 598 pages. 2002. 0-7808-0376-0. $78.

ALSO AVAILABLE: Allergies Sourcebook, 1st Edition. Edited by Allan R. Cook. 611 pages. 1997. 0-7808-0036-2. $78.

"This book brings a great deal of useful material together. . . . This is an excellent addition to public and consumer health library collections."
— *American Reference Books Annual, 2003*

"This second edition would be useful to laypersons with little or advanced knowledge of the subject matter. This book would also serve as a resource for nursing and other health care professions students. It would be useful in public, academic, and hospital libraries with consumer health collections."　　— *E-Streams, Jul '02*

■

Alternative Medicine Sourcebook, 2nd Edition

Basic Consumer Health Information about Alternative and Complementary Medical Practices, Including Acupuncture, Chiropractic, Herbal Medicine, Homeopathy, Naturopathic Medicine, Mind-Body Interventions, Ayurveda, and Other Non-Western Medical Traditions

Along with Facts about such Specific Therapies as Massage Therapy, Aromatherapy, Qigong, Hypnosis, Prayer, Dance, and Art Therapies, a Glossary, and Resources for Further Information

Edited by Dawn D. Matthews. 618 pages. 2002. 0-7808-0605-0. $78.

ALSO AVAILABLE: Alternative Medicine Sourcebook, 1st Edition. Edited by Allan R. Cook. 737 pages. 1999. 0-7808-0200-4. $78.

"Recommended for public, high school, and academic libraries that have consumer health collections. Hospital libraries that also serve the public will find this to be a useful resource."　　— *E-Streams, Feb '03*

"Recommended reference source."
— *Booklist, American Library Association, Jan '03*

"An important alternate health reference."
— *MBR Bookwatch, Oct '02*

"A great addition to the reference collection of every type of library." — *American Reference Books Annual, 2000*

Alzheimer's Disease Sourcebook, 2nd Edition

Basic Consumer Health Information about Alzheimer's Disease, Related Disorders, and Other Dementias, Including Multi-Infarct Dementia, AIDS-Related Dementia, Alcoholic Dementia, Huntington's Disease, Delirium, and Confusional States

Along with Reports Detailing Current Research Efforts in Prevention and Treatment, Long-Term Care Issues, and Listings of Sources for Additional Help and Information

Edited by Karen Bellenir. 524 pages. 1999. 0-7808-0223-3. $78.

ALSO AVAILABLE: Alzheimer's, Stroke & 29 Other Neurological Disorders Sourcebook, 1st Edition. Edited by Frank E. Bair. 579 pages. 1993. 1-55888-748-2. $78.

"Provides a wealth of useful information not otherwise available in one place. This resource is recommended for all types of libraries."
— *American Reference Books Annual, 2000*

"Recommended reference source."
— *Booklist, American Library Association, Oct '99*

SEE ALSO Brain Disorders Sourcebook

■

Arthritis Sourcebook

Basic Consumer Health Information about Specific Forms of Arthritis and Related Disorders, Including Rheumatoid Arthritis, Osteoarthritis, Gout, Polymyalgia Rheumatica, Psoriatic Arthritis, Spondyloarthropathies, Juvenile Rheumatoid Arthritis, and Juvenile Ankylosing Spondylitis

Along with Information about Medical, Surgical, and Alternative Treatment Options, and Including Strategies for Coping with Pain, Fatigue, and Stress

Edited by Allan R. Cook. 550 pages. 1998. 0-7808-0201-2. $78.

". . . accessible to the layperson."
— *Reference and Research Book News, Feb '99*

■

Asthma Sourcebook

Basic Consumer Health Information about Asthma, Including Symptoms, Traditional and Nontraditional Remedies, Treatment Advances, Quality-of-Life Aids, Medical Research Updates, and the Role of Allergies, Exercise, Age, the Environment, and Genetics in the Development of Asthma

Along with Statistical Data, a Glossary, and Directories of Support Groups, and Other Resources for Further Information

Edited by Annemarie S. Muth. 628 pages. 2000. 0-7808-0381-7. $78.

"A worthwhile reference acquisition for public libraries and academic medical libraries whose readers desire a quick introduction to the wide range of asthma information." — *Choice, Association of College & Research Libraries, Jun '01*

"Recommended reference source."
— *Booklist, American Library Association, Feb '01*

"Highly recommended." — *The Bookwatch, Jan '01*

"There is much good information for patients and their families who deal with asthma daily."
— *American Medical Writers Association Journal, Winter '01*

"This informative text is recommended for consumer health collections in public, secondary school, and community college libraries and the libraries of universities with a large undergraduate population."
— *American Reference Books Annual, 2001*

■

Attention Deficit Disorder Sourcebook

Basic Consumer Health Information about Attention Deficit/Hyperactivity Disorder in Children and Adults, Including Facts about Causes, Symptoms, Diagnostic Criteria, and Treatment Options Such as Medications, Behavior Therapy, Coaching, and Homeopathy

Along with Reports on Current Research Initiatives, Legal Issues, and Government Regulations, and Featuring a Glossary of Related Terms, Internet Resources, and a List of Additional Reading Material

Edited by Dawn D. Matthews. 470 pages. 2002. 0-7808-0624-7. $78.

"Recommended reference source."
— *Booklist, American Library Association, Jan '03*

"This book is recommended for all school libraries and the reference or consumer health sections of public libraries." — *American Reference Books Annual, 2003*

■

Back & Neck Disorders Sourcebook

Basic Information about Disorders and Injuries of the Spinal Cord and Vertebrae, Including Facts on Chiropractic Treatment, Surgical Interventions, Paralysis, and Rehabilitation

Along with Advice for Preventing Back Trouble

Edited by Karen Bellenir. 548 pages. 1997. 0-7808-0202-0. $78.

"The strength of this work is its basic, easy-to-read format. Recommended."
— *Reference and User Services Quarterly, American Library Association, Winter '97*

■

Blood & Circulatory Disorders Sourcebook

Basic Information about Blood and Its Components, Anemias, Leukemias, Bleeding Disorders, and Circulatory Disorders, Including Aplastic Anemia, Thalassemia, Sickle-Cell Disease, Hemochromatosis, Hemophilia, Von Willebrand Disease, and Vascular Diseases

Along with a Special Section on Blood Transfusions and Blood Supply Safety, a Glossary, and Source Listings for Further Help and Information

Edited by Karen Bellenir and Linda M. Shin. 554 pages. 1998. 0-7808-0203-9. $78.

"Recommended reference source."
— *Booklist, American Library Association, Feb '99*

"An important reference sourcebook written in simple language for everyday, non-technical users. "
— *Reviewer's Bookwatch, Jan '99*

■

Brain Disorders Sourcebook

Basic Consumer Health Information about Strokes, Epilepsy, Amyotrophic Lateral Sclerosis (ALS/Lou Gehrig's Disease), Parkinson's Disease, Brain Tumors, Cerebral Palsy, Headache, Tourette Syndrome, and More

Along with Statistical Data, Treatment and Rehabilitation Options, Coping Strategies, Reports on Current Research Initiatives, a Glossary, and Resource Listings for Additional Help and Information

Edited by Karen Bellenir. 481 pages. 1999. 0-7808-0229-2. $78.

"Belongs on the shelves of any library with a consumer health collection." — *E-Streams, Mar '00*

"Recommended reference source."
— *Booklist, American Library Association, Oct '99*

SEE ALSO *Alzheimer's Disease Sourcebook*

■

Breast Cancer Sourcebook

Basic Consumer Health Information about Breast Cancer, Including Diagnostic Methods, Treatment Options, Alternative Therapies, Self-Help Information, Related Health Concerns, Statistical and Demographic Data, and Facts for Men with Breast Cancer

Along with Reports on Current Research Initiatives, a Glossary of Related Medical Terms, and a Directory of Sources for Further Help and Information

Edited by Edward J. Prucha and Karen Bellenir. 580 pages. 2001. 0-7808-0244-6. $78.

"It would be a useful reference book in a library or on loan to women in a support group."
— *Cancer Forum, Mar '03*

"Recommended reference source."
— *Booklist, American Library Association, Jan '02*

"This reference source is highly recommended. It is quite informative, comprehensive and detailed in nature, and yet it offers practical advice in easy-to-read language. It could be thought of as the 'bible' of breast cancer for the consumer." — *E-Streams, Jan '02*

"The broad range of topics covered in lay language make the *Breast Cancer Sourcebook* an excellent addition to public and consumer health library collections."
— *American Reference Books Annual 2002*

"From the pros and cons of different screening methods and results to treatment options, *Breast Cancer Sourcebook* provides the latest information on the subject."
— *Library Bookwatch, Dec '01*

"This thoroughgoing, very readable reference covers all aspects of breast health and cancer. . . . Readers will find much to consider here. Recommended for all public and patient health collections."
— *Library Journal, Sep '01*

SEE ALSO *Cancer Sourcebook for Women, Women's Health Concerns Sourcebook*

■

Breastfeeding Sourcebook

Basic Consumer Health Information about the Benefits of Breastmilk, Preparing to Breastfeed, Breastfeeding as a Baby Grows, Nutrition, and More, Including Information on Special Situations and Concerns Such as Mastitis, Illness, Medications, Allergies, Multiple Births, Prematurity, Special Needs, and Adoption

Along with a Glossary and Resources for Additional Help and Information

Edited by Jenni Lynn Colson. 388 pages. 2002. 0-7808-0332-9. $78.

SEE ALSO *Pregnancy & Birth Sourcebook*

"Particularly useful is the information about professional lactation services and chapters on breastfeeding when returning to work. . . . *Breastfeeding Sourcebook* will be useful for public libraries, consumer health libraries, and technical schools offering nurse assistant training, especially in areas where Internet access is problematic."
— *American Reference Books Annual, 2003*

■

Burns Sourcebook

Basic Consumer Health Information about Various Types of Burns and Scalds, Including Flame, Heat, Cold, Electrical, Chemical, and Sun Burns

Along with Information on Short-Term and Long-Term Treatments, Tissue Reconstruction, Plastic Surgery, Prevention Suggestions, and First Aid

Edited by Allan R. Cook. 604 pages. 1999. 0-7808-0204-7. $78.

"This is an exceptional addition to the series and is highly recommended for all consumer health collections, hospital libraries, and academic medical centers."
— *E-Streams, Mar '00*

"This key reference guide is an invaluable addition to all health care and public libraries in confronting this ongoing health issue."
— *American Reference Books Annual, 2000*

"Recommended reference source."
— *Booklist, American Library Association, Dec '99*

SEE ALSO *Skin Disorders Sourcebook*

Cancer Sourcebook, 4th Edition

Basic Consumer Health Information about Major Forms and Stages of Cancer, Featuring Facts about Head and Neck Cancers, Lung Cancers, Gastrointestinal Cancers, Genitourinary Cancers, Lymphomas, Blood Cell Cancers, Endocrine Cancers, Skin Cancers, Bone Cancers, Sarcomas, and Others, and Including Information about Cancer Treatments and Therapies, Identifying and Reducing Cancer Risks, and Strategies for Coping with Cancer and the Side Effects of Treatment

Along with a Cancer Glossary, Statistical and Demographic Data, and a Directory of Sources for Additional Help and Information

Edited by Karen Bellenir. 1,119 pages. 2003. 0-7808-0633-6. $78.

ALSO AVAILABLE: *Cancer Sourcebook, 1st Edition.* Edited by Frank E. Bair. 932 pages. 1990. 1-55888-888-8. $78.

New Cancer Sourcebook, 2nd Edition. Edited by Allan R. Cook. 1,313 pages. 1996. 0-7808-0041-9. $78.

Cancer Sourcebook, 3rd Edition. Edited by Edward J. Prucha. 1,069 pages. 2000. 0-7808-0227-6. $78.

"This title is recommended for health sciences and public libraries with consumer health collections."
— *E-Streams, Feb '01*

". . . can be effectively used by cancer patients and their families who are looking for answers in a language they can understand. Public and hospital libraries should have it on their shelves."
— *American Reference Books Annual, 2001*

"Recommended reference source."
— *Booklist, American Library Association, Dec '00*

Cited in *Reference Sources for Small and Medium-Sized Libraries, American Library Association, 1999*

"The amount of factual and useful information is extensive. The writing is very clear, geared to general readers. Recommended for all levels." — *Choice, Association of College & Research Libraries, Jan '97*

SEE ALSO *Breast Cancer Sourcebook, Cancer Sourcebook for Women, Pediatric Cancer Sourcebook, Prostate Cancer Sourcebook*

■

Cancer Sourcebook for Women, 2nd Edition

Basic Consumer Health Information about Gynecologic Cancers and Related Concerns, Including Cervical Cancer, Endometrial Cancer, Gestational Trophoblastic Tumor, Ovarian Cancer, Uterine Cancer, Vaginal Cancer, Vulvar Cancer, Breast Cancer, and Common Non-Cancerous Uterine Conditions, with Facts about Cancer Risk Factors, Screening and Prevention, Treatment Options, and Reports on Current Research Initiatives

Along with a Glossary of Cancer Terms and a Directory of Resources for Additional Help and Information

Edited by Karen Bellenir. 604 pages. 2002. 0-7808-0226-8. $78.

"An excellent addition to collections in public, consumer health, and women's health libraries."
— *American Reference Books Annual, 2003*

"Overall, the information is excellent, and complex topics are clearly explained. As a reference book for the consumer it is a valuable resource to assist them to make informed decisions about cancer and its treatments." — *Cancer Forum, Nov '02*

"Highly recommended for academic and medical reference collections." — *Library Bookwatch, Sep '02*

"This is a highly recommended book for any public or consumer library, being reader friendly and containing accurate and helpful information."
— *E-Streams, Aug '02*

"Recommended reference source."
— *Booklist, American Library Association, Jul '02*

SEE ALSO *Breast Cancer Sourcebook, Women's Health Concerns Sourcebook*

Cardiovascular Diseases & Disorders Sourcebook, 1st Edition

SEE *Heart Diseases & Disorders Sourcebook, 2nd Edition*

Caregiving Sourcebook

Basic Consumer Health Information for Caregivers, Including a Profile of Caregivers, Caregiving Responsibilities and Concerns, Tips for Specific Conditions, Care Environments, and the Effects of Caregiving

Along with Facts about Legal Issues, Financial Information, and Future Planning, a Glossary, and a Listing of Additional Resources

Edited by Joyce Brennfleck Shannon. 600 pages. 2001. 0-7808-0331-0. $78.

"Essential for most collections."
— *Library Journal, Apr 1, 2002*

"An ideal addition to the reference collection of any public library. Health sciences information professionals may also want to acquire the *Caregiving Sourcebook* for their hospital or academic library for use as a ready reference tool by health care workers interested in aging and caregiving." — *E-Streams, Jan '02*

"Recommended reference source."
— *Booklist, American Library Association, Oct '01*

Childhood Diseases & Disorders Sourcebook

Basic Consumer Health Information about Medical Problems Often Encountered in Pre-Adolescent Children, Including Respiratory Tract Ailments, Ear Infections, Sore Throats, Disorders of the Skin and Scalp,

Digestive and Genitourinary Diseases, Infectious Diseases, Inflammatory Disorders, Chronic Physical and Developmental Disorders, Allergies, and More

Along with Information about Diagnostic Tests, Common Childhood Surgeries, and Frequently Used Medications, with a Glossary of Important Terms and Resource Directory

Edited by Chad T. Kimball. 662 pages. 2003. 0-7808-0458-9. $78.

Colds, Flu & Other Common Ailments Sourcebook

Basic Consumer Health Information about Common Ailments and Injuries, Including Colds, Coughs, the Flu, Sinus Problems, Headaches, Fever, Nausea and Vomiting, Menstrual Cramps, Diarrhea, Constipation, Hemorrhoids, Back Pain, Dandruff, Dry and Itchy Skin, Cuts, Scrapes, Sprains, Bruises, and More

Along with Information about Prevention, Self-Care, Choosing a Doctor, Over-the-Counter Medications, Folk Remedies, and Alternative Therapies, and Including a Glossary of Important Terms and a Directory of Resources for Further Help and Information

Edited by Chad T. Kimball. 638 pages. 2001. 0-7808-0435-X. $78.

"A good starting point for research on common illnesses. It will be a useful addition to public and consumer health library collections."
— *American Reference Books Annual 2002*

"Will prove valuable to any library seeking to maintain a current, comprehensive reference collection of health resources. . . . Excellent reference."
— *The Bookwatch, Aug '01*

"Recommended reference source."
— *Booklist, American Library Association, July '01*

Communication Disorders Sourcebook

Basic Information about Deafness and Hearing Loss, Speech and Language Disorders, Voice Disorders, Balance and Vestibular Disorders, and Disorders of Smell, Taste, and Touch

Edited by Linda M. Ross. 533 pages. 1996. 0-7808-0077-X. $78.

"This is skillfully edited and is a welcome resource for the layperson. It should be found in every public and medical library." — *Booklist Health Sciences Supplement, American Library Association, Oct '97*

Congenital Disorders Sourcebook

Basic Information about Disorders Acquired during Gestation, Including Spina Bifida, Hydrocephalus, Cerebral Palsy, Heart Defects, Craniofacial Abnormalities, Fetal Alcohol Syndrome, and More

Along with Current Treatment Options and Statistical Data

Edited by Karen Bellenir. 607 pages. 1997. 0-7808-0205-5. $78.

"Recommended reference source."
—*Booklist, American Library Association, Oct '97*

SEE ALSO Pregnancy & Birth Sourcebook

Consumer Issues in Health Care Sourcebook

Basic Information about Health Care Fundamentals and Related Consumer Issues, Including Exams and Screening Tests, Physician Specialties, Choosing a Doctor, Using Prescription and Over-the-Counter Medications Safely, Avoiding Health Scams, Managing Common Health Risks in the Home, Care Options for Chronically or Terminally Ill Patients, and a List of Resources for Obtaining Help and Further Information

Edited by Karen Bellenir. 618 pages. 1998. 0-7808-0221-7. $78.

"Both public and academic libraries will want to have a copy in their collection for readers who are interested in self-education on health issues."
—*American Reference Books Annual, 2000*

"The editor has researched the literature from government agencies and others, saving readers the time and effort of having to do the research themselves. Recommended for public libraries."
—*Reference and User Services Quarterly, American Library Association, Spring '99*

"Recommended reference source."
—*Booklist, American Library Association, Dec '98*

Contagious & Non-Contagious Infectious Diseases Sourcebook

Basic Information about Contagious Diseases like Measles, Polio, Hepatitis B, and Infectious Mononucleosis, and Non-Contagious Infectious Diseases like Tetanus and Toxic Shock Syndrome, and Diseases Occurring as Secondary Infections Such as Shingles and Reye Syndrome

Along with Vaccination, Prevention, and Treatment Information, and a Section Describing Emerging Infectious Disease Threats

Edited by Karen Bellenir and Peter D. Dresser. 566 pages. 1996. 0-7808-0075-3. $78.

Death & Dying Sourcebook

Basic Consumer Health Information for the Layperson about End-of-Life Care and Related Ethical and Legal Issues, Including Chief Causes of Death, Autopsies, Pain Management for the Terminally Ill, Life Support Systems, Insurance, Euthanasia, Assisted Suicide, Hospice Programs, Living Wills, Funeral Planning, Counseling, Mourning, Organ Donation, and Physician Training

Along with Statistical Data, a Glossary, and Listings of Sources for Further Help and Information

Edited by Annemarie S. Muth. 641 pages. 1999. 0-7808-0230-6. $78.

"Public libraries, medical libraries, and academic libraries will all find this sourcebook a useful addition to their collections."
—*American Reference Books Annual, 2001*

"An extremely useful resource for those concerned with death and dying in the United States."
—*Respiratory Care, Nov '00*

"Recommended reference source."
—*Booklist, American Library Association, Aug '00*

"This book is a definite must for all those involved in end-of-life care." —*Doody's Review Service, 2000*

Depression Sourcebook

Basic Consumer Health Information about Unipolar Depression, Bipolar Disorder, Postpartum Depression, Seasonal Affective Disorder, and Other Types of Depression in Children, Adolescents, Women, Men, the Elderly, and Other Selected Populations

Along with Facts about Causes, Risk Factors, Diagnostic Criteria, Treatment Options, Coping Strategies, Suicide Prevention, a Glossary, and a Directory of Sources for Additional Help and Information

Edited by Karen Belleni. 602 pages. 2002. 0-7808-0611-5. $78.

"Invaluable reference for public and school library collections alike." —*Library Bookwatch, Apr '03*

"Recommended for purchase."
—*American Reference Books Annual, 2003*

Diabetes Sourcebook, 3rd Edition

Basic Consumer Health Information about Type 1 Diabetes (Insulin-Dependent or Juvenile-Onset Diabetes), Type 2 Diabetes (Noninsulin-Dependent or Adult-Onset Diabetes), Gestational Diabetes, Impaired Glucose Tolerance (IGT), and Related Complications, Such as Amputation, Eye Disease, Gum Disease, Nerve Damage, and End-Stage Renal Disease, Including Facts about Insulin, Oral Diabetes Medications, Blood Sugar Testing, and the Role of Exercise and Nutrition in the Control of Diabetes

Along with a Glossary and Resources for Further Help and Information

Edited by Dawn D. Matthews. 622 pages. 2003. 0-7808-0629-8. $78.

ALSO AVAILABLE: *Diabetes Sourcebook, 1st Edition.* Edited by Karen Bellenir and Peter D. Dresser. 827 pages. 1994. 1-55888-751-2. $78.

Diabetes Sourcebook, 2nd Edition. Edited by Karen Bellenir. 688 pages. 1998. 0-7808-0224-1. $78.

"An invaluable reference." —*Library Journal, May '00*

Selected as one of the 250 "Best Health Sciences Books of 1999." — *Doody's Rating Service, Mar-Apr 2000*

"This comprehensive book is an excellent addition for high school, academic, medical, and public libraries. This volume is highly recommended."
— *American Reference Books Annual, 2000*

"Provides useful information for the general public."
— *Healthlines, University of Michigan Health Management Research Center, Sep/Oct '99*

". . . provides reliable mainstream medical information . . . belongs on the shelves of any library with a consumer health collection." — *E-Streams, Sep '99*

"Recommended reference source."
— *Booklist, American Library Association, Feb '99*

▪

Diet & Nutrition Sourcebook, 2nd Edition

Basic Consumer Health Information about Dietary Guidelines, Recommended Daily Intake Values, Vitamins, Minerals, Fiber, Fat, Weight Control, Dietary Supplements, and Food Additives

Along with Special Sections on Nutrition Needs throughout Life and Nutrition for People with Such Specific Medical Concerns as Allergies, High Blood Cholesterol, Hypertension, Diabetes, Celiac Disease, Seizure Disorders, Phenylketonuria (PKU), Cancer, and Eating Disorders, and Including Reports on Current Nutrition Research and Source Listings for Additional Help and Information

Edited by Karen Bellenir. 650 pages. 1999. 0-7808-0228-4. $78.

ALSO AVAILABLE: Diet & Nutrition Sourcebook, 1st Edition. Edited by Dan R. Harris. 662 pages. 1996. 0-7808-0084-2. $78.

"This book is an excellent source of basic diet and nutrition information." — *Booklist Health Sciences Supplement, American Library Association, Dec '00*

"This reference document should be in any public library, but it would be a very good guide for beginning students in the health sciences. If the other books in this publisher's series are as good as this, they should all be in the health sciences collections."
— *American Reference Books Annual, 2000*

"This book is an excellent general nutrition reference for consumers who desire to take an active role in their health care for prevention. Consumers of all ages who select this book can feel confident they are receiving current and accurate information." — *Journal of Nutrition for the Elderly, Vol. 19, No. 4, '00*

"Recommended reference source."
— *Booklist, American Library Association, Dec '99*

SEE ALSO Digestive Diseases & Disorders Sourcebook, Eating Disorders Sourcebook, Gastrointestinal Diseases & Disorders Sourcebook, Vegetarian Sourcebook

Digestive Diseases & Disorders Sourcebook

Basic Consumer Health Information about Diseases and Disorders that Impact the Upper and Lower Digestive System, Including Celiac Disease, Constipation, Crohn's Disease, Cyclic Vomiting Syndrome, Diarrhea, Diverticulosis and Diverticulitis, Gallstones, Heartburn, Hemorrhoids, Hernias, Indigestion (Dyspepsia), Irritable Bowel Syndrome, Lactose Intolerance, Ulcers, and More

Along with Information about Medications and Other Treatments, Tips for Maintaining a Healthy Digestive Tract, a Glossary, and Directory of Digestive Diseases Organizations

Edited by Karen Bellenir. 335 pages. 2000. 0-7808-0327-2. $78.

"This title would be an excellent addition to all public or patient-research libraries."
— *American Reference Books Annual, 2001*

"This title is recommended for public, hospital, and health sciences libraries with consumer health collections." — *E-Streams, Jul-Aug '00*

"Recommended reference source."
— *Booklist, American Library Association, May '00*

SEE ALSO Diet & Nutrition Sourcebook, Eating Disorders Sourcebook, Gastrointestinal Diseases & Disorders Sourcebook

▪

Disabilities Sourcebook

Basic Consumer Health Information about Physical and Psychiatric Disabilities, Including Descriptions of Major Causes of Disability, Assistive and Adaptive Aids, Workplace Issues, and Accessibility Concerns

Along with Information about the Americans with Disabilities Act, a Glossary, and Resources for Additional Help and Information

Edited by Dawn D. Matthews. 616 pages. 2000. 0-7808-0389-2. $78.

"It is a must for libraries with a consumer health section." — *American Reference Books Annual 2002*

"A much needed addition to the Omnigraphics *Health Reference Series*. A current reference work to provide people with disabilities, their families, caregivers or those who work with them, a broad range of information in one volume, has not been available until now. . . . It is recommended for all public and academic library reference collections." — *E-Streams, May '01*

"An excellent source book in easy-to-read format covering many current topics; highly recommended for all libraries." — *Choice, Association of College and Research Libraries, Jan '01*

"Recommended reference source."
— *Booklist, American Library Association, Jul '00*

Domestic Violence & Child Abuse Sourcebook

Basic Consumer Health Information about Spousal/ Partner, Child, Sibling, Parent, and Elder Abuse, Covering Physical, Emotional, and Sexual Abuse, Teen Dating Violence, and Stalking; Includes Information about Hotlines, Safe Houses, Safety Plans, and Other Resources for Support and Assistance, Community Initiatives, and Reports on Current Directions in Research and Treatment

Along with a Glossary, Sources for Further Reading, and Governmental and Non-Governmental Organizations Contact Information

Edited by Helene Henderson. 1,064 pages. 2001. 0-7808-0235-7. $78.

"Interested lay persons should find the book extremely beneficial. . . . A copy of *Domestic Violence and Child Abuse Sourcebook* should be in every public library in the United States."
— *Social Science & Medicine, No. 56, 2003*

"This is important information. The Web has many resources but this sourcebook fills an important societal need. I am not aware of any other resources of this type." — *Doody's Review Service, Sep '01*

"Recommended for all libraries, scholars, and practitioners." — *Choice, Association of College & Research Libraries, Jul '01*

"Recommended reference source." — *Booklist, American Library Association, Apr '01*

"Important pick for college-level health reference libraries." — *The Bookwatch, Mar '01*

"Because this problem is so widespread and because this book includes a lot of issues within one volume, this work is recommended for all public libraries." — *American Reference Books Annual, 2001*

Drug Abuse Sourcebook

Basic Consumer Health Information about Illicit Substances of Abuse and the Diversion of Prescription Medications, Including Depressants, Hallucinogens, Inhalants, Marijuana, Narcotics, Stimulants, and Anabolic Steroids

Along with Facts about Related Health Risks, Treatment Issues, and Substance Abuse Prevention Programs, a Glossary of Terms, Statistical Data, and Directories of Hotline Services, Self-Help Groups, and Organizations Able to Provide Further Information

Edited by Karen Bellenir. 629 pages. 2000. 0-7808-0242-X. $78.

"Containing a wealth of information . . . . This resource belongs in libraries that serve a lower-division undergraduate or community college clientele as well as the general public." — *Choice, Association of College and Research Libraries, Jun '01*

"Recommended reference source."
— *Booklist, American Library Association, Feb '01*

"Highly recommended." — *The Bookwatch, Jan '01*

"Even though there is a plethora of books on drug abuse, this volume is recommended for school, public, and college libraries."
— *American Reference Books Annual, 2001*

SEE ALSO *Alcoholism Sourcebook, Substance Abuse Sourcebook*

Ear, Nose & Throat Disorders Sourcebook

Basic Information about Disorders of the Ears, Nose, Sinus Cavities, Pharynx, and Larynx, Including Ear Infections, Tinnitus, Vestibular Disorders, Allergic and Non-Allergic Rhinitis, Sore Throats, Tonsillitis, and Cancers That Affect the Ears, Nose, Sinuses, and Throat

Along with Reports on Current Research Initiatives, a Glossary of Related Medical Terms, and a Directory of Sources for Further Help and Information

Edited by Karen Bellenir and Linda M. Shin. 576 pages. 1998. 0-7808-0206-3. $78.

"Overall, this sourcebook is helpful for the consumer seeking information on ENT issues. It is recommended for public libraries."
— *American Reference Books Annual, 1999*

"Recommended reference source."
— *Booklist, American Library Association, Dec '98*

Eating Disorders Sourcebook

Basic Consumer Health Information about Eating Disorders, Including Information about Anorexia Nervosa, Bulimia Nervosa, Binge Eating, Body Dysmorphic Disorder, Pica, Laxative Abuse, and Night Eating Syndrome

Along with Information about Causes, Adverse Effects, and Treatment and Prevention Issues, and Featuring a Section on Concerns Specific to Children and Adolescents, a Glossary, and Resources for Further Help and Information

Edited by Dawn D. Matthews. 322 pages. 2001. 0-7808-0335-3. $78.

"Recommended for health science libraries that are open to the public, as well as hospital libraries. This book is a good resource for the consumer who is concerned about eating disorders." — *E-Streams, Mar '02*

"This volume is another convenient collection of excerpted articles. Recommended for school and public library patrons; lower-division undergraduates; and two-year technical program students." — *Choice, Association of College & Research Libraries, Jan '02*

"Recommended reference source." — *Booklist, American Library Association, Oct '01*

SEE ALSO *Diet & Nutrition Sourcebook, Digestive Diseases & Disorders Sourcebook, Gastrointestinal Diseases & Disorders Sourcebook*

Emergency Medical Services Sourcebook

Basic Consumer Health Information about Preventing, Preparing for, and Managing Emergency Situations, When and Who to Call for Help, What to Expect in the Emergency Room, the Emergency Medical Team, Patient Issues, and Current Topics in Emergency Medicine

Along with Statistical Data, a Glossary, and Sources of Additional Help and Information

Edited by Jenni Lynn Colson. 494 pages. 2002. 0-7808-0420-1. $78.

"Handy and convenient for home, public, school, and college libraries. Recommended."
— *Choice, Association of College and Research Libraries, Apr '03*

"This reference can provide the consumer with answers to most questions about emergency care in the United States, or it will direct them to a resource where the answer can be found."
— *American Reference Books Annual, 2003*

"Recommended reference source."
— *Booklist, American Library Association, Feb '03*

▪

Endocrine & Metabolic Disorders Sourcebook

Basic Information for the Layperson about Pancreatic and Insulin-Related Disorders Such as Pancreatitis, Diabetes, and Hypoglycemia; Adrenal Gland Disorders Such as Cushing's Syndrome, Addison's Disease, and Congenital Adrenal Hyperplasia; Pituitary Gland Disorders Such as Growth Hormone Deficiency, Acromegaly, and Pituitary Tumors; Thyroid Disorders Such as Hypothyroidism, Graves' Disease, Hashimoto's Disease, and Goiter; Hyperparathyroidism; and Other Diseases and Syndromes of Hormone Imbalance or Metabolic Dysfunction

Along with Reports on Current Research Initiatives

Edited by Linda M. Shin. 574 pages. 1998. 0-7808-0207-1. $78.

"Omnigraphics has produced another needed resource for health information consumers."
— *American Reference Books Annual, 2000*

"Recommended reference source."
— *Booklist, American Library Association, Dec '98*

▪

Environmental Health Sourcebook, 2nd Edition

Basic Consumer Health Information about the Environment and Its Effect on Human Health, Including the Effects of Air Pollution, Water Pollution, Hazardous Chemicals, Food Hazards, Radiation Hazards, Biological Agents, Household Hazards, Such as Radon, Asbestos, Carbon Monoxide, and Mold, and Information about Associated Diseases and Disorders, Including Cancer, Allergies, Respiratory Problems, and Skin Disorders

Along with Information about Environmental Concerns for Specific Populations, a Glossary of Related Terms, and Resources for Further Help and Information

Edited by Dawn D. Matthews. 673 pages. 2003. 0-7808-0632-8. $78.

ALSO AVAILABLE: *Environmentally Induced Disorders Sourcebook, 1st Edition.* Edited by Allan R. Cook. 620 pages. 1997. 0-7808-0083-4. $78.

"Recommended reference source."
— *Booklist, American Library Association, Sep '98*

"This book will be a useful addition to anyone's library." — *Choice Health Sciences Supplement, Association of College and Research Libraries, May '98*

". . . a good survey of numerous environmentally induced physical disorders . . . a useful addition to anyone's library."
— *Doody's Health Sciences Book Reviews, Jan '98*

". . . provide[s] introductory information from the best authorities around. Since this volume covers topics that potentially affect everyone, it will surely be one of the most frequently consulted volumes in the *Health Reference Series*." — *Rettig on Reference, Nov '97*

▪

Environmentally Induced Disorders Sourcebook, 1st Edition

SEE *Environmental Health Sourcebook, 2nd Edition*

▪

Ethnic Diseases Sourcebook

Basic Consumer Health Information for Ethnic and Racial Minority Groups in the United States, Including General Health Indicators and Behaviors, Ethnic Diseases, Genetic Testing, the Impact of Chronic Diseases, Women's Health, Mental Health Issues, and Preventive Health Care Services

Along with a Glossary and a Listing of Additional Resources

Edited by Joyce Brennfleck Shannon. 664 pages. 2001. 0-7808-0336-1. $78.

"Recommended for health sciences libraries where public health programs are a priority."
— *E-Streams, Jan '02*

"Not many books have been written on this topic to date, and the *Ethnic Diseases Sourcebook* is a strong addition to the list. It will be an important introductory resource for health consumers, students, health care personnel, and social scientists. It is recommended for public, academic, and large hospital libraries."
— *American Reference Books Annual 2002*

"Recommended reference source."
— *Booklist, American Library Association, Oct '01*

"Will prove valuable to any library seeking to maintain a current, comprehensive reference collection of health resources. . . . An excellent source of health information about genetic disorders which affect particular ethnic and racial minorities in the U.S."
— *The Bookwatch, Aug '01*

Eye Care Sourcebook, 2nd Edition

Basic Consumer Health Information about Eye Care and Eye Disorders, Including Facts about the Diagnosis, Prevention, and Treatment of Common Refractive Problems Such as Myopia, Hyperopia, Astigmatism, and Presbyopia, and Eye Diseases, Including Glaucoma, Cataract, Age-Related Macular Degeneration, and Diabetic Retinopathy

Along with a Section on Vision Correction and Refractive Surgeries, Including LASIK and LASEK, a Glossary, and Directories of Resources for Additional Help and Information

Edited by Amy L. Sutton. 543 pages. 2003. 0-7808-0635-2. $78.

ALSO AVAILABLE: Ophthalmic Disorders Sourcebook, 1st Edition. Edited by Linda M. Ross. 631 pages. 1996. 0-7808-0081-8. $78.

Family Planning Sourcebook

Basic Consumer Health Information about Planning for Pregnancy and Contraception, Including Traditional Methods, Barrier Methods, Hormonal Methods, Permanent Methods, Future Methods, Emergency Contraception, and Birth Control Choices for Women at Each Stage of Life

Along with Statistics, a Glossary, and Sources of Additional Information

Edited by Amy Marcaccio Keyzer. 520 pages. 2001. 0-7808-0379-5. $78.

"Recommended for public, health, and undergraduate libraries as part of the circulating collection."
—E-Streams, Mar '02

"Information is presented in an unbiased, readable manner, and the sourcebook will certainly be a necessary addition to those public and high school libraries where Internet access is restricted or otherwise problematic." —American Reference Books Annual 2002

"Recommended reference source."
—Booklist, American Library Association, Oct '01

"Will prove valuable to any library seeking to maintain a current, comprehensive reference collection of health resources. . . . Excellent reference."
—The Bookwatch, Aug '01

SEE ALSO Pregnancy & Birth Sourcebook

Fitness & Exercise Sourcebook, 2nd Edition

Basic Consumer Health Information about the Fundamentals of Fitness and Exercise, Including How to Begin and Maintain a Fitness Program, Fitness as a Lifestyle, the Link between Fitness and Diet, Advice for Specific Groups of People, Exercise as It Relates to Specific Medical Conditions, and Recent Research in Fitness and Exercise

Along with a Glossary of Important Terms and Resources for Additional Help and Information

Edited by Kristen M. Gledhill. 646 pages. 2001. 0-7808-0334-5. $78.

ALSO AVAILABLE: Fitness & Exercise Sourcebook, 1st Edition. Edited by Dan R. Harris. 663 pages. 1996. 0-7808-0186-5. $78.

"This work is recommended for all general reference collections."
—American Reference Books Annual 2002

"Highly recommended for public, consumer, and school grades fourth through college."
—E-Streams, Nov '01

"Recommended reference source." —Booklist, American Library Association, Oct '01

"The information appears quite comprehensive and is considered reliable. . . . This second edition is a welcomed addition to the series."
—Doody's Review Service, Sep '01

"This reference is a valuable choice for those who desire a broad source of information on exercise, fitness, and chronic-disease prevention through a healthy lifestyle." —American Medical Writers Association Journal, Fall '01

"Will prove valuable to any library seeking to maintain a current, comprehensive reference collection of health resources. . . . Excellent reference."
—The Bookwatch, Aug '01

Food & Animal Borne Diseases Sourcebook

Basic Information about Diseases That Can Be Spread to Humans through the Ingestion of Contaminated Food or Water or by Contact with Infected Animals and Insects, Such as Botulism, E. Coli, Hepatitis A, Trichinosis, Lyme Disease, and Rabies

Along with Information Regarding Prevention and Treatment Methods, and Including a Special Section for International Travelers Describing Diseases Such as Cholera, Malaria, Travelers' Diarrhea, and Yellow Fever, and Offering Recommendations for Avoiding Illness

Edited by Karen Bellenir and Peter D. Dresser. 535 pages. 1995. 0-7808-0033-8. $78.

"Targeting general readers and providing them with a single, comprehensive source of information on selected topics, this book continues, with the excellent caliber of its predecessors, to catalog topical information on health matters of general interest. Readable and thorough, this valuable resource is highly recommended for all libraries."
—Academic Library Book Review, Summer '96

"A comprehensive collection of authoritative information." —Emergency Medical Services, Oct '95

Food Safety Sourcebook

Basic Consumer Health Information about the Safe Handling of Meat, Poultry, Seafood, Eggs, Fruit Juices, and Other Food Items, and Facts about Pesticides, Drinking Water, Food Safety Overseas, and the Onset, Duration, and Symptoms of Foodborne Illnesses, Including Types of Pathogenic Bacteria, Parasitic Protozoa, Worms, Viruses, and Natural Toxins

Along with the Role of the Consumer, the Food Handler, and the Government in Food Safety; a Glossary, and Resources for Additional Help and Information

Edited by Dawn D. Matthews. 339 pages. 1999. 0-7808-0326-4. $78.

"This book is recommended for public libraries and universities with home economic and food science programs." — *E-Streams, Nov '00*

"Recommended reference source."
—*Booklist, American Library Association, May '00*

"This book takes the complex issues of food safety and foodborne pathogens and presents them in an easily understood manner. [It does] an excellent job of covering a large and often confusing topic."
—*American Reference Books Annual, 2000*

Forensic Medicine Sourcebook

Basic Consumer Information for the Layperson about Forensic Medicine, Including Crime Scene Investigation, Evidence Collection and Analysis, Expert Testimony, Computer-Aided Criminal Identification, Digital Imaging in the Courtroom, DNA Profiling, Accident Reconstruction, Autopsies, Ballistics, Drugs and Explosives Detection, Latent Fingerprints, Product Tampering, and Questioned Document Examination

Along with Statistical Data, a Glossary of Forensics Terminology, and Listings of Sources for Further Help and Information

Edited by Annemarie S. Muth. 574 pages. 1999. 0-7808-0232-2. $78.

"Given the expected widespread interest in its content and its easy to read style, this book is recommended for most public and all college and university libraries."
— *E-Streams, Feb '01*

"Recommended for public libraries."
—*Reference & User Services Quarterly, American Library Association, Spring 2000*

"Recommended reference source."
—*Booklist, American Library Association, Feb '00*

"A wealth of information, useful statistics, references are up-to-date and extremely complete. This wonderful collection of data will help students who are interested in a career in any type of forensic field. It is a great resource for attorneys who need information about types of expert witnesses needed in a particular case. It also offers useful information for fiction and nonfiction writers whose work involves a crime. A fascinating compilation. All levels." — *Choice, Association of College and Research Libraries, Jan 2000*

"There are several items that make this book attractive to consumers who are seeking certain forensic data. . . . This is a useful current source for those seeking general forensic medical answers."
—*American Reference Books Annual, 2000*

Gastrointestinal Diseases & Disorders Sourcebook

Basic Information about Gastroesophageal Reflux Disease (Heartburn), Ulcers, Diverticulosis, Irritable Bowel Syndrome, Crohn's Disease, Ulcerative Colitis, Diarrhea, Constipation, Lactose Intolerance, Hemorrhoids, Hepatitis, Cirrhosis, and Other Digestive Problems, Featuring Statistics, Descriptions of Symptoms, and Current Treatment Methods of Interest for Persons Living with Upper and Lower Gastrointestinal Maladies

Edited by Linda M. Ross. 413 pages. 1996. 0-7808-0078-8. $78.

". . . very readable form. The successful editorial work that brought this material together into a useful and understandable reference makes accessible to all readers information that can help them more effectively understand and obtain help for digestive tract problems."
— *Choice, Association of College & Research Libraries, Feb '97*

SEE ALSO *Diet & Nutrition Sourcebook, Digestive Diseases & Disorders, Eating Disorders Sourcebook*

Genetic Disorders Sourcebook, 2nd Edition

Basic Consumer Health Information about Hereditary Diseases and Disorders, Including Cystic Fibrosis, Down Syndrome, Hemophilia, Huntington's Disease, Sickle Cell Anemia, and More; Facts about Genes, Gene Research and Therapy, Genetic Screening, Ethics of Gene Testing, Genetic Counseling, and Advice on Coping and Caring

Along with a Glossary of Genetic Terminology and a Resource List for Help, Support, and Further Information

Edited by Kathy Massimini. 768 pages. 2001. 0-7808-0241-1. $78.

ALSO AVAILABLE: *Genetic Disorders Sourcebook, 1st Edition.* Edited by Karen Bellenir. 642 pages. 1996. 0-7808-0034-6. $78.

"Recommended for public libraries and medical and hospital libraries with consumer health collections."
— *E-Streams, May '01*

"Recommended reference source."
— *Booklist, American Library Association, Apr '01*

"Important pick for college-level health reference libraries." — *The Bookwatch, Mar '01*

"Provides essential medical information to both the general public and those diagnosed with a serious or fatal genetic disease or disorder." —*Choice, Association of College and Research Libraries, Jan '97*

Head Trauma Sourcebook

Basic Information for the Layperson about Open-Head and Closed-Head Injuries, Treatment Advances, Recovery, and Rehabilitation

Along with Reports on Current Research Initiatives

Edited by Karen Bellenir. 414 pages. 1997. 0-7808-0208-X. $78.

Headache Sourcebook

Basic Consumer Health Information about Migraine, Tension, Cluster, Rebound and Other Types of Headaches, with Facts about the Cause and Prevention of Headaches, the Effects of Stress and the Environment, Headaches during Pregnancy and Menopause, and Childhood Headaches

Along with a Glossary and Other Resources for Additional Help and Information

Edited by Dawn D. Matthews. 362 pages. 2002. 0-7808-0337-X. $78.

"Highly recommended for academic and medical reference collections." — *Library Bookwatch, Sep '02*

Health Insurance Sourcebook

Basic Information about Managed Care Organizations, Traditional Fee-for-Service Insurance, Insurance Portability and Pre-Existing Conditions Clauses, Medicare, Medicaid, Social Security, and Military Health Care

Along with Information about Insurance Fraud

Edited by Wendy Wilcox. 530 pages. 1997. 0-7808-0222-5. $78.

"Particularly useful because it brings much of this information together in one volume. This book will be a handy reference source in the health sciences library, hospital library, college and university library, and medium to large public library." — *Medical Reference Services Quarterly, Fall '98*

Awarded "Books of the Year Award" — *American Journal of Nursing, 1997*

"The layout of the book is particularly helpful as it provides easy access to reference material. A most useful addition to the vast amount of information about health insurance. The use of data from U.S. government agencies is most commendable. Useful in a library or learning center for healthcare professional students." — *Doody's Health Sciences Book Reviews, Nov '97*

Health Reference Series Cumulative Index 1999

A Comprehensive Index to the Individual Volumes of the Health Reference Series, Including a Subject Index, Name Index, Organization Index, and Publication Index

Along with a Master List of Acronyms and Abbreviations

Edited by Edward J. Prucha, Anne Holmes, and Robert Rudnick. 990 pages. 2000. 0-7808-0382-5. $78.

"This volume will be most helpful in libraries that have a relatively complete collection of the Health Reference Series." — *American Reference Books Annual, 2001*

"Essential for collections that hold any of the numerous *Health Reference Series* titles."
— *Choice, Association of College and Research Libraries, Nov '00*

Healthy Aging Sourcebook

Basic Consumer Health Information about Maintaining Health through the Aging Process, Including Advice on Nutrition, Exercise, and Sleep, Help in Making Decisions about Midlife Issues and Retirement, and Guidance Concerning Practical and Informed Choices in Health Consumerism

Along with Data Concerning the Theories of Aging, Different Experiences in Aging by Minority Groups, and Facts about Aging Now and Aging in the Future; and Featuring a Glossary, a Guide to Consumer Help, Additional Suggested Reading, and Practical Resource Directory

Edited by Jenifer Swanson. 536 pages. 1999. 0-7808-0390-6. $78.

"Recommended reference source."
— *Booklist, American Library Association, Feb '00*

SEE ALSO *Physical & Mental Issues in Aging Sourcebook*

Healthy Heart Sourcebook for Women

Basic Consumer Health Information about Cardiac Issues Specific to Women, Including Facts about Major Risk Factors and Prevention, Treatment and Control Strategies, and Important Dietary Issues

Along with a Special Section Regarding the Pros and Cons of Hormone Replacement Therapy and Its Impact on Heart Health, and Additional Help, Including Recipes, a Glossary, and a Directory of Resources

Edited by Dawn D. Matthews. 336 pages. 2000. 0-7808-0329-9. $78.

"A good reference source and recommended for all public, academic, medical, and hospital libraries."
— *Medical Reference Services Quarterly, Summer '01*

"Because of the lack of information specific to women on this topic, this book is recommended for public libraries and consumer libraries."
— *American Reference Books Annual, 2001*

"Contains very important information about coronary artery disease that all women should know. The information is current and presented in an easy-to-read format. The book will make a good addition to any library." — *American Medical Writers Association Journal, Summer '00*

"Important, basic reference."
— *Reviewer's Bookwatch, Jul '00*

SEE ALSO *Heart Diseases & Disorders Sourcebook, Women's Health Concerns Sourcebook*

Heart Diseases & Disorders Sourcebook, 2nd Edition

Basic Consumer Health Information about Heart Attacks, Angina, Rhythm Disorders, Heart Failure, Valve Disease, Congenital Heart Disorders, and More, Including Descriptions of Surgical Procedures and Other Interventions, Medications, Cardiac Rehabilitation, Risk Identification, and Prevention Tips

Along with Statistical Data, Reports on Current Research Initiatives, a Glossary of Cardiovascular Terms, and Resource Directory

Edited by Karen Bellenir. 612 pages. 2000. 0-7808-0238-1. $78.

ALSO AVAILABLE: *Cardiovascular Diseases & Disorders Sourcebook, 1st Edition.* Edited by Karen Bellenir and Peter D. Dresser. 683 pages. 1995. 0-7808-0032-X. $78.

"This work stands out as an imminently accessible resource for the general public. It is recommended for the reference and circulating shelves of school, public, and academic libraries."
—*American Reference Books Annual, 2001*

"Recommended reference source."
—*Booklist, American Library Association, Dec '00*

"Provides comprehensive coverage of matters related to the heart. This title is recommended for health sciences and public libraries with consumer health collections."
—*E-Streams, Oct '00*

SEE ALSO *Healthy Heart Sourcebook for Women*

Household Safety Sourcebook

Basic Consumer Health Information about Household Safety, Including Information about Poisons, Chemicals, Fire, and Water Hazards in the Home

Along with Advice about the Safe Use of Home Maintenance Equipment, Choosing Toys and Nursery Furniture, Holiday and Recreation Safety, a Glossary, and Resources for Further Help and Information

Edited by Dawn D. Matthews. 606 pages. 2002. 0-7808-0338-8. $78.

"This work will be useful in public libraries with large consumer health and wellness departments."
—*American Reference Books Annual, 2003*

"As a sourcebook on household safety this book meets its mark. It is encyclopedic in scope and covers a wide range of safety issues that are commonly seen in the home."
—*E-Streams, Jul '02*

Immune System Disorders Sourcebook

Basic Information about Lupus, Multiple Sclerosis, Guillain-Barré Syndrome, Chronic Granulomatous Disease, and More

Along with Statistical and Demographic Data and Reports on Current Research Initiatives

Edited by Allan R. Cook. 608 pages. 1997. 0-7808-0209-8. $78.

Infant & Toddler Health Sourcebook

Basic Consumer Health Information about the Physical and Mental Development of Newborns, Infants, and Toddlers, Including Neonatal Concerns, Nutrition Recommendations, Immunization Schedules, Common Pediatric Disorders, Assessments and Milestones, Safety Tips, and Advice for Parents and Other Caregivers

Along with a Glossary of Terms and Resource Listings for Additional Help

Edited by Jenifer Swanson. 585 pages. 2000. 0-7808-0246-2. $78.

"As a reference for the general public, this would be useful in any library."
—*E-Streams, May '01*

"Recommended reference source."
—*Booklist, American Library Association, Feb '01*

"This is a good source for general use."
—*American Reference Books Annual, 2001*

Injury & Trauma Sourcebook

Basic Consumer Health Information about the Impact of Injury, the Diagnosis and Treatment of Common and Traumatic Injuries, Emergency Care, and Specific Injuries Related to Home, Community, Workplace, Transportation, and Recreation

Along with Guidelines for Injury Prevention, a Glossary, and a Directory of Additional Resources

Edited by Joyce Brennfleck Shannon. 696 pages. 2002. 0-7808-0421-X. $78.

"This publication is the most comprehensive work of its kind about injury and trauma."
—*American Reference Books Annual, 2003*

"This sourcebook provides concise, easily readable, basic health information about injuries. . . . This book is well organized and an easy to use reference resource suitable for hospital, health sciences and public libraries with consumer health collections."
—*E-Streams, Nov '02*

"Practitioners should be aware of guides such as this in order to facilitate their use by patients and their families."
—*Doody's Health Sciences Book Review Journal, Sep-Oct '02*

"Recommended reference source."
—*Booklist, American Library Association, Sep '02*

"Highly recommended for academic and medical reference collections."
—*Library Bookwatch, Sep '02*

Kidney & Urinary Tract Diseases & Disorders Sourcebook

Basic Information about Kidney Stones, Urinary Incontinence, Bladder Disease, End Stage Renal Disease, Dialysis, and More

Along with Statistical and Demographic Data and Reports on Current Research Initiatives

Edited by Linda M. Ross. 602 pages. 1997. 0-7808-0079-6. $78.

Learning Disabilities Sourcebook, 2nd Edition

Basic Consumer Health Information about Learning Disabilities, Including Dyslexia, Developmental Speech and Language Disabilities, Non-Verbal Learning Disorders, Developmental Arithmetic Disorder, Developmental Writing Disorder, and Other Conditions That Impede Learning Such as Attention Deficit/ Hyperactivity Disorder, Brain Injury, Hearing Impairment, Klinefelter Syndrome, Dyspraxia, and Tourette Syndrome

Along with Facts about Educational Issues and Assistive Technology, Coping Strategies, a Glossary of Related Terms, and Resources for Further Help and Information

Edited by Dawn D. Matthews. 621 pages. 2003. 0-7808-0626-3. $78.

ALSO AVAILABLE: *Learning Disabilities Sourcebook, 1st Edition.* Edited by Linda M. Shin. 579 pages. 1998. 0-7808-0210-1. $78.

"Teachers as well as consumers will find this an essential guide to understanding various syndromes and their latest treatments. [An] invaluable reference for public and school library collections alike."
— Library Bookwatch, Apr '03

Named "Outstanding Reference Book of 1999."
— New York Public Library, Feb 2000

"An excellent candidate for inclusion in a public library reference section. It's a great source of information. Teachers will also find the book useful. Definitely worth reading."
— Journal of Adolescent & Adult Literacy, Feb 2000

"Readable . . . provides a solid base of information regarding successful techniques used with individuals who have learning disabilities, as well as practical suggestions for educators and family members. Clear language, concise descriptions, and pertinent information for contacting multiple resources add to the strength of this book as a useful tool." *— Choice, Association of College and Research Libraries, Feb '99*

"Recommended reference source."
— Booklist, American Library Association, Sep '98

"A useful resource for libraries and for those who don't have the time to identify and locate the individual publications." *— Disability Resources Monthly, Sep '98*

Leukemia Sourcebook

Basic Consumer Health Information about Adult and Childhood Leukemias, Including Acute Lymphocytic Leukemia (ALL), Chronic Lymphocytic Leukemia (CLL), Acute Myelogenous Leukemia (AML), Chronic Myelogenous Leukemia (CML), and Hairy Cell Leukemia, and Treatments Such as Chemotherapy, Radiation Therapy, Peripheral Blood Stem Cell and Marrow Transplantation, and Immunotherapy

Along with Tips for Life During and After Treatment, a Glossary, and Directories of Additional Resources

Edited by Joyce Brennfleck Shannon. 588 pages. 2003. 0-7808-0627-1. $78.

Liver Disorders Sourcebook

Basic Consumer Health Information about the Liver and How It Works; Liver Diseases, Including Cancer, Cirrhosis, Hepatitis, and Toxic and Drug Related Diseases; Tips for Maintaining a Healthy Liver; Laboratory Tests, Radiology Tests, and Facts about Liver Transplantation

Along with a Section on Support Groups, a Glossary, and Resource Listings

Edited by Joyce Brennfleck Shannon. 591 pages. 2000. 0-7808-0383-3. $78.

"A valuable resource."
—American Reference Books Annual, 2001

"This title is recommended for health sciences and public libraries with consumer health collections."
— E-Streams, Oct '00

"Recommended reference source."
—Booklist, American Library Association, Jun '00

Lung Disorders Sourcebook

Basic Consumer Health Information about Emphysema, Pneumonia, Tuberculosis, Asthma, Cystic Fibrosis, and Other Lung Disorders, Including Facts about Diagnostic Procedures, Treatment Strategies, Disease Prevention Efforts, and Such Risk Factors as Smoking, Air Pollution, and Exposure to Asbestos, Radon, and Other Agents

Along with a Glossary and Resources for Additional Help and Information

Edited by Dawn D. Matthews. 678 pages. 2002. 0-7808-0339-6. $78.

"This title is a great addition for public and school libraries because it provides concise health information on the lungs."
—American Reference Books Annual, 2003

"Highly recommended for academic and medical reference collections." *— Library Bookwatch, Sep '02*

Medical Tests Sourcebook

Basic Consumer Health Information about Medical Tests, Including Periodic Health Exams, General Screening Tests, Tests You Can Do at Home, Findings of the U.S. Preventive Services Task Force, X-ray and Radiology Tests, Electrical Tests, Tests of Blood and Other Body Fluids and Tissues, Scope Tests, Lung Tests, Genetic Tests, Pregnancy Tests, Newborn Screening Tests, Sexually Transmitted Disease Tests, and Computer Aided Diagnoses

Along with a Section on Paying for Medical Tests, a Glossary, and Resource Listings

Edited by Joyce Brennfleck Shannon. 691 pages. 1999. 0-7808-0243-8. $78.

"Recommended for hospital and health sciences libraries with consumer health collections."
— E-Streams, Mar '00

"This is an overall excellent reference with a wealth of general knowledge that may aid those who are reluctant to get vital tests performed."
— Today's Librarian, Jan 2000

"A valuable reference guide."
— American Reference Books Annual, 2000

Men's Health Concerns Sourcebook

Basic Information about Health Issues That Affect Men, Featuring Facts about the Top Causes of Death in Men, Including Heart Disease, Stroke, Cancers, Prostate Disorders, Chronic Obstructive Pulmonary Disease, Pneumonia and Influenza, Human Immunodeficiency Virus and Acquired Immune Deficiency Syndrome, Diabetes Mellitus, Stress, Suicide, Accidents and Homicides, and Facts about Common Concerns for Men, Including Impotence, Contraception, Circumcision, Sleep Disorders, Snoring, Hair Loss, Diet, Nutrition, Exercise, Kidney and Urological Disorders, and Backaches

Edited by Allan R. Cook. 738 pages. 1998. 0-7808-0212-8. $78.

"This comprehensive resource and the series are highly recommended."
— American Reference Books Annual, 2000

"Recommended reference source."
— Booklist, American Library Association, Dec '98

Mental Health Disorders Sourcebook, 2nd Edition

Basic Consumer Health Information about Anxiety Disorders, Depression and Other Mood Disorders, Eating Disorders, Personality Disorders, Schizophrenia, and More, Including Disease Descriptions, Treatment Options, and Reports on Current Research Initiatives

Along with Statistical Data, Tips for Maintaining Mental Health, a Glossary, and Directory of Sources for Additional Help and Information

Edited by Karen Bellenir. 605 pages. 2000. 0-7808-0240-3. $78.

ALSO AVAILABLE: *Mental Health Disorders Sourcebook, 1st Edition.* Edited by Karen Bellenir. 548 pages. 1995. 0-7808-0040-0. $78.

"Well organized and well written."
— American Reference Books Annual, 2001

"Recommended reference source."
— Booklist, American Library Association, Jun '00

Mental Retardation Sourcebook

Basic Consumer Health Information about Mental Retardation and Its Causes, Including Down Syndrome, Fetal Alcohol Syndrome, Fragile X Syndrome, Genetic Conditions, Injury, and Environmental Sources

Along with Preventive Strategies, Parenting Issues, Educational Implications, Health Care Needs, Employment and Economic Matters, Legal Issues, a Glossary, and a Resource Listing for Additional Help and Information

Edited by Joyce Brennfleck Shannon. 642 pages. 2000. 0-7808-0377-9. $78.

"Public libraries will find the book useful for reference and as a beginning research point for students, parents, and caregivers."
— American Reference Books Annual, 2001

"The strength of this work is that it compiles many basic fact sheets and addresses for further information in one volume. It is intended and suitable for the general public. This sourcebook is relevant to any collection providing health information to the general public."
— E-Streams, Nov '00

"From preventing retardation to parenting and family challenges, this covers health, social and legal issues and will prove an invaluable overview."
— Reviewer's Bookwatch, Jul '00

Movement Disorders Sourcebook

Basic Consumer Health Information about Neurological Movement Disorders, Including Essential Tremor, Parkinson's Disease, Dystonia, Cerebral Palsy, Huntington's Disease, Myasthenia Gravis, Multiple Sclerosis, and Other Early-Onset and Adult-Onset Movement Disorders, Their Symptoms and Causes, Diagnostic Tests, and Treatments

Along with Mobility and Assistive Technology Information, a Glossary, and a Directory of Additional Resources

Edited by Joyce Brennfleck Shannon. 655 pages. 2003. 0-7808-0628-X. $78.

Obesity Sourcebook

Basic Consumer Health Information about Diseases and Other Problems Associated with Obesity, and Including Facts about Risk Factors, Prevention Issues, and Management Approaches

Along with Statistical and Demographic Data, Information about Special Populations, Research Updates, a Glossary, and Source Listings for Further Help and Information

Edited by Wilma Caldwell and Chad T. Kimball. 376 pages. 2001. 0-7808-0333-7. $78.

"The book synthesizes the reliable medical literature on obesity into one easy-to-read and useful resource for the general public."
—American Reference Books Annual 2002

"This is a very useful resource book for the lay public."
—Doody's Review Service, Nov '01

"Well suited for the health reference collection of a public library or an academic health science library that serves the general population." —E-Streams, Sep '01

"Recommended reference source."
—Booklist, American Library Association, Apr '01

" Recommended pick both for specialty health library collections and any general consumer health reference collection." —The Bookwatch, Apr '01

■

Ophthalmic Disorders Sourcebook, 1st Edition

SEE Eye Care Sourcebook, 2nd Edition

■

Oral Health Sourcebook

Basic Information about Diseases and Conditions Affecting Oral Health, Including Cavities, Gum Disease, Dry Mouth, Oral Cancers, Fever Blisters, Canker Sores, Oral Thrush, Bad Breath, Temporomandibular Disorders, and other Craniofacial Syndromes

Along with Statistical Data on the Oral Health of Americans, Oral Hygiene, Emergency First Aid, Information on Treatment Procedures and Methods of Replacing Lost Teeth

Edited by Allan R. Cook. 558 pages. 1997. 0-7808-0082-6. $78.

"Unique source which will fill a gap in dental sources for patients and the lay public. A valuable reference tool even in a library with thousands of books on dentistry. Comprehensive, clear, inexpensive, and easy to read and use. It fills an enormous gap in the health care literature." —Reference and User Services Quarterly, American Library Association, Summer '98

"Recommended reference source."
—Booklist, American Library Association, Dec '97

■

Osteoporosis Sourcebook

Basic Consumer Health Information about Primary and Secondary Osteoporosis and Juvenile Osteoporosis and Related Conditions, Including Fibrous Dysplasia, Gaucher Disease, Hyperthyroidism, Hypophosphatasia, Myeloma, Osteopetrosis, Osteogenesis Imperfecta, and Paget's Disease

Along with Information about Risk Factors, Treatments, Traditional and Non-Traditional Pain Management, a Glossary of Related Terms, and a Directory of Resources

Edited by Allan R. Cook. 584 pages. 2001. 0-7808-0239-X. $78.

"This would be a book to be kept in a staff or patient library. The targeted audience is the layperson, but the therapist who needs a quick bit of information on a particular topic will also find the book useful."
—Physical Therapy, Jan '02

"This resource is recommended as a great reference source for public, health, and academic libraries, and is another triumph for the editors of Omnigraphics."
—American Reference Books Annual 2002

"Recommended for all public libraries and general health collections, especially those supporting patient education or consumer health programs."
—E-Streams, Nov '01

"Will prove valuable to any library seeking to maintain a current, comprehensive reference collection of health resources. . . . From prevention to treatment and associated conditions, this provides an excellent survey."
—The Bookwatch, Aug '01

"Recommended reference source."
—Booklist, American Library Association, July '01

SEE ALSO Women's Health Concerns Sourcebook

■

Pain Sourcebook, 2nd Edition

Basic Consumer Health Information about Specific Forms of Acute and Chronic Pain, Including Muscle and Skeletal Pain, Nerve Pain, Cancer Pain, and Disorders Characterized by Pain, Such as Fibromyalgia, Shingles, Angina, Arthritis, and Headaches

Along with Information about Pain Medications and Management Techniques, Complementary and Alternative Pain Relief Options, Tips for People Living with Chronic Pain, a Glossary, and a Directory of Sources for Further Information

Edited by Karen Bellenir. 670 pages. 2002. 0-7808-0612-3. $78.

ALSO AVAILABLE: Pain Sourcebook, 1st Edition. Edited by Allan R. Cook. 667 pages. 1997. 0-7808-0213-6. $78.

"A source of valuable information. . . . This book offers help to nonmedical people who need information about pain and pain management. It is also an excellent reference for those who participate in patient education."
—Doody's Review Service, Sep '02

"The text is readable, easily understood, and well indexed. This excellent volume belongs in all patient education libraries, consumer health sections of public libraries, and many personal collections."
—American Reference Books Annual, 1999

"A beneficial reference." —Booklist Health Sciences Supplement, American Library Association, Oct '98

"The information is basic in terms of scholarship and is appropriate for general readers. Written in journalistic style . . . intended for non-professionals. Quite thorough in its coverage of different pain conditions and summarizes the latest clinical information regarding pain treatment." — *Choice, Association of College and Research Libraries, Jun '98*

"Recommended reference source."
—*Booklist, American Library Association, Mar '98*

Pediatric Cancer Sourcebook

Basic Consumer Health Information about Leukemias, Brain Tumors, Sarcomas, Lymphomas, and Other Cancers in Infants, Children, and Adolescents, Including Descriptions of Cancers, Treatments, and Coping Strategies

Along with Suggestions for Parents, Caregivers, and Concerned Relatives, a Glossary of Cancer Terms, and Resource Listings

Edited by Edward J. Prucha. 587 pages. 1999. 0-7808-0245-4. $78.

"An excellent source of information. Recommended for public, hospital, and health science libraries with consumer health collections." — *E-Streams, Jun '00*

"Recommended reference source."
— *Booklist, American Library Association, Feb '00*

"A valuable addition to all libraries specializing in health services and many public libraries."
—*American Reference Books Annual, 2000*

Physical & Mental Issues in Aging Sourcebook

Basic Consumer Health Information on Physical and Mental Disorders Associated with the Aging Process, Including Concerns about Cardiovascular Disease, Pulmonary Disease, Oral Health, Digestive Disorders, Musculoskeletal and Skin Disorders, Metabolic Changes, Sexual and Reproductive Issues, and Changes in Vision, Hearing, and Other Senses

Along with Data about Longevity and Causes of Death, Information on Acute and Chronic Pain, Descriptions of Mental Concerns, a Glossary of Terms, and Resource Listings for Additional Help

Edited by Jenifer Swanson. 660 pages. 1999. 0-7808-0233-0. $78.

"This is a treasure of health information for the layperson." — *Choice Health Sciences Supplement, Association of College & Research Libraries, May 2000*

"Recommended for public libraries."
—*American Reference Books Annual, 2000*

"Recommended reference source."
— *Booklist, American Library Association, Oct '99*

SEE ALSO *Healthy Aging Sourcebook*

Podiatry Sourcebook

Basic Consumer Health Information about Foot Conditions, Diseases, and Injuries, Including Bunions, Corns, Calluses, Athlete's Foot, Plantar Warts, Hammertoes and Clawtoes, Clubfoot, Heel Pain, Gout, and More

Along with Facts about Foot Care, Disease Prevention, Foot Safety, Choosing a Foot Care Specialist, a Glossary of Terms, and Resource Listings for Additional Information

Edited by M. Lisa Weatherford. 380 pages. 2001. 0-7808-0215-2. $78.

"Recommended reference source."
— *Booklist, American Library Association, Feb '02*

"There is a lot of information presented here on a topic that is usually only covered sparingly in most larger comprehensive medical encyclopedias."
—*American Reference Books Annual 2002*

Pregnancy & Birth Sourcebook

Basic Information about Planning for Pregnancy, Maternal Health, Fetal Growth and Development, Labor and Delivery, Postpartum and Perinatal Care, Pregnancy in Mothers with Special Concerns, and Disorders of Pregnancy, Including Genetic Counseling, Nutrition and Exercise, Obstetrical Tests, Pregnancy Discomfort, Multiple Births, Cesarean Sections, Medical Testing of Newborns, Breastfeeding, Gestational Diabetes, and Ectopic Pregnancy

Edited by Heather E. Aldred. 737 pages. 1997. 0-7808-0216-0. $78.

"A well-organized handbook. Recommended."
— *Choice, Association of College and Research Libraries, Apr '98*

"Recommended reference source."
— *Booklist, American Library Association, Mar '98*

"Recommended for public libraries."
— *American Reference Books Annual, 1998*

SEE ALSO *Congenital Disorders Sourcebook, Family Planning Sourcebook*

Prostate Cancer Sourcebook

Basic Consumer Health Information about Prostate Cancer, Including Information about the Associated Risk Factors, Detection, Diagnosis, and Treatment of Prostate Cancer

Along with Information on Non-Malignant Prostate Conditions, and Featuring a Section Listing Support and Treatment Centers and a Glossary of Related Terms

Edited by Dawn D. Matthews. 358 pages. 2001. 0-7808-0324-8. $78.

"Recommended reference source."
— *Booklist, American Library Association, Jan '02*

"A valuable resource for health care consumers seeking information on the subject. . . .All text is written in a clear, easy-to-understand language that avoids technical jargon. Any library that collects consumer health resources would strengthen their collection with the addition of the *Prostate Cancer Sourcebook."*

— *American Reference Books Annual 2002*

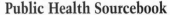

Public Health Sourcebook

Basic Information about Government Health Agencies, Including National Health Statistics and Trends, Healthy People 2000 Program Goals and Objectives, the Centers for Disease Control and Prevention, the Food and Drug Administration, and the National Institutes of Health

Along with Full Contact Information for Each Agency

Edited by Wendy Wilcox. 698 pages. 1998. 0-7808-0220-9. $78.

"Recommended reference source."
— *Booklist, American Library Association, Sep '98*

"This consumer guide provides welcome assistance in navigating the maze of federal health agencies and their data on public health concerns."
— *SciTech Book News, Sep '98*

Reconstructive & Cosmetic Surgery Sourcebook

Basic Consumer Health Information on Cosmetic and Reconstructive Plastic Surgery, Including Statistical Information about Different Surgical Procedures, Things to Consider Prior to Surgery, Plastic Surgery Techniques and Tools, Emotional and Psychological Considerations, and Procedure-Specific Information

Along with a Glossary of Terms and a Listing of Resources for Additional Help and Information

Edited by M. Lisa Weatherford. 374 pages. 2001. 0-7808-0214-4. $78.

"An excellent reference that addresses cosmetic and medically necessary reconstructive surgeries. . . . The style of the prose is calm and reassuring, discussing the many positive outcomes now available due to advances in surgical techniques."
— *American Reference Books Annual 2002*

"Recommended for health science libraries that are open to the public, as well as hospital libraries that are open to the patients. This book is a good resource for the consumer interested in plastic surgery."
— *E-Streams, Dec '01*

"Recommended reference source."
— *Booklist, American Library Association, July '01*

Rehabilitation Sourcebook

Basic Consumer Health Information about Rehabilitation for People Recovering from Heart Surgery, Spinal Cord Injury, Stroke, Orthopedic Impairments, Amputation, Pulmonary Impairments, Traumatic Injury, and More, Including Physical Therapy, Occupational Therapy, Speech/ Language Therapy, Massage

Therapy, Dance Therapy, Art Therapy, and Recreational Therapy

Along with Information on Assistive and Adaptive Devices, a Glossary, and Resources for Additional Help and Information

Edited by Dawn D. Matthews. 531 pages. 1999. 0-7808-0236-5. $78.

"This is an excellent resource for public library reference and health collections."
— *American Reference Books Annual, 2001*

"Recommended reference source."
— *Booklist, American Library Association, May '00*

Respiratory Diseases & Disorders Sourcebook

Basic Information about Respiratory Diseases and Disorders, Including Asthma, Cystic Fibrosis, Pneumonia, the Common Cold, Influenza, and Others, Featuring Facts about the Respiratory System, Statistical and Demographic Data, Treatments, Self-Help Management Suggestions, and Current Research Initiatives

Edited by Allan R. Cook and Peter D. Dresser. 771 pages. 1995. 0-7808-0037-0. $78.

"Designed for the layperson and for patients and their families coping with respiratory illness. . . . an extensive array of information on diagnosis, treatment, management, and prevention of respiratory illnesses for the general reader." — *Choice, Association of College and Research Libraries, Jun '96*

"A highly recommended text for all collections. It is a comforting reminder of the power of knowledge that good books carry between their covers."
— *Academic Library Book Review, Spring '96*

"A comprehensive collection of authoritative information presented in a nontechnical, humanitarian style for patients, families, and caregivers."
— *Association of Operating Room Nurses, Sep/Oct '95*

SEE ALSO Lung Disorders Sourcebook

Sexually Transmitted Diseases Sourcebook, 2nd Edition

Basic Consumer Health Information about Sexually Transmitted Diseases, Including Information on the Diagnosis and Treatment of Chlamydia, Gonorrhea, Hepatitis, Herpes, HIV, Mononucleosis, Syphilis, and Others

Along with Information on Prevention, Such as Condom Use, Vaccines, and STD Education; And Featuring a Section on Issues Related to Youth and Adolescents, a Glossary, and Resources for Additional Help and Information

Edited by Dawn D. Matthews. 538 pages. 2001. 0-7808-0249-7. $78.

ALSO AVAILABLE: Sexually Transmitted Diseases Sourcebook, 1st Edition. Edited by Linda M. Ross. 550 pages. 1997. 0-7808-0217-9. $78.

Skin Disorders Sourcebook

Basic Information about Common Skin and Scalp Conditions Caused by Aging, Allergies, Immune Reactions, Sun Exposure, Infectious Organisms, Parasites, Cosmetics, and Skin Traumas, Including Abrasions, Cuts, and Pressure Sores

Along with Information on Prevention and Treatment

Edited by Allan R. Cook. 647 pages. 1997. 0-7808-0080-X. $78.

SEE ALSO Burns Sourcebook

Sleep Disorders Sourcebook

Basic Consumer Health Information about Sleep and Its Disorders, Including Insomnia, Sleepwalking, Sleep Apnea, Restless Leg Syndrome, and Narcolepsy

Along with Data about Shiftwork and Its Effects, Information on the Societal Costs of Sleep Deprivation, Descriptions of Treatment Options, a Glossary of Terms, and Resource Listings for Additional Help

Edited by Jenifer Swanson. 439 pages. 1998. 0-7808-0234-9. $78.

Sports Injuries Sourcebook, 2nd Edition

Basic Consumer Health Information about the Diagnosis, Treatment, and Rehabilitation of Common Sports-Related Injuries in Children and Adults

Along with Suggestions for Conditioning and Training, Information and Prevention Tips for Injuries Frequently Associated with Specific Sports and Special Populations, a Glossary, and a Directory of Additional Resources

Edited by Joyce Brennfleck Shannon. 614 pages. 2002. 0-7808-0604-2. $78.

ALSO AVAILABLE: Sports Injuries Sourcebook, 1st Edition. Edited by Heather E. Aldred. 624 pages. 1999. 0-7808-0218-7. $78.

Stress-Related Disorders Sourcebook

Basic Consumer Health Information about Stress and Stress-Related Disorders, Including Stress Origins and Signals, Environmental Stress at Work and Home, Mental and Emotional Stress Associated with Depression, Post-Traumatic Stress Disorder, Panic Disorder, Suicide, and the Physical Effects of Stress on the Cardiovascular, Immune, and Nervous Systems

Along with Stress Management Techniques, a Glossary, and a Listing of Additional Resources

Edited by Joyce Brennfleck Shannon. 610 pages. 2002. 0-7808-0560-7. $78.

Stroke Sourcebook

Basic Consumer Health Information about Stroke, Including Ischemic, Hemorrhagic, Transient Ischemic Attack (TIA), and Pediatric Stroke, Stroke Triggers and Risks, Diagnostic Tests, Treatments, and Rehabilitation Information

Along with Stroke Prevention Guidelines, Legal and Financial Information, a Glossary, and a Directory of Additional Resources

Edited by Joyce Brennfleck Shannon. 606 pages. 2003. 0-7808-0630-1. $78.

Substance Abuse Sourcebook

Basic Health-Related Information about the Abuse of Legal and Illegal Substances Such as Alcohol, Tobacco, Prescription Drugs, Marijuana, Cocaine, and Heroin; and Including Facts about Substance Abuse Prevention Strategies, Intervention Methods, Treatment and Recovery Programs, and a Section Addressing the Special Problems Related to Substance Abuse during Pregnancy

Edited by Karen Bellenir. 573 pages. 1996. 0-7808-0038-9. $78.

"A valuable addition to any health reference section. Highly recommended."
— The Book Report, Mar/Apr '97

". . . a comprehensive collection of substance abuse information that's both highly readable and compact. Families and caregivers of substance abusers will find the information enlightening and helpful, while teachers, social workers and journalists should benefit from the concise format. Recommended."
— Drug Abuse Update, Winter '96/'97

SEE ALSO *Alcoholism Sourcebook, Drug Abuse Sourcebook*

Surgery Sourcebook

Basic Consumer Health Information about Inpatient and Outpatient Surgeries, Including Cardiac, Vascular, Orthopedic, Ocular, Reconstructive, Cosmetic, Gynecologic, and Ear, Nose, and Throat Procedures and More

Along with Information about Operating Room Policies and Instruments, Laser Surgery Techniques, Hospital Errors, Statistical Data, a Glossary, and Listings of Sources for Further Help and Information

Edited by Annemarie S. Muth and Karen Bellenir. 596 pages. 2002. 0-7808-0380-9. $78.

"Invaluable reference for public and school library collections alike."
— Library Bookwatch, Apr '03

Transplantation Sourcebook

Basic Consumer Health Information about Organ and Tissue Transplantation, Including Physical and Financial Preparations, Procedures and Issues Relating to Specific Solid Organ and Tissue Transplants, Rehabilitation, Pediatric Transplant Information, the Future of Transplantation, and Organ and Tissue Donation

Along with a Glossary and Listings of Additional Resources

Edited by Joyce Brennfleck Shannon. 628 pages. 2002. 0-7808-0322-1. $78.

"Along with these advances [in transplantation technology] have come a number of daunting questions for potential transplant patients, their families, and their health care providers. This reference text is the best single tool to address many of these questions. . . . It will be a much-needed addition to the reference collections in health care, academic, and large public libraries."
— American Reference Books Annual, 2003

"Recommended for libraries with an interest in offering consumer health information." *— E-Streams, Jul '02*

"This is a unique and valuable resource for patients facing transplantation and their families."
— Doody's Review Service, Jun '02

Traveler's Health Sourcebook

Basic Consumer Health Information for Travelers, Including Physical and Medical Preparations, Transportation Health and Safety, Essential Information about Food and Water, Sun Exposure, Insect and Snake Bites, Camping and Wilderness Medicine, and Travel with Physical or Medical Disabilities

Along with International Travel Tips, Vaccination Recommendations, Geographical Health Issues, Disease Risks, a Glossary, and a Listing of Additional Resources

Edited by Joyce Brennfleck Shannon. 613 pages. 2000. 0-7808-0384-1. $78.

"Recommended reference source."
— Booklist, American Library Association, Feb '01

"This book is recommended for any public library, any travel collection, and especially any collection for the physically disabled."
— American Reference Books Annual, 2001

Vegetarian Sourcebook

Basic Consumer Health Information about Vegetarian Diets, Lifestyle, and Philosophy, Including Definitions of Vegetarianism and Veganism, Tips about Adopting Vegetarianism, Creating a Vegetarian Pantry, and Meeting Nutritional Needs of Vegetarians, with Facts Regarding Vegetarianism's Effect on Pregnant and Lactating Women, Children, Athletes, and Senior Citizens

Along with a Glossary of Commonly Used Vegetarian Terms and Resources for Additional Help and Information

Edited by Chad T. Kimball. 360 pages. 2002. 0-7808-0439-2. $78.

"Organizes into one concise volume the answers to the most common questions concerning vegetarian diets and lifestyles. This title is recommended for public and secondary school libraries." *— E-Streams, Apr '03*

"Invaluable reference for public and school library collections alike." *— Library Bookwatch, Apr '03*

"The articles in this volume are easy to read and come from authoritative sources. The book does not necessarily support the vegetarian diet but instead provides the pros and cons of this important decision. The *Vegetarian Sourcebook* is recommended for public libraries and consumer health libraries."
— American Reference Books Annual, 2003

670

Women's Health Concerns Sourcebook

Basic Information about Health Issues That Affect Women, Featuring Facts about Menstruation and Other Gynecological Concerns, Including Endometriosis, Fibroids, Menopause, and Vaginitis; Reproductive Concerns, Including Birth Control, Infertility, and Abortion; and Facts about Additional Physical, Emotional, and Mental Health Concerns Prevalent among Women Such as Osteoporosis, Urinary Tract Disorders, Eating Disorders, and Depression

Along with Tips for Maintaining a Healthy Lifestyle

Edited by Heather E. Aldred. 567 pages. 1997. 0-7808-0219-5. $78.

"Handy compilation. There is an impressive range of diseases, devices, disorders, procedures, and other physical and emotional issues covered . . . well organized, illustrated, and indexed." — Choice, Association of College and Research Libraries, Jan '98

SEE ALSO Breast Cancer Sourcebook, Cancer Sourcebook for Women, Healthy Heart Sourcebook for Women, Osteoporosis Sourcebook

■

Workplace Health & Safety Sourcebook

Basic Consumer Health Information about Workplace Health and Safety, Including the Effect of Workplace Hazards on the Lungs, Skin, Heart, Ears, Eyes, Brain, Reproductive Organs, Musculoskeletal System, and Other Organs and Body Parts

Along with Information about Occupational Cancer, Personal Protective Equipment, Toxic and Hazardous Chemicals, Child Labor, Stress, and Workplace Violence

Edited by Chad T. Kimball. 626 pages. 2000. 0-7808-0231-4. $78.

"As a reference for the general public, this would be useful in any library." —E-Streams, Jun '01

"Provides helpful information for primary care physicians and other caregivers interested in occupational medicine. . . . General readers; professionals." — Choice, Association of College & Research Libraries, May '01

"Recommended reference source." — Booklist, American Library Association, Feb '01

"Highly recommended." — The Bookwatch, Jan '01

■

Worldwide Health Sourcebook

Basic Information about Global Health Issues, Including Malnutrition, Reproductive Health, Disease Dispersion and Prevention, Emerging Diseases, Risky Health Behaviors, and the Leading Causes of Death

Along with Global Health Concerns for Children, Women, and the Elderly, Mental Health Issues, Research and Technology Advancements, and Economic, Environmental, and Political Health Implications, a

Glossary, and a Resource Listing for Additional Help and Information

Edited by Joyce Brennfleck Shannon. 614 pages. 2001. 0-7808-0330-2. $78.

"Named an Outstanding Academic Title." —Choice, Association of College & Research Libraries, Jan '02

"Yet another handy but also unique compilation in the extensive Health Reference Series, this is a useful work because many of the international publications reprinted or excerpted are not readily available. Highly recommended." —Choice, Association of College & Research Libraries, Nov '01

"Recommended reference source." —Booklist, American Library Association, Oct '01

671

Teen Health Series

Helping Young Adults Understand, Manage,
and Avoid Serious Illness

Diet Information for Teens
Health Tips about Diet and Nutrition

Including Facts about Nutrients, Dietary Guidelines, Breakfasts, School Lunches, Snacks, Party Food, Weight Control, Eating Disorders, and More

Edited by Karen Bellenir. 399 pages. 2001. 0-7808-0441-4. $58.

"Full of helpful insights and facts throughout the book. ... An excellent resource to be placed in public libraries or even in personal collections."
—*American Reference Books Annual 2002*

"Recommended for middle and high school libraries and media centers as well as academic libraries that educate future teachers of teenagers. It is also a suitable addition to health science libraries that serve patrons who are interested in teen health promotion and education."
—*E-Streams, Oct '01*

"This comprehensive book would be beneficial to collections that need information about nutrition, dietary guidelines, meal planning, and weight control. ... This reference is so easy to use that its purchase is recommended."
—*The Book Report, Sep-Oct '01*

"This book is written in an easy to understand format describing issues that many teens face every day, and then provides thoughtful explanations so that teens can make informed decisions. This is an interesting book that provides important facts and information for today's teens."
—*Doody's Health Sciences Book Review Journal, Jul-Aug '01*

"A comprehensive compendium of diet and nutrition. The information is presented in a straightforward, plain-spoken manner. This title will be useful to those working on reports on a variety of topics, as well as to general readers concerned about their dietary health."
—*School Library Journal, Jun '01*

Drug Information for Teens
Health Tips about the Physical and Mental Effects of Substance Abuse

Including Facts about Alcohol, Anabolic Steroids, Club Drugs, Cocaine, Depressants, Hallucinogens, Herbal Products, Inhalants, Marijuana, Narcotics, Stimulants, Tobacco, and More

Edited by Karen Bellenir. 452 pages. 2002. 0-7808-0444-9. $58.

"The chapters are quick to make a connection to their teenage reading audience. The prose is straightforward and the book lends itself to spot reading. It should be useful both for practical information and for research, and it is suitable for public and school libraries."
—*American Reference Books Annual, 2003*

"Recommended reference source."
—*Booklist, American Library Association, Feb '03*

"This is an excellent resource for teens and their parents. Education about drugs and substances is key to discouraging teen drug abuse and this book provides this much needed information in a way that is interesting and factual."
—*Doody's Review Service, Dec '02*

Mental Health Information for Teens
Health Tips about Mental Health and Mental Illness

Including Facts about Anxiety, Depression, Suicide, Eating Disorders, Obsessive-Compulsive Disorders, Panic Attacks, Phobias, Schizophrenia, and More

Edited by Karen Bellenir. 406 pages. 2001. 0-7808-0442-2. $58.

"In both language and approach, this user-friendly entry in the *Teen Health Series* is on target for teens needing information on mental health concerns." —*Booklist, American Library Association, Jan '02*

"Readers will find the material accessible and informative, with the shaded notes, facts, and embedded glossary insets adding appropriately to the already interesting and succinct presentation."
—*School Library Journal, Jan '02*

"This title is highly recommended for any library that serves adolescents and parents/caregivers of adolescents." —*E-Streams, Jan '02*

"Recommended for high school libraries and young adult collections in public libraries. Both health professionals and teenagers will find this book useful."
—*American Reference Books Annual 2002*

"This is a nice book written to enlighten the society, primarily teenagers, about common teen mental health issues. It is highly recommended to teachers and parents as well as adolescents."
—*Doody's Review Service, Dec '01*

Sexual Health Information for Teens
Health Tips about Sexual Development, Human Reproduction, and Sexually Transmitted Diseases

Including Facts about Puberty, Reproductive Health, Chlamydia, Human Papillomavirus, Pelvic Inflam-

matory Disease, Herpes, AIDS, Contraception, Pregnancy, and More

Edited by Deborah A. Stanley. 400 pages. 2003. 0-7808-0445-7. $58.

Skin Health Information For Teens
Health Tips about Dermatological Concerns and Skin Cancer Risks

Including Facts about Acne, Warts, Hives, and Other Conditions and Lifestyle Choices, Such as Tanning, Tattooing, and Piercing, That Affect the Skin, Nails, Scalp, and Hair

Edited by Robert Aquinas McNally. 430 pages. 2003. 0-7808-0446-5. $58.

Health Reference Series

Adolescent Health Sourcebook

AIDS Sourcebook, 1st Edition

AIDS Sourcebook, 2nd Edition

AIDS Sourcebook, 3rd Edition

Alcoholism Sourcebook

Allergies Sourcebook, 1st Edition

Allergies Sourcebook, 2nd Edition

Alternative Medicine Sourcebook, 1st Edition

Alternative Medicine Sourcebook, 2nd Edition

Alzheimer's, Stroke & 29 Other Neurological Disorders Sourcebook, 1st Edition

Alzheimer's Disease Sourcebook, 2nd Edition

Arthritis Sourcebook

Asthma Sourcebook

Attention Deficit Disorder Sourcebook

Back & Neck Disorders Sourcebook

Blood & Circulatory Disorders Sourcebook

Brain Disorders Sourcebook

Breast Cancer Sourcebook

Breastfeeding Sourcebook

Burns Sourcebook

Cancer Sourcebook, 1st Edition

Cancer Sourcebook (New), 2nd Edition

Cancer Sourcebook, 3rd Edition

Cancer Sourcebook for Women, 1st Edition

Cancer Sourcebook for Women, 2nd Edition

Cardiovascular Diseases & Disorders Sourcebook, 1st Edition

Caregiving Sourcebook

Childhood Diseases & Disorders Sourcebook

Colds, Flu & Other Common Ailments Sourcebook

Communication Disorders Sourcebook

Congenital Disorders Sourcebook

Consumer Issues in Health Care Sourcebook

Contagious & Non-Contagious Infectious Diseases Sourcebook

Death & Dying Sourcebook

Depression Sourcebook

Diabetes Sourcebook, 1st Edition

Diabetes Sourcebook, 2nd Edition

Diabetes Sourcebook, 3rd Edition

Diet & Nutrition Sourcebook, 1st Edition

Diet & Nutrition Sourcebook, 2nd Edition

Digestive Diseases & Disorder Sourcebook

Disabilities Sourcebook

Domestic Violence & Child Abuse Sourcebook

Drug Abuse Sourcebook

Ear, Nose & Throat Disorders Sourcebook

Eating Disorders Sourcebook

Emergency Medical Services Sourcebook

Endocrine & Metabolic Disorders Sourcebook

Environmentally Induced Disorders Sourcebook

Ethnic Diseases Sourcebook

Eye Care Sourcebook, 2nd Edition

Family Planning Sourcebook

Fitness & Exercise Sourcebook, 1st Edition

Fitness & Exercise Sourcebook, 2nd Edition

Food & Animal Borne Diseases Sourcebook

Food Safety Sourcebook

Forensic Medicine Sourcebook

Gastrointestinal Diseases & Disorders Sourcebook